# MOTIVATIONAL YOGA

## 100 Lessons for Strength, Energy, and Transformation

### Nancy Gerstein

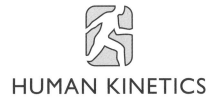

HUMAN KINETICS

**Library of Congress Cataloging-in-Publication Data**

Names: Gerstein, Nancy, 1958- author.
Title: Motivational yoga : 100 lessons for strength, energy, and
    transformation / Nancy Gerstein.
Other titles: Guiding yoga's light
Description: Revised edition. | Champaign, IL : Human Kinetics, [2020] |
    "Revised edition of Guiding Yoga's Light: Lessons for Yoga Teachers,
    Second Edition, published in 2008 by Human Kinetics." | Includes index.
Identifiers: LCCN 2019005193 (print) | LCCN 2019006800 (ebook) | ISBN
    9781492588276 (epub) | ISBN 9781492588252 (PDF) | ISBN 9781492588207
    (print)
Subjects:  LCSH: Hatha yoga--Study and teaching.
Classification: LCC RA781.7 (ebook) | LCC RA781.7 .G44 2020 (print) | DDC
    613.7/046--dc23
LC record available at https://lccn.loc.gov/2019005193

ISBN: 978-1-4925-8820-7 (print)

This publication is written and published to provide accurate and authoritative information relevant to the subject matter presented. It is published and sold with the understanding that the author and publisher are not engaged in rendering legal, medical, or other professional services by reason of their authorship or publication of this work. If medical or other expert assistance is required, the services of a competent professional person should be sought.

The web addresses cited in this text were current as of February 2019, unless otherwise noted.

**Senior Acquisitions Editor:** Michelle Maloney; **Managing Editor:** Miranda K. Baur; **Copyeditor:** Joanna Hatzopoulos; **Permissions Manager:** Martha Gullo; **Graphic Designer:** Julie L. Denzer; **Cover Designer:** Keri Evans; **Cover Design Associate:** Susan Rothermel Allen; **Photographs (cover and interior):** Jason Allen/© Human Kinetics, unless otherwise noted; **Photo Asset Manager:** Laura Fitch; **Photo Production Coordinator:** Amy M. Rose; **Photo Production Manager:** Jason Allen; **Senior Art Manager:** Kelly Hendren; **Illustrations:** © Human Kinetics; **Printer:** Sheridan Books

Printed in the United States of America    10 9 8 7 6 5 4 3 2 1

The paper in this book is certified under a sustainable forestry program.

**Human Kinetics**
P.O. Box 5076
Champaign, IL 61825-5076
Website: www.HumanKinetics.com

In the United States, email info@hkusa.com or call 800-747-4457.
In Canada, email info@hkcanada.com.
In the United Kingdom/Europe, email hk@hkeurope.com.

For information about Human Kinetics' coverage in other areas of the world,
please visit our website: **www.HumanKinetics.com**

E7531

**Tell us what you think!**
Human Kinetics would love to hear what we
can do to improve the customer experience.
Use this QR code to take our brief survey.

To Max and Grace, the lights of my life.

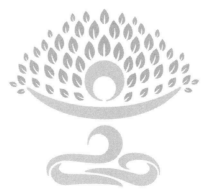

*One moment can change a day,*
*one day can change a life,*
*and one life can change the world.*
Buddha

# Contents

# Preface

*Whatever words we utter should be chosen with care for people will hear them and be influenced by them for good or ill.*

Buddha

*Motivational Yoga* defines the limitless potential of yoga. This mindful practice brings clarity to the mind and the body, influencing the way you make decisions and take action. With a dedicated, consistent, and disciplined practice, you can incorporate the teachings of yoga into your personal consciousness. The practices can permeate how you live, affecting how you choose to handle life's inevitable ups and downs.

This book is for the curious and introspective yoga teacher, the serious yoga student, or the fitness instructor who wants to step out of the bounds of teaching asana only. While asana is an excellent tool for holistic health and wellness, yoga's mental and spiritual benefits far outweigh the physical exercises that have become synonymous with the practice. *Motivational Yoga* distills the principles of yoga's science and philosophy, offering yogis the tools to empower their own decisions and personalize their results. It encourages practitioners to move forward, be inquisitive, and discover their unlimited potential by going after the life they desire.

*Motivational Yoga* interprets yoga's 5,000-year-old philosophy in a way that inspires yoga teachers and students to dig deeper into their physical practice and take control of their own progress. Each lesson includes the relevant and systematic practices of yoga on and off the mat, while teaching accessible strategies for lasting lifestyle changes. On a universal scale, the palpable message of *Motivational Yoga* is that the discipline of yoga practice influences all aspects of the collective consciousness.

No matter how you feel today or any other day, *Motivational Yoga* demonstrates that as long as you can get up, you can show up. This empowerment is *yoga fuel for life.*

*Motivational Yoga*'s lessons use the following five-step format:

1. **Intention** defines the meaning of the class and creates awareness of a specific yogic experience.

2. **Lesson** is the core and script of the class.

3. **Asanas for Deepening** features postures that demonstrate the lesson through body stretch, movement, and sensation. Note that the postures are suggestions only; include the movements that work best for your teaching style and student level.

4. **Motivation Off the Mat** includes suggestions for homework assignments, reminders, and topics for discussion to help students integrate the lesson into their personal journey.

5. **Wise Words** and **Teacher Tips** present advice and proverbs within the context of each lesson.

The lessons of *Motivational Yoga* are organized so that new students can begin their journey by first understanding the fundamentals of hatha practice. The beginning lessons focus on body and breath awareness, describing the benefits of yoga, basic postures, and diaphragmatic breathing. The succeeding chapters introduce the yogi to the principles of Motivational Yoga, which encompass the yamas and niyamas as well as lessons of relaxation, the heart center, chakras, emotions, and mindfulness.

The motivational yogi is inquisitive and passionate, asking *Is what I'm doing today making a difference for the world tomorrow?* The motivational yogi doesn't settle for mediocre; we aim to lead, love, and learn while dedicating our lives to fulfilling a meaningful journey.

May you always find what makes you feel alive!

Namaste.

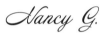

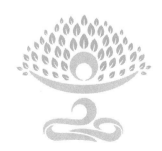

# Acknowledgments

This work is dedicated to the radiant spirits of the yoga community—the teachers, students, and sages who have guided my path to where I am today.

My deepest gratitude extends to the brilliant team at Human Kinetics who made this new yoga teaching book a reality. A colossal thank you to acquisitions editor Michelle Maloney, who sought to reenergize these lessons for a new age of yogis.

I hold my hands in prayer and bow in gratitude to the divine souls who have helped me stay on my yoga path, reminding me to shine my light even during the darkest of times. You have been my spiritual mentors and emotional charges. You have taught me that through your support, encouragement, and laughter, the prana of love can cure almost anything. Thank you from the bottom of my big, glowing, emerald green heart center to Judy, Donny, Judith, Allan, Helen, Marcie, Mike, Mindy, Gigi, Deb, Megan, Ricky, and the many other wise souls along the way. I love you all.

Thank you to Bobbie and Louie who gave me life, love, and the blessings of roots and wings.

To Jon, the most positive person in my universe. Your understanding, love, and support have helped ferry me through this excursion. You're the farmer in the *Good Luck, Bad Luck* story, the pragmatic mind who understands that things aren't always what they seem. Thank you for stimulating my thinking, encouraging adventure, and giving me permission to shut my door and write. My love for you is beyond words.

Finally, to Max and Grace (and Kelsey, too), who will always have the cutest little asanas I know. I love you this much.

# Introduction

*If you light a lamp for somebody, it will also brighten your path.*

Buddha

I have a love affair with yoga. While the practice is time consuming and laborious, it's often serendipitous and packed with revelation. It's at once a celebration of movement and curious adventure, a momentous disclosure, and a quiet day trip to my inner world. Each instant on this yogic path holds the opportunity to feel spacious, connected, and more alive.

Since the beginning of my journey into yoga, I've cherished the ancient yoga teachings and ideas that apply to modern living. I've learned that practicing the yoga of life is invaluable at work; at leisure; in your role as a parent, partner, neighbor, and friend; and especially during the challenges of our ongoing celebrations and traumas. Perhaps this love affair with yoga is grounded in the eternal love of life itself.

The ultimate reward of the motivational yoga life is that you feel better at every level of your consciousness. Yoga fosters mindfulness and silences chattering thoughts; its potential impact is infinite. No matter what your role is in the world—teacher, parent, daughter, friend, CEO, student, coach, or something else—the motivational yoga life will help you lead others, communicate clearly, and foster creativity and flexibility.

This book is a starting point, a tool for bringing yoga's abundant teachings into the daily lives of yoga teachers and students. Over the years, I've recorded my lesson plans to track where I have been as a teacher, and where the path has taken me as a student. These lessons have evolved into scores of inspirational journals that guide my goals for my own practice and progress.

My objective is not to shape all yoga classes with the same physical practices; rather, I offer a template to explore each yoga lesson wherever it may lead. Equipped with the knowledge passed down from yogic ancestors, my intention is to create an experience that is vital and current to modern life while sustaining yoga's deep traditional roots. It is with great joy and love that I venture into *Motivational Yoga* as a tiny step toward meeting that end.

## TEACHING WHAT YOU NEED TO LEARN

*Your greatest value is the effect you have on others. As a yoga teacher and leader, your responsibility is to remain present, clear, and confident so that you can motivate, teach, and inspire those around you.*

Yoga induces a relaxed state that alleviates stress. It builds a mind–body partnership by helping you identify your own negative behaviors and thinking patterns. I've seen students (myself included) target the specific paradigm that was holding them back from joy, love, and courage. Making the changes needed for a contented life *and* having them endure is the core of Motivational Yoga. I call it the *yoga fuel for life*.

The benefits of this yoga fuel are not exclusive to your students; they apply to you too. A daily yoga ritual develops a disciplined, reflective mind that forms a deep connection to the supreme self. Yoga teaches you how to shift the direction of your energies and, in so doing, your entire physiology. It teaches that life is full of possibilities, many of which are within your control. When you understand how to empower your *own* life with these teachings, you're better able to pass them on to your students.

To help you on your teaching and learning journey, use the following guidelines:

○ *Remain a student.* The hidden perk of teaching yoga is that your sad old stories, daily stresses, and changes in your personal life often work themselves out in your classes. The most inspirational teachers I've encountered have been able to brave through their darkest places by virtue of their yoga journey.

   Before I even had one anxiety attack, I spent years teaching students how to recognize and subsequently calm them. Once I was "blessed" with my own episodes of anxiety, I scoured my yoga toolbox in search of the methods that would help me. When I found the right tools, I had this epiphany: Until you've walked through a particular hell, you're not qualified to give advice on the territory.

○ *Learn and teach calming techniques.* Learning how to calm yourself down is of benefit to anyone, from toddlers to seniors. Try two-to-one breathing (lengthening the exhalation to twice as long as the inhalation) and short vinyasas such as five rounds of downward dog to upward dog to child's pose to help yourself and your students return to a centered mind.

○ *Practice patience, one of the highest forms of wisdom.* Move slowly and deliberately, using the powerful mantra, *Life moves at its own pace.* When impatience arises, be mindful of it, hold on to the moment, and accept that everything evolves in its own time.

○ *Abandon self-criticism.* Free yourself of negative thoughts and sensations. If you criticize yourself during class, notice the judgment, then ask yourself if it's related to your emotions, your body, or your breath. Teaching yoga is not about instructing perfect positions—it's about feeling the potential comfort that's possible in any asana when you teach with acceptance.

○ *Face your fears.* Asana and pranayama are two of the most vigorous practices for releasing fear lodged in the body's tissues. For instance, if you're feeling a lack of courage, remember that backbends loosen the armor around the solar plexus and heart, stimulate the circulation in the spine, and make you feel more vital, alive, and brave.

○ *Keep mild depression in check.* My go-to practice for easing malaise is to begin my practice with the "Gratitude of Heart" meditation: Visualize someone or something you appreciate, such as your children, parents, or spouse; or having a roof over your head and food to eat. As you breathe, feel the emotion, not just the thought. Hold on to it for several minutes. Remember to send appreciation to your amazing body; it's a living miracle.

## TIPS FROM THE FRONT OF THE ROOM

Yoga practice begins every time you take a conscious breath, movement, or thought. Whether you're a new or seasoned teacher, what you learn along the road of life influences your impact as a leader.

○ *Maintain a relaxed presence.* Until you feel calm as a teacher, simultaneously take and teach your class. Make the lesson part of your learning experience. You're guiding the way, and nothing is more motivating than a clear, meaningful presence.

○ *Enjoy the day's lesson.* Discover what the lesson means to you so that you can put your heart into it.

○ *Radiate your light and love.* On low-energy days when you feel you have nothing to give, your physical being, smile, and voice are enough to make a difference. Never underestimate the power of simply being you.

○ *Take a lesson from the student.* Just as you ask students to focus on their own practice rather than compare themselves with others, don't compare yourself to other teachers. Everyone has their own light and their reasons for walking their yoga path.

○ *Remember that teaching is a joy and privilege.* Do your best to help others find healing, self-discipline, and inner peace. Make every class count.

# EIGHT LIMBS OF RAJA YOGA

The word *raja* means "royal." Raja yoga describes the path of yoga in its highest, most comprehensive form.

Gathered by the sage Patanjali Maharishi in his *Yoga Sutras* written around 400 AD, the eight limbs of yoga are a progressive series of disciplines that purify the body, mind, and spirit, leading the yogi to enlightenment and liberation from suffering. The sutras describe how to be your true self and appreciate every moment.

### First Limb: Yamas (Moral Disciplines and Restraints)

Ahimsa—Nonharming, nonviolence; not *wishing or performing* mental or physical harm on any living creature, including oneself.

Satya—Nonlying, truthfulness; telling the highest truth but without harm.

Asteya—Nonstealing, noncovetousness; disinterest in wanting more than one has, or what another has.

Brahmacharya—Self-control; moderation in all things; not wasting one's energy on unnecessary indulgences.

Aparigraha—Nonpossessiveness; letting go of all attachment to one's possessions; nongreed, nongrasping, nonindulgence.

### Second Limb: Niyamas (Observances)

Saucha—Purity; cleanliness of internal and external worlds, including bodies, thoughts, and environment.

Santosha—Contentment; acceptance of the present moment, no matter how difficult.

Tapas—Determined effort; the discipline, heat, and enthusiasm of practice.

Svadhyaya—Self-study, introspection, turning inward; questioning one's motives, speeches, and actions.

Ishvara Pranidhana—Surrender to the divine light; the celebration and respect for all of life within the universe.

### Third Limb: Asana (Seat)

Creating and maintaining a steady and comfortable posture.

### Fourth Limb: Pranayama (Breathing Practices)

Regulation and control of prana, the body's lifeforce.

### Fifth Limb: Pratyahara (Sense Withdrawal)

Closing one's mind to the sensory world.

### Sixth Limb: Dharana (Concentration)

Introspective focus and one-pointedness of mind on a particular inner state, subject, or topic.

### Seventh Limb: Dhyana (Meditation)

The yoga state of interrupted stream of continuous thought about an object of concentration.

### Eighth Limb: Samadhi (Integration or Absorption)

The superconscious state in which the yogi perceives the identity of one's soul as spirit.

Many Western yoga students step onto the eight-limbed path by learning the disciplines of hatha, the physical yoga practices intended to eliminate distractions from the mind by stilling the body. The lessons in *Motivational Yoga* begin with the discovery of body and breath awareness, preparing the student for yoga's more advanced practices. Once the body's energies are awakened, the student is equipped to learn the deeper elements of the eight limbs—right and mindful living, care of the body through asana, and the remaining internal steps that lead to meditation and the superconscious state.

*Your yoga begins when you leave the classroom.*
*It's how you connect to people and how you relate to the world.*
*Your yoga is the giving and receiving.*
*It's the wellness between inner and outer worlds.*
*Your yoga is living the purpose of your life.*
*Your yoga is to spread peace, one person at a time.*
*The light and love in me*
*bows to the light and love in you.*
*Om.*
*Shanti, shanti, shanti*

# Beginning
# Lessons

*Words have the power to both destroy and heal.*
*When words are both true and kind, they can*
*change our world.*

—Buddha

As a yogic guide, you have a lot to teach your new students during the first few classes.

For absolute beginners, the primary focus is on body awareness through asanas (postures) and opening the body—the outermost layer of consciousness. This opening, strengthening, and ultimate aligning of the body, clears the nadis (the body's subtle energy channels) and enhances the flow of prana (lifeforce). Guided by mind and breath, this heightened flow of prana creates changes on the physical, emotional, and spiritual levels. Most students feel the effects of the yoga practice after their first time on the mat.

For experienced yogis, the practice is often more substantial than attaining a strong core or flexible hamstrings as it profoundly affects the mental and spiritual layers of consciousness by calming the mind and awakening the body's higher intelligence. Within these layers, the yogi experiences a deeper understanding of his essential nature, inner powers, and the world. A simple, mindful practice can be a ticket to transforming an ordinary life into one that is more fulfilling and awakened.

Whether your class consists of new or experienced yogis, always consider the following points when structuring your lesson plans.

*Hatha yoga is more than an exercise system.* It's a 5,000-year-old holistic path of health and self-development that begins by using the body to influence all aspects of one's being.

*Never underestimate breath awareness while practicing and teaching asana.* The breath is the link between body and mind. Demonstrate and teach the practice during every class. Mindful breathing makes the difference between achieving the holistic effects of asana and a glorified exercise class.

*Practice is individualistic and systematic.* Encourage students to challenge themselves to begin the process of change but to back off the physical practice when they feel pain. Students who tend to be competitive should be reminded not to force asana or breath. This balance requires inner listening.

*Maintain "beginner's mind"—an open mind.* Just as every day is new, every experience on the yoga mat is different. As the Japanese Zen monk Suzuki said, "In the beginner's mind, there are many possibilities; in the expert's mind, there are few."

*Teach from the heart while you teach the lessons you want to learn.* Find your voice, and have fun with your lesson plans.

*The teacher always remains a student, even in her own class.* A hidden perk of yoga teaching is that class is where old baggage, daily stresses, and changes in your personal life work themselves out. The best teachers are often those who have braved the darkest places and, through their teaching and studies, have come out the other side glowing with inner joy and a new appreciation for life.

# BEGINNER'S FLOW

The primary focus is on feeling the energy and changes in the body and breath.

1. Reclining stretch. Extend the arms over the head, and interlace the thumbs; flex the feet.

2. Knees to chest/feet to the sky. As you exhale, bring the knees to the chest; as you inhale, extend the feet to the sky. Repeat the movement 5 times.

3. Head to knees/reclining mountain. As you exhale, curl into a ball; bring the forehead toward the knees, keeping the shoulders down away from the ears, and chin tucked toward the chest; as you inhale, reach the arms over the head, and extend the legs and feet to the ground. Repeat the movement 3 times.

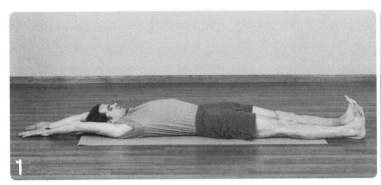

1

Reclining stretch

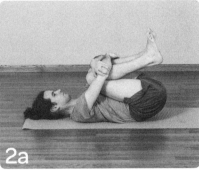

2a

Knees to chest

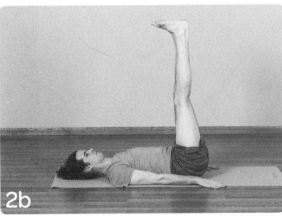

2b

Feet to sky

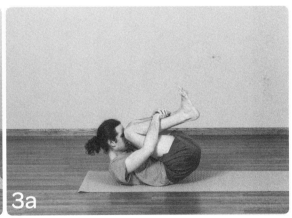

3a

Head to knees

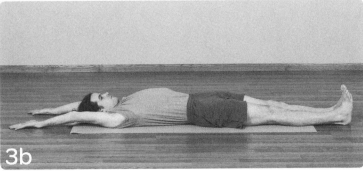

3b

Reclining mountain

*(continued)*

4. Reclining twist. Lower the knees and feet to the ground on one side of the body (or on a block if the knees don't meet the ground), extend the arms to a T shape, reaching from the shoulders.

5. Breathing bridge. As you inhale, press the feet into the earth as you move energy up the legs into the pelvic center, lifting the low back off the mat; as you exhale, lower the back to the ground. Repeat the movement 4 times.

6. Rocking chair. Hug the knees to the chest, and rock up and back along the spine several times to stimulate the back's meridians.

7. Easy pose. Pause and experience the energy radiating along the spine, the heat in the body, and the after-effects of the stretches.

8. Savasana (corpse pose). Pause. This resting pose is a state of being; feel the expression of a relaxing body.

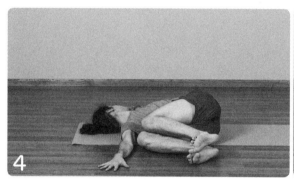

Reclining twist

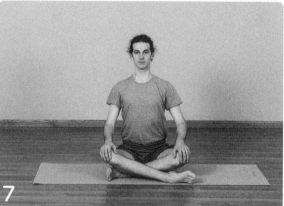

Breathing bridge

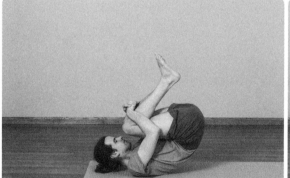

Rocking chair

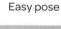

Easy pose

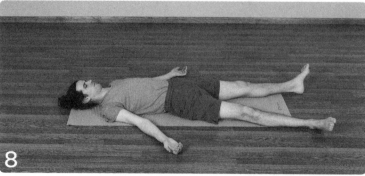

Savasana

# FIRST CLASS FACTS

## Intention

To introduce the foundation of yoga.

## Lesson

Welcome to the ancient science and practice of yoga. Before we begin, I want to mention a few things to make your experience in class the best it can be.

- Yoga is practiced in bare feet, so please take off your shoes and socks. Your feet have tiny receptors on the bottom; when you're in bare feet, you can feel the earth beneath you and sense your feet and legs plugging into the earth's energy. Practicing yoga in bare feet also helps improve your balance.

- Come to class on an empty stomach. Wait about 2 or 3 hours after a big meal, or about 1 hour after a snack. If you've just eaten, you'll quickly find out why you shouldn't have!

- Please silence your phones.

- Arrive a few minutes early. Consider being prompt a part of your practice.

- Let me know if you have any preexisting injuries or special conditions so that I can help you through variations of postures. No matter what physical limitations you have, there are many ways to practice a pose.

- Yoga philosophy asks you to let go of any competitive mind-set you bring to your practice. We can all be quite competitive, even with ourselves. Consider shifting those thoughts to remember that yoga is not just a workout, it's a spiritual practice that makes the body and mind stronger, more flexible, and generally healthier. The aim is to calm the mind, open the heart, and stimulate the spiritual evolution. Practicing yoga is a process. It's not about getting poses picture-perfect. It's about being sensitive to your body and quiet enough to hear your inner voice. So, get out of your own way and let the practice be your guide.

- Yoga has been praised for its stress-reducing properties. Essentially, the process works like this: Stress and tension cause the body to tighten up. Tension blocks energy flow. In yoga, we use asanas (the postures), and mindful breathing to open constricted areas of the body and mind. This helps to release and erase tension. As the body relaxes and opens, the mind becomes calm and quiet. When the mind is quiet, negative feelings like anxiety, fear, and anger melt and lose their control over you. Suddenly, you're thinking with clarity and making decisions by acting instead of *re*acting. And if that's not enough inspiration, consider that when the mind is open, it's available for achieving positive results such as patience, acceptance, and compassion.

- The one ground rule we have is to stay within your physical limitations. This means listening carefully to what your body is telling you, making decisions during your practice by honoring your body's messages, and erring on the side of safety. If you want to grow and heal, you have to take responsibility for listening to yourself.

- And most of all, have fun! This practice should feel good.

- [Follow this introduction with a lesson on diaphragmatic breathing. See the next lesson.]

## Asanas for Deepening

These opening asanas allow beginning students to awaken their bodies through gentle and subtle methods. Because this may be their first lesson in body awareness, concentrate on the most prominent points of beginning practice, such as opening the back and sensing the spine, feeling the feet on the earth, and stretching the breathing anatomy where breath is naturally blocked—the rib cage and intercostal muscles, waist, and hips. These movements ultimately help the student feel and release the breath.

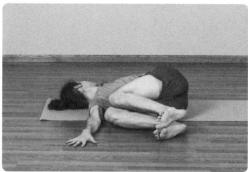
Reclining twist

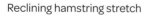
Reclining twist with eagle legs

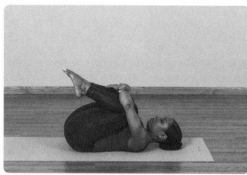
Knees to chest

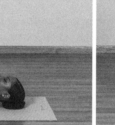
Leg cradle

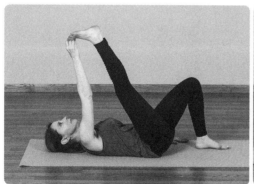
Reclining hamstring stretch

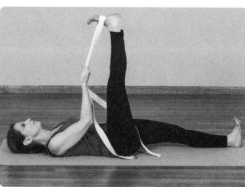
Hamstring stretch variation with strap

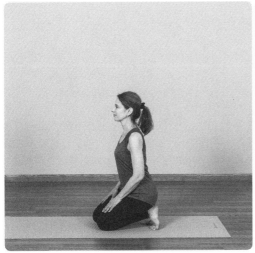
Sitting on toes

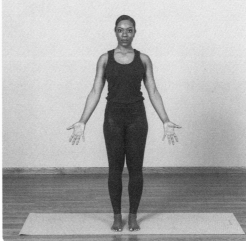
Mountain pose

## Motivation Off the Mat

At any given moment, keep your attention on what you're doing. When your mind wanders off to matters of the past or the future, like work, family, or old shadow stories, bring it back to the present moment.

## WISE WORDS

Your inner teacher holds all the answers. Listen.

Sensation is the language of the body. What's your body telling you now?

Yoga is a time-tested path for developing a deeper experience of yourself and the world.

Be kind and loving to yourself, accept all your flaws as well as your strengths. Many people are physically stressed because they believe their minds and bodies are separate. It's time to change that belief system.

## Teacher Tip

Smile and shine your light. Show your students the healing power of yoga.

# LEARNING DIAPHRAGMATIC BREATHING

## Intention

To educate students about the importance of diaphragmatic breathing.

## Lesson

Contrary to what you may have heard about modern-day yoga classes, perfecting a pose is not the intention or goal of yoga. The foundation of this yoga class is learning to breathe properly and completely. To do so, you need to learn a deep breathing technique called diaphragmatic breathing. Taking full and complete breaths allows you to slow down the heart rate, lower the blood pressure, clear the mind, and relax the muscles. In fact, it's the single most important thing you can do to reduce everyday stress. When you're not breathing fully, blood pressure rises, heart rate increases, muscles become tense, and thinking becomes scattered.

Breathing properly is not just the foundation of yoga; it's the foundation of life itself. Think about it: It's the first thing you do when you're born and the last thing you do before you die. You can actually live a few weeks without food, but you can only survive a few minutes without breathing.

Let's learn how to breathe diaphragmatically. Lie on your back with your feet about 12 inches (30 cm) apart, your arms at your sides, and palms up. Take a moment to sweep away any random thoughts other than being here in this room. Leave your past and your future. Keep your attention here in the present moment, feeling the weight of your body on the ground. When other thoughts pop into your mind, push them away and focus on these two words: *Just. This*. That's it. *Just. This*. This is your time to look inward and take care of your well-being. In doing so, you'll become highly adept at handling life's challenges.

Close your eyes and focus on your breath. As you breathe through your nose, bring all your awareness to your breathing. Notice if your breathing is shallow or noisy. Is your inhalation the same duration as your exhalation? Bring your focus to the space between your nostrils. Feel the coolness of the inhalation, the warmth of the exhalation. By focusing here, you're starting to turn inside.

The idea is to slide into an awareness of the breath—gently. No forcing. No pushing. Just remain present to the coming and going of breath. When the mind wanders off to work, family or responsibilities, simply bring it back to the breath. *Just. This*. Back to the breath. *Just. This*.

Now make sure that you're breathing from the diaphragm. First, soften the belly. Consciously release any tension you may be holding there. Then, place your right hand on your abdomen and your left hand in the middle of your chest. If you're breathing diaphragmatically, your right hand will move up and down as your abdomen naturally extends out on the inhalation and lowers on the exhalation. Your left hand should stay relatively still. [Pause long enough for students to take three to five breaths.] If only your left hand is moving, you're breathing from your chest, and getting about a third to half of the oxygen you'd get from diaphragmatic breathing. [Pause and walk the room to observe the students.] Think about your torso as a balloon, filling up with air, light, and energy from your belly on the inhalation. On the exhalation, releasing toxins and tensions from the pelvic floor to the crown of the head.

If you're not getting it today, keep trying; it will come naturally. Breathe diaphragmatically through the nose throughout class. Breathing through a posture helps you relax through it.

The deeper you breathe, the more relaxed and focused you become. Every inhalation brings in fresh prana, or lifeforce. Every exhalation releases the tension within the muscles as well as the mind.

Being sensitive to the whole body, breathe in; being sensitive to the whole body, breathe out. No striving, no forcing.

## Asanas for Deepening

○ *Reclining side stretch and sitting side stretch.* These poses open the intercostal muscles between the ribs, broadening the diaphragmatic breath.

○ *Clam.* Gently loosen the groin, low back, and hips.

○ *Crocodile.* Feel the inhalation fill the lower back as the abdomen presses to the ground.

○ *Standing forward bend.* Sense how the breath creates a waterfall vibration within the torso.

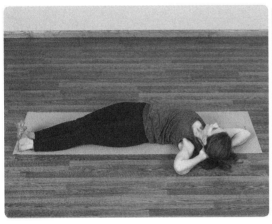
Reclining side stretch

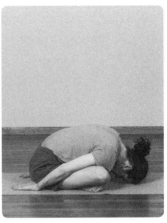
Sitting side stretch

Clam

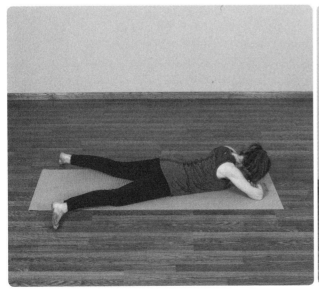
Crocodile

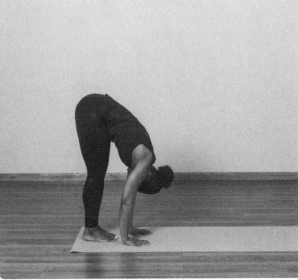
Standing forward bend

## Motivation Off the Mat

In crocodile or on your back, practice diaphragmatic breathing for 5 minutes a day. When you use the diaphragmatic breath to keep your emotions in check, you'll discover the supreme value of breath awareness.

## WISE WORDS

Gently nudge your tight areas with breath.

Diaphragmatic breathing is innate. We're born breathing this way; babies do it without any training. Later in life, when stress sneaks into the consciousness, we forget how to relax and simply breathe.

Yoga is preparation for living. It piques your curiosity and enthusiasm for life.

Breathing diaphragmatically awakens the body's relaxation response.

## Teacher Tip

Keep it simple; too many instructions confuse the outcome.

# BENEFITS OF YOGA

## Intention

Discovering the benefits of yoga practice.

## Lesson

Lie on your back with your feet about 12 inches (30 cm) apart, your arms at your sides, and your palms up. Rock your head from side to side until you find the flat part on your skull. Rest your head there.

Feel your abdomen rise and fall with each breath. Imagine your lungs as a pair of balloons, filling as you inhale and emptying as you exhale. As they fill, they become longer and rounder, growing in all directions. Feel the air in the back, the chest, sideways down the waist, each breath elongating the spine.

Yoga is a practical philosophy and science that involves every aspect of being. It teaches both self-discipline and self-awareness. At the physical level, yoga provides relief from many illnesses and diseases. The postures strengthen and stretch the body, and create a feeling of well-being. Yoga sharpens the intellect and improves concentration. Breathing practices calm the mind. Spiritually, yoga introduces you to yourself and your inner world, and gives you the gift of stillness.

Yoga is a time-tested path toward inner peace. Begin your journey by assigning meaning to every movement, breath, and thought, bringing you completely into the present moment.

## Asanas for Deepening

○ *Cat–cow.* Be aware of the whole body breathing, from the top of the head to the soles of the feet. Move with the breath. Inhaling at the navel center, pull the pubic bone toward the back of the room letting the belly hang loose *(photo a)*; as you exhale, round the spine, drawing the navel in *(photo b)*.

○ *Hip openers.* These poses uncover blocks of trapped energy that cause tension through the back and hamstrings. While practicing the reclining hip openers, focus on the physical and emotional edges of the stretch. Relax into the limitation, and see if you can stay with the pose for one more breath. Notice what's stretching; is it your muscles or your patience?

○ *Spinal rocks.* The spinal rock and roll presents an exhilarating approach to soothe and awaken the torso. Roll several times, building momentum with the breath. Exhale up to a seated position *(photo a)*, and inhale as you roll back *(photo b)*. Enjoy the tingling sensation along the spine.

## CAT–COW

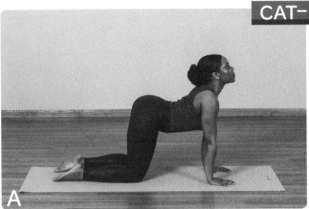

A

Inhaling, lift the abdomen and heart center (cow)

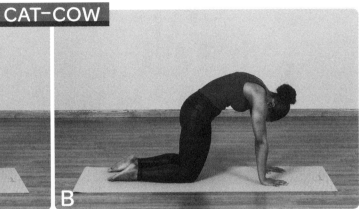

B

Exhaling, round the back, pulling the navel toward the spine (cat)

## HIP OPENERS

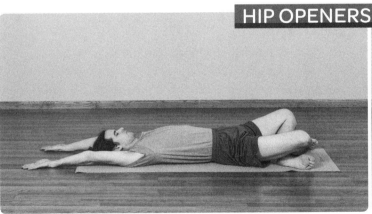

Reclining easy pose

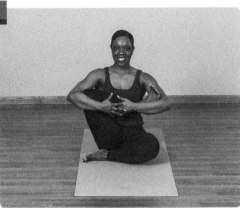

Leg cradle

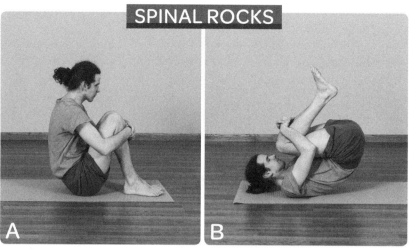

**SPINAL ROCKS**

A — Exhaling, sit up

B — Inhaling, roll back

## Motivation Off the Mat

Notice the subtle changes happening in your life. Do you sleep better after yoga practice? Are you more aware of your breath and how it relates to your emotions?

The next time you're in a tense situation, pause, drop your shoulders, and establish your diaphragmatic breath. Notice the positive effects of mindfully working stress out of your body.

## WISE WORDS

Learn what every posture has to teach you.

Listen to the sound of your breath, feel it in every cell, and imagine that the breath is stretching you.

Every emotion leaves an imprint on the physical body.

Watch your body alignment so that you can release trapped negative energy.

Experience gratitude for your body, including how it moves and the miracles it performs.

## Teacher Tip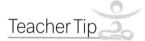

The real practice is showing up. Remember to give your students a world of credit and respect for coming to class. At the end of class, I always add, "Thank you for joining me today."

# SOFTENING THE EDGES

## Intention

Training the body and mind to surrender to the practice.

## Lesson

Lie on your back. Take a few minutes to relax and settle the body, especially the abdominal area. Then gently focus your attention on your breath.

The breath is loose and unrestricted. With each exhalation, let the weight of your body surrender to the floor, every muscle releasing its grip on the bones. Feel your eyes relax and soften, and your facial muscles release.

During today's practice, we'll use the definition of yoga (union) to guide movement. Yoga is about being integrated and connected to your breath, body, and mind. From this integration comes liberation, and that's when yoga happens. The breath creates this connection. By staying linked with the breath, you can direct prana (lifeforce) into areas that are tight, shallow, or shut down. You can then gently build an asana out of the breath's vibration, letting the breath move you.

When you work with this purpose, the pose comes alive. It's easy and fluid, rather than forced, stiff, or breathless. Roughness or shortness of breath is a symptom that you're forcing things instead of softening first and letting the breath do its job.

Be patient with yourself, and your tight edges will slowly open. Instead of trying to get into an asana first, connect with the breath and then flow into the asana; let your breath be the leader. Follow your in-breath and your out-breath. Join with the breath before you begin to move your body.

## Asanas for Deepening

○ *Reclining side stretch.* This stretch softens the ribs and each side of the back to help release into the postures that follow.

○ *Twisting triangle.* Stand with your feet 3 to 4 feet (about 1 meter) apart. Line up the toes and heels. Bring one hand toward the opposite leg, ankle, or foot; and reach the opposite arm toward the sky. Twist, using your hips and arms to expand the sensation. Spread your shoulder blades wide. Soften the pose one breath at a time. Welcome the subtle openings from hamstrings and groin to shoulders and fingertips.

○ *Standing yoga mudra.* Interlace the hands behind the back, cascading the torso toward the floor while draining the tension from the upper back, shoulders, and neck.

○ *Butterfly.* While sitting upright, press the soles of the feet together and soften the hips, inner thighs, and buttocks. Pause for 3 to 5 breaths before lengthening through the crown of your head, bending at the hips, and pouring the torso forward over the legs.

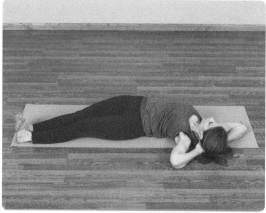
Reclining side stretch

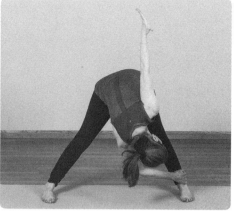
Twisting triangle

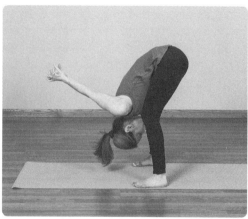
Standing yoga mudra

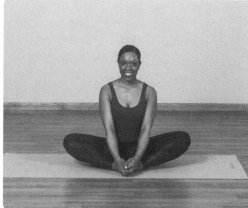
Butterfly

## Motivation Off the Mat

When you say or think negative thoughts about yourself, it has a small but measurable effect that takes root in your body and your mind . Think about what you think as well as what you say.

Stop beating yourself up and experience the freedom of your positive intentions. Focus on what's right in your life, not what's wrong with it.

## WISE WORDS

Empower creativity in each posture. Do them over and over again with the intention of activating different body parts and energy centers.

For your body, every day is a new beginning.

Give your muscles *permission* to soften and lengthen.

You've allocated this time for yoga class. Make the most of it by staying in the present moment.

Acknowledge rather than resist your limitations. Think to yourself, *It's okay to be exactly who I am.*

Speak the truth when speaking to yourself. If you can't be truthful to yourself, who can you be truthful with?

New teacher jitters? Sit quietly and breathe before class, gradually lengthening your exhalations to activate the relaxation state and engage your teacher clarity.

# BODY TENSION

## Intention

To discover the roots of tension.

## Lesson

Today, with awareness of breath and body, let's work through tension.

From a yogic perspective, every tension has a cause. Scan your body from head to toe and notice areas of obvious discomfort. Get clear and descriptive about the places where discomfort is living right now. Then, ask yourself what may be causing it in this area of your body. Be honest and objective with your answer.

Tension can originate from anything—relationships, work, anger, fatigue, caffeine, even an incident that happened years ago that's still lingering and taking up precious space in your body and mind. Muscle tension blocks the natural flow of lymph, hormones, nerve impulses, blood, and pranic energy. Eventually these blockages affect other parts of the body, creating weaknesses and lowering resistance to disease and infections. It's a ripple effect; when one thing is out of balance, it throws other body parts out of balance.

Tension may also be caused by excess like food, exercise, work, even rest; or spending too much time doing something that isn't productive, like staying in the presence of someone you don't like. Oftentimes people don't do anything about it except get angry or disappointed in themselves or others, and wish that person would change. The first step in dissolving tension is to get clear about what *is* out of balance.

Yoga practices teach us how to use body tension as a learning tool to guide us into the areas that we need to work on most.

Lie down on your back. Tune into the body on the ground, feeling the parts of the body that touch the ground. Pay close attention to the breath. This task is difficult if the mind is busy because the breath may feel awkwardly slow compared to the speed of your thoughts. Acknowledge this imbalance without judgment. Stay on track; keep practicing and watching.

In your mind's eye, search inside yourself for tight areas. Explore where you hold tension and what may be causing it. If your shoulders and neck are tight, ask them why. Keep your eyes closed, and let your mind open for the answers. A few simple words or visuals may come to you. Take the time to look clearly at what's there.

## Asanas for Deepening

Practice approaching poses with tension.

○ *Triangle.* Take the pose with exaggerated shoulder tension, then consciously remove the tension by spreading the shoulder blades across the back. Note the relief of letting go.

- *Superman.* Long, deep breathing in superman pose releases a central acupressure point located between the navel and the breastbone that helps free body tension. Hold the posture for 3 breaths.
- *Shoulder openers.* Shoulder movements free up tension in the shoulders and upper back. These movements are especially effective for students who sit all day at desk jobs.
- *Neck rolls.* Begin with the head, neck, and trunk in alignment. Notice any tension that may be present in your muscles, especially the trapezius, located on top of your shoulders. Stay in a pain-free range of movement. Do not drop your head back.

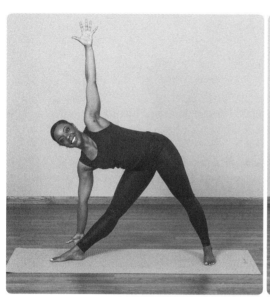

Triangle

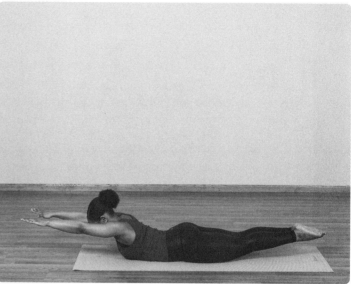

Superman

## SHOULDER OPENERS

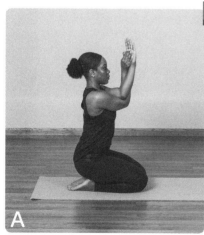

A

Eagle arms

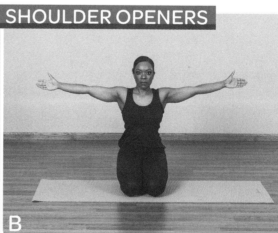

B

Arm swing wide

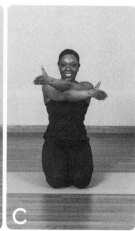

C

Arm swing across

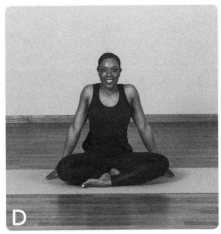

D

Shoulders tense

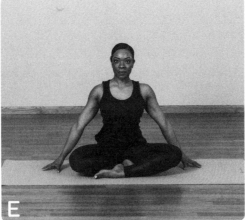

E

Shoulders release

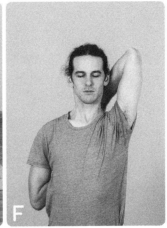

F

Cow face arms

## NECK ROLLS

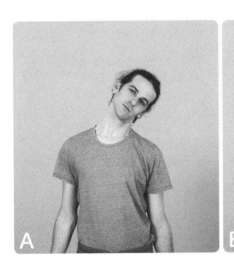

A

Ear to shoulder

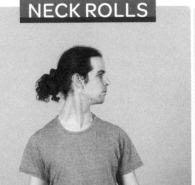

B

Look over shoulder

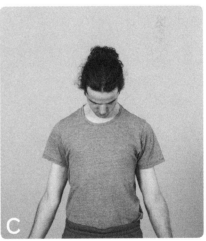

C

Chin to chest

## Motivation Off the Mat

Be open to all the benefits of yoga. The rewards may come at any time during your day.

What triggers your anger? Uncontrolled emotions use up a lot of spiritual fuel. A few minutes of anger can cost more energy than a day of physical labor. Have compassion for yourself.

*You will not be punished for your anger; you will be punished by your anger.*

—Buddha

A pose can be heavy, clogged, and uncomfortable or bright, light, and full of inner expression. Which one do you choose?

The wise yogi lets go of all results, whether good or bad, and stays focused on the action alone.

### Teacher Tip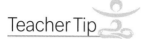

Words are like seeds that take root; make sure you're planting good ones.

# LENGTHENING THE EXHALATION

## Intention

To learn how to relax during stressful life events.

## Lesson

[Begin class with neck and shoulder rolls.] Lie on your back and take a few minutes to relax and settle the body. Next, focus your attention on your exhalation, following it to flow all the way down into the pause at the end of the breath. Intently focus on watching your breath for a few minutes.

With each exhalation, feel the weight of the body surrender to the floor, the muscles releasing their grip on the bones. Gradually begin to lengthen your exhalation. If you feel any shortness of breath, return to even breathing. If it helps, open your mouth on the exhalation.

Continue until you find a comfortable rhythm, sensing inner calm and relief. As you enter a deeper state of relaxation, let go of any control of your breathing and simply watch the spontaneous breathing pattern that's now happening.

Notice how you feel. Can you sense more clarity in the mind? Do the muscles feel more relaxed? This ability to willfully relax is only a few exhalations away.

In today's practice, use this gift of lengthening the exhalation to facilitate healing.

## Asanas for Deepening

Observe the cleansing power of the exhalation within each asana.

- *Downward dog.* Move into the posture with a long exhalation, squeezing the navel toward the spine as you pull the heels toward the earth.

- *Head to knee.* Moving with the breath, exhale to bend forward. As you inhale, rise up slightly, with the chest opening and lifting away from the pelvis. Discover any tight or stuck spots and breathe into those areas, releasing tension with the exhalation.

- *Twisted chair.* In chair pose, bring the palms together at the heart, twist to one side, and place the opposite elbow on the outside of the knee. Drop the sit bones, and pull back through the spine to experience a tenacious, relaxed effort.

- *Dancing warrior II.* Ground the back foot and straighten the leg. On an exhalation, bend the front knee and widen the arms, reaching from the heart *(photo a)*. Inhale to straighten the bent knee, moving the arms up to the sky *(photo b)*. Repeat the movement 3 times.

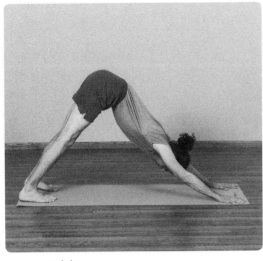

Downward dog

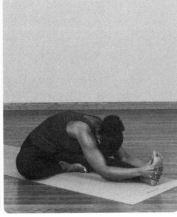

Head to knee

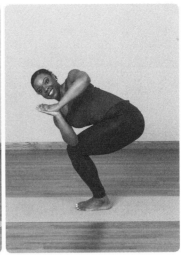

Twisted chair

## DANCING WARRIOR II

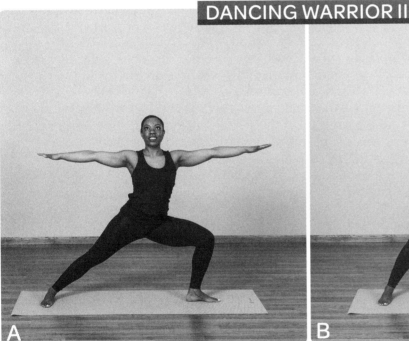

**A**

Lengthen the arms and ground the feet

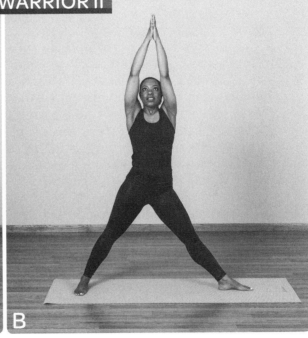

**B**

Straighten the legs and reach to the sky

## Motivation Off the Mat

During stressful times, take long, conscious exhalations, imagining the tension and dark emotions leaving your body through every pore of your body.

## WISE WORDS

Asana pulls your attention to the present moment, a practice that leads to a sense of self-study and inner peace.

By being attentive to every thought and sensation, observe how the mind constantly influences asana.

Scan your body and objectively notice where you feel stuck or open, strong or weak.

## Intention

To define the components of the word *hatha*.

## Lesson

The balance of body, breath, mind, and spirit is not easy to achieve. From day to day and minute to minute, you could find yourself emotionally swinging back and forth. However, when you use yoga techniques to actively calm the body and mind, you can more easily accept and adapt to life's changes and challenges. This resilience is an essential component to living a more satisfied, joyous, and balanced life.

Fundamentally, the concept of hatha yoga is bringing opposites into balance. The word *yoga* means "union," "yoking," or "joining together." The root word *ha* in the term *hatha* means "sun," and *tha* means "moon", which are polar opposites. These opposites include attributes like hot and cold, dark and light, physical and mental, hard and soft, left and right, and male and female. Hatha yoga acknowledges these opposing factors and brings them together in an effort to reach mental, physical, and spiritual balance.

The physical practice of executing specific postures with proper breathing is the primary stepping stone on the path to harmony among body, breath, mind, and spirit.

According to the ancient yogis, asana was originally developed as a prerequisite to dharana (concentration) and dhyana (meditation). The body was seen as a vehicle to the soul, and meditation was the process to get there. However, to sit in meditation for long periods of time, the body needs to be free of tension and sufficiently flexible to sit without discomfort, and the mind should be quiet and able to concentrate.

The body is the vehicle to the soul, so treat it with respect. Feel your boundaries. Sense your limitations. At the same time, expect and allow yourself to expand, to get better, stronger, and experience a calm heart.

While seated or lying on your back, bring all your awareness to your breathing, establishing the diaphragmatic breath. As the abdomen rises and falls with each breath, feel it taking in life. Observe the natural flow in and out of your body. Let the breath be the link between the mind and the body.

## Asanas for Deepening

Remember to balance *ha* and *tha* by combining easy with challenging, relaxing with invigorating, and stretching with strengthening.

○ *Serpent.* Press the toes toward the forehead. Note the difference in flexibility from one side to the other.

○ *Tree.* Is it possible to find equal balance between the right and left sides?

○ *Hatha flow.* Move from triangle pose *(photo 1)* to pyramid pose *(photo 2)* to high-lunge twist *(photo 3)*, taking three complete breaths in each pose. Feel the sensation of left versus right or stronger versus weaker. Are you feeling warmth on one side? Are you off balance? Now try the sequence with your eyes closed.

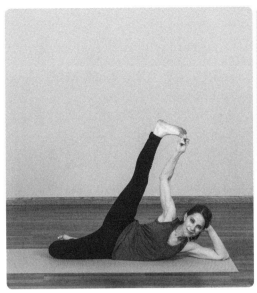
Serpent

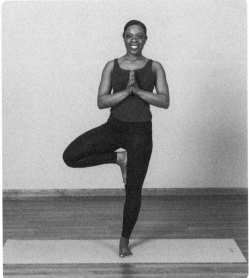
Tree

## HATHA FLOW

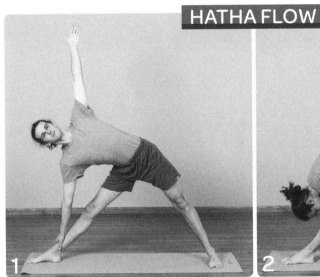
**1** Triangle

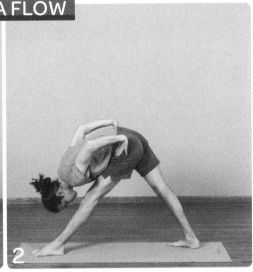
**2** Pyramid

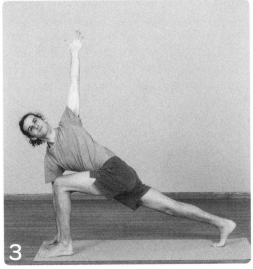
**3** High lunge twist

## Motivation Off the Mat

Experiencing pleasure requires focus on what you're doing and how you are doing it. Stay present, living consciously in each moment.

Life balance is acknowledging that what you're doing right now is the right choice for what you need *today*. It's common to feel gloomy or irritated when you work, sleep, eat, or drink too much (or too little). If you're sensing an imbalance, contemplate this question: *What would a balanced day look like?*

## WISE WORDS

A posture isn't an asana unless you're breathing through it and mentally connecting to it.

Yoga isn't measured by the depth of a forward bend or the flexibility of the hamstrings. It's not about how your postures look; it's how they feel when you're in them.

A calm approach to your yoga frees the mind to experience a deeper awareness of the moment. This is the highest form of practice.

Lengthen your subtle lines of energy by visualizing them filled with light, air, and intention.

When a posture becomes effortless, it becomes meditation.

## Teacher Tip

Prior to the start of class, go inside of your energetic self and review the day's lesson. Speak from the heart. Speak your truth. If you don't get it, your students won't either.

# SETTING AN INTENTION

## Intention

To create a dedicated purpose to hatha yoga practice.

## Lesson

Before we begin asana, sit quietly and set an intention for your yoga practice. Setting an intention narrows the focus of your practice by working with a defined objective. Your clear intention makes the difference between a powerful, progressive form of conscious physical and mental action, and just a limited exercise experience.

An intention can come from any number of mind-sets. It can be simple, such as *To create relief in my neck,* or it can be more complex, such as *I'm moving out of a bad relationship, so my intention is to find inner strength.* An intention can be a blessing, a prayer for someone you love, affirmation, or a doorway to begin a process of change. What do you want to manifest?

Keep your intention concrete and specific, and word it in a positive manner. Instead of saying "I don't want to be lonely," you might reframe it to say "I feel the love and support of my friends." Intentions amplify our mental clarity and focus, as well as our emotional state and perspective.

Revisit your intention throughout class to keep it at the top of your mind. In this way, you can hold it in your heart from now through the end of class.

Bring your hands together to prayer position to seal in the purpose for today's practice, as if you were holding your intention at your heart center. Hold this position as a reminder of your intention. See yourself in complete mindfulness, holding space for your intention, before taking the first conscious breath.

## Asanas for Deepening

- *Spinal rocks.* Wake up the energy in the spine.
- *Seated arm stretch.* Embrace movement by using a loving experience rather than by muscular power. Think of reaching out to a loved one. Notice how intention matters.
- *Inverted plank.* Relax into the full expression of the pose, observing the responses and fluctuations among the outer body, will, and ego.
- *Hidden lotus or easy pose.* Take lotus (or easy pose) to the knees, and slowly walk the hands forward until the abdomen is on the ground. Spread the hips wide open.
- *Intention vinyasa.* Begin in active child's pose with the arms stretched and elbows off the ground *(photo 1)*. Holding your intention in mind, exhale into table twist. Inhale to reach one arm to the sky *(photo 2)*, then exhale to lower the arm to table pose, and lift your hips to downward dog *(photo 3)*. Inhale into upward dog *(photo 4)*, and exhale back to child's pose *(photo 5)*. Move with your words of intention, synchronizing the breath with the movement.

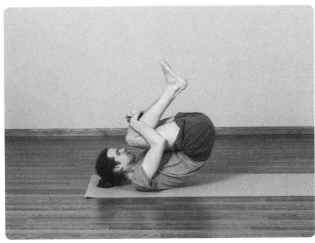

Spinal rocks

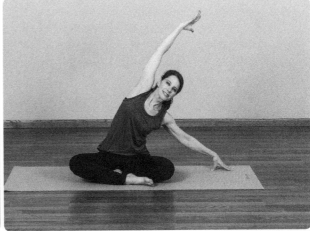

Seated arm stretch

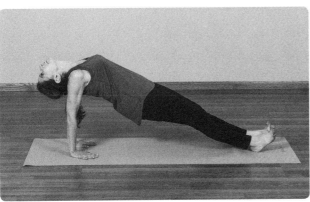

Inverted plank

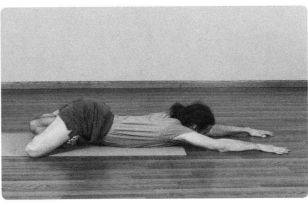

Hidden lotus

# INTENTION VINYASA

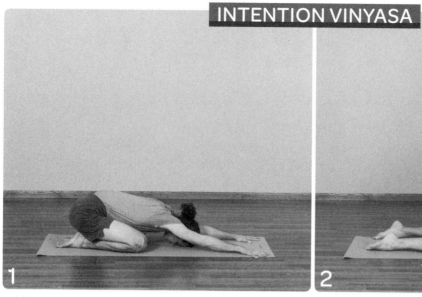

**1** Child's pose

**2** Table twist

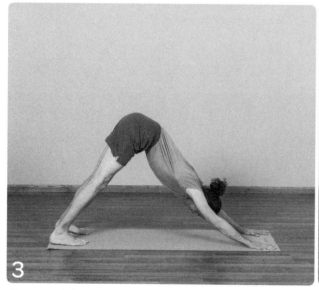

**3** Downward dog

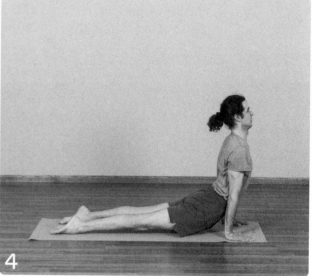

**4** Upward dog

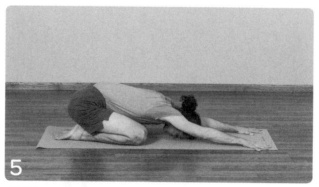

**5** Child's pose

## Motivation Off the Mat

Set a daily intention every morning. Before you begin, pause for a moment to breathe self-acceptance into your eyes, skin, muscles, bones, and heart. Feel yourself alive! Breathe and receive.

## WISE WORDS

Notice your physical sensations, the quality of your natural breath, and your state of mind. Concentrate on how the body's sensations contribute to your mental strength.

By applying mindful intention, you can practice the same pose every day for 10 years and have a different experience every time you do it.

## Teacher Tip

Create classes and themes to benefit your students, not you. Feel the energy in the room, and ask your students what they need today. Teach your class with mindful intention.

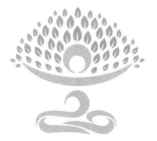

# Breathing Practices

*To enjoy good health, to bring true happiness to one's family, to bring peace to all, one must first discipline and control one's own mind.*

—Buddha

This chapter is intended to advance your practice and teaching of complete breathing. At their core, these techniques are the most effective tools for better health, better living, and better awareness.

The lessons in this chapter reveal that the healthiest breathing skill is mastering the complete diaphragmatic breath. If the breath is shallow or uneven, these exercises will be inefficient and may even cause dizziness or lightheadedness.

Focusing on the breath is a decision to live in the moment. Take a mindful breath now as you embark on the training for a more gratifying and yogic life.

# SMILING BREATH VINYASA

In most yogic traditions, pranayama is an essential part of yoga classes. Treat your students to the allure of pranayama practices, and they'll not only relish the physical postures, they'll appreciate the aftereffects that pranayama adds to their class experience.

1. Seated. Begin by putting a gentle smile on your face.
2. Scrape the barrel. Move the torso in a clockwise direction, planting the sit bones while taking one complete breath for each rotation. Repeat the movement 3 times, then reverse the rotation.
3. Seated twist. Take one complete breath on each side. Repeat the sequence 3 times.
4. Cat–cow. As you exhale, round the spine and tuck in the tailbone; as you inhale, lift the sit bones, relax the belly, and lift the head. Repeat the sequence 3 times.
5. Cat–downward dog–cow. From the cat position, exhale, squeezing all the air out of the lungs, round the back, and aim the navel center toward the spine. Next, hold the

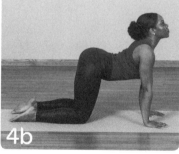
1 Seated

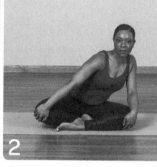
2 Scrape the barrel

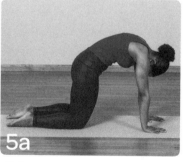
3 Seated twist

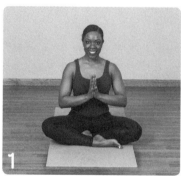
4a Cat

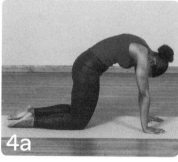
4b Cow

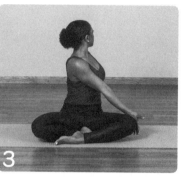
5a Cat

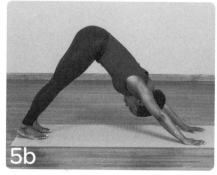
5b Downward dog

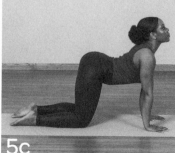
5c Cow

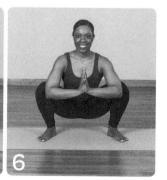
6 Squat

breath out and lift your pelvis into downward dog. As you inhale, gently lower the knees to the ground, lifting the sit bones and heart. Repeat the sequence 3 times.

6. *Squats.* Squats free up sukha (good space) in the body. Bend and straighten the legs 3 times, inhaling on the squat as you rise up to standing.

# TWO-TO-ONE BREATHING

## Intention

To feel the cleansing and releasing power of the exhalation during asana.

## Lesson

Please take a seated position. Keep your attention in the now, gradually leaving your past and your future. Become intimate with the sensitivity of your body on the ground, the sound of my voice, and the awareness of your own breath. When your attention is focused, your mind is focused.

Establish your diaphragmatic breath, feeling your navel rise and fall. Allowing the breathing to be free and easy.

When people feel stressed, our natural fight or flight reaction is for the breath to become shallow, resulting in breathing from the chest rather than the belly. The inhalation becomes longer than the exhalation, eventually causing waste and tension to build up, ultimately making people vulnerable to more anxiety and stress.

The practice of two-to-one breathing lengthens the exhalation to twice as long as the inhalation to quickly calm the body, release mental tension, and induce a natural state of relaxation. It's like taking a big sigh, and it's an indispensable skill to have in your yoga toolbox.

Try it now. Gradually slow down the exhalation until you're exhaling to a silent count of *4, 3, 2, 1;* and inhale to a silent count of *1, 2.* Exhale *4, 3, 2, 1;* inhale *1, 2.* Continue this tempo as you pull in the navel slightly to get a longer exhalation. Don't force the breath on either the inhalation or exhalation; you're simply changing the rhythm of breath. [Pause 1 to 3 minutes.] Now return to normal diaphragmatic breathing.

While using the two-to-one breath in asana practice today, stay connected to the quality and length of your breathing.

## Asanas for Deepening

Practice any pose using two-to-one breathing. Observe how the torso moves and loosens with each exhalation, developing patience and mental clarity.

○ *Pyramid.* Use an elongated, soothing exhale to soften the hamstrings and the lower back.

○ *Butterfly.* Sitting tall, press the soles of the feet together. On the inhalation, extend through the crown of the head; on a long exhalation, release the head, neck, and trunk forward and down.

○ *Woodchopper.* Inhale lifting your "ax" to chop wood *(photo a)*; exhale bending forward while visualizing chopping the wood *(photo b)*.

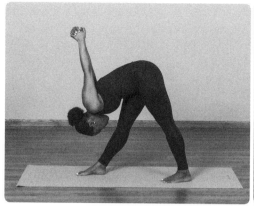

Pyramid

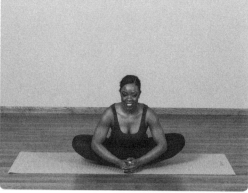

Butterfly

## WOODCHOPPER

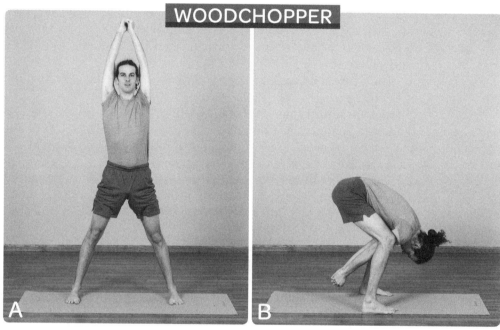

A — Arms above head

B — Arms between legs

## Motivation Off the Mat

The technique of exhaling as long or longer than you inhale helps release stress, anxiety, and fear, allowing you to act instead of react.

Counting the duration of the breath helps focus a scattered mind and prepares us for dharana (concentration).

Breathing practices are *meant* to be taken off the mat. Try it to ease your next anxiety-producing experience like going to a job interview, meeting new people, or getting caught in a traffic jam.

## Teacher Tip

Your teaching style changes shape and direction as you do. Embrace the progress of inevitable change.

# THREE-PART EXHALATION

## Intention

To release built-up tension by enhancing the exhalation while stimulating the inhalation.

## Lesson

Today we're going to change our thinking patterns by consciously altering our breathing pattern. One way to make this happen is through lengthening the exhalation by dividing it into three equal parts, and pausing briefly between each exhalation.

This exercise produces a longer exhalation than you might usually take. The three-part exhalation breath is useful if you have trouble releasing stress, falling asleep, or when you have a buildup of tension, which is common during menstruation and menopause.

Please take a comfortable seated position. Begin by taking a normal breath in, then divide the exhalation into three equal parts so that you're emptying the breath from the bottom of the torso—the pelvic floor, to the top—the throat center.

First inhale completely, then exhale from the pelvic floor to the navel center. Pause. Then exhale from the navel center to the heart center. Pause. Finally, exhale from the heart center to the throat. Pause. Inhale again, and repeat the process. Let each part of the exhalation be of equal length. The pauses between the sections of exhalation should feel like a calm moment of hesitation rather than holding the breath.

Take two to three normal breaths, then repeat the three-part exhalation breath. Visualize walking up a tall staircase, exhaling as you step up and pausing at each step before ascending further.

Try 10 breath cycles, then return to normal diaphragmatic breathing.

## Asanas for Deepening

Use the three-part exhalation to help ease into and out of the pose.

○ *Seated twist.* Take a simple twist *(photo a)* or sage twist *(photo b).* Use the three-part exhalation to move into the pose, twisting farther with each exhalation. Feel how the exhalation strengthens the depth of the pose.

○ *Extended standing forward bend.* Follow your three-part exhalation downward to take the pose outward through the crown of your head. Note how a relaxed breath helps to unwind and brighten the pose. Inhaling, fill your posture with breath. Exhaling, melt the crown toward the ground.

○ *Bridge.* Release the back of the torso with a three-part exhalation, feeling each section of vertebrae touch the earth.

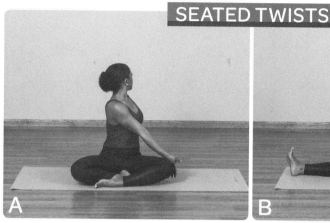

## SEATED TWISTS

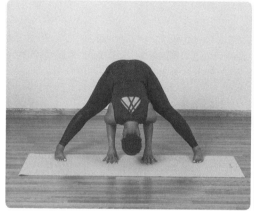

A — Simple twist

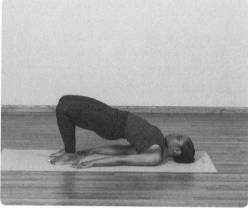

B — Sage twist

Extended standing forward bend

Bridge

## Motivation Off the Mat

Consider your time on the mat as a means to sweep through your energy field, erasing mental and physical debris. Get clear about what you want to remove. Use your concentrated thoughts to weed out that debris, creating more space for personal growth. Feel the lightness as the weight of your worries is lifted from your consciousness.

## WISE WORDS

A focused mind directs prana.

When you have the ability to direct your own prana, you'll discover that you're in control of your own lifeforce.

When you're filled with toxins, tensions, and closed-down body parts, you leave no room to store prana.

Invite your mind to breathe into every part of the body.

It's wise to practice your class lesson when you feel overwhelmed to ensure that what you're delivering to your students is useful to *you*.

# UJJAYI BREATH

## Intention

To use the breath to focus on the deeper physical awareness of the postures.

## Lesson

Today we're learning ujjayi breath. The word *ujjayi* means "victory" and it's often referred to as the victorious breath. Unlike normal diaphragmatic breathing, in which the throat is relaxed and the breath is silent, ujjayi uses an audible vibration with purposeful tension.

Through sound, this type of breathing during asana and some pranayama practices, draws attention to the breath and internalizes awareness. It also helps develop consciousness of the subtle body and psychic sensitivity. Using ujjayi breath during asana practice is an excellent preparation for meditation. It also helps you prepare for more advanced breathing exercises by reducing body tension and generating heat.

Ujjayi requires breathing against the resistance of a constricted glottis, the aperture in the throat just behind the Adam's apple that opens and closes when you hold your breath. Closing the glottis allows pressure to build up before you cough, and permits liquid to stay in your mouth without running down your throat, as when you gargle.

The distinct sound of ujjayi breath is similar to the sound of ocean waves, and it's often called *ocean breath*. [Demonstrate the breath, walking around to each student so that they can hear the sound.] As you can hear, the breath is deeper than usual. To learn this breath, whisper "ha" with the mouth open on the exhalation, and whisper "ah" on the inhale. Then, gradually close the mouth. You'll begin to feel the air on the back of your throat.

Sometimes you'll notice a short pause in the sound of ujjayi after inhalation and exhalation, but don't allow a pause in the breathing itself. Each inhalation flows into the next exhalation. The easiest way to deepen the breath is to expand the abdomen fully during inhalation and to contract it completely during exhalation.

Be attentive to the soothing effects on the mind and the nervous system. We'll work with ujjayi during our asana practice. If you feel dizzy or out of breath during this practice, please return to normal diaphragmatic breathing.

## Asanas for Deepening

Ujjayi breath leads to a deeper awareness of the posture by internalizing the attention.

○ *Lotus.* Breathe with ujjayi breath, sensing the air move up and down the spine. Mentally repeat the mantra of the sound of the breath, *so hum.* As you inhale and feel the breath move down the spine, mentally repeat *so.* As you exhale and feel the breath move up the spine, mentally repeat the sound *hum.*

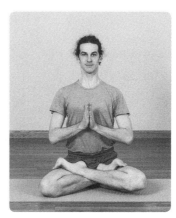

Lotus

○ *Lunge series.* Work with full, deep ujjayi breaths through a series of lunge variations, including hip openers such as heel to hip *(photo a)*, dragon pose *(photo b)*, and lunge twist *(photo c)*.

○ *Upward dog–downward dog.* Inhaling in upward dog pose, spread the collar bones wide *(photo a)*; moving to downward dog pose, exhale a long, audible *ha* breath *(photo b)*.

## LUNGE SERIES

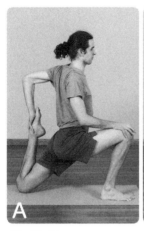 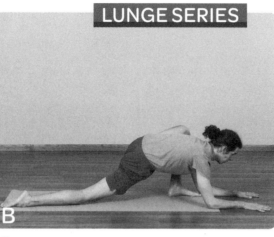 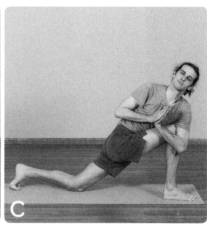

A — Heel to hip

B — Dragon

C — Lunge twist

## UPWARD DOG–DOWNWARD DOG

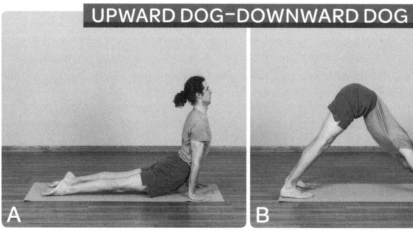 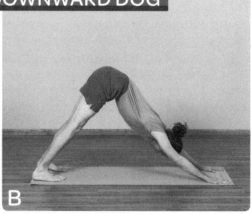

A — Upward dog

B — Downward dog with audible *ha* breath

## Motivation Off the Mat

As with any yoga pose, let life unfold naturally. Resist the temptation to dominate a situation or the body.

Experience the sweetness of now within each breath.

## WISE WORDS

Ujjayi promotes the embodiment of the senses.

As the breath becomes more refined, so does the posture.

If you forget ujjayi after a few breaths, be patient. Continued practice will allow you to stay inside the posture and the breath.

Ujjayi is a combination of two Sanskrit words: *ud*, meaning "up," and *jayi*, meaning "victory." Experience yourself victorious!

Typically, beginning yoga students don't like to bring attention to themselves by making audible breathing noises. When my classes get too quiet, I raise my voice and say, "Remind your fellow yogis to use ujjayi breath by breathing loud enough so that *everyone* can hear it!"

# NADI SHODHANA

## Intention

To learn alternate-nostril breathing and its benefits.

## Lesson

[Practice this lesson at the beginning, middle, or end of class.] Our pranayama practices are intended to control prana, the vital energy force within all of us. There are over 72,000 nadis (subtle energy channels) within the body through which prana flows. If the nadis are blocked, prana can't readily move through the body, which inhibits consciousness and clarity, and makes it difficult to find meaning in daily life. This kind of blockage results in the manifestations of suffering—distraction, dullness, anger, fear, anxiety, sleepiness, and depression. But there's good news. As the nadis are purified and cleansed, prana can travel freely and consciousness is restored. It's a lot like having your air ducts freed of debris.

*Nadi shodhana* means "nadi cleansing," or alternate-nostril breathing. It's a breathing exercise that helps anchor the wandering mind as it purifies the nadis. The focus is on the two main nadis, called the *pingala* and the *ida,* which begin at the base of the spine. Pingala ends at the right nostril; ida ends at the left.

Pingala (the right nostril) embodies the sun. It has a yang, or heating effect on the body. It's described as male energy and linked to left-brain function associated with active external energy, intellectual pursuits, and rational reasoning. When this nostril is open, the pathways to logical thinking are open as well. It's a good time to do some bookkeeping, make a business presentation, or socialize. Right-nostril dominance also gives you the warming power to digest food.

Ida (the left nostril) represents the moon and has a yin, or cooling effect on the body. It's described as feminine energy and linked to the right side of the brain and internal energy. Left-nostril dominance is connected to imagination, intuitive thinking, introspection, and subjective decisions. When this nostril is open, it's a good time for creative thinking, writing, listening to music, or meditating.

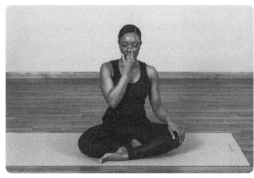

Pingala (right-nostril) breathing

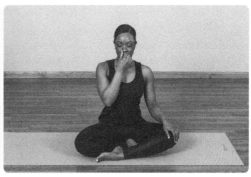

Ida (left-nostril) breathing

In nadi shodhana, the breath alternates between the right and left nostrils, seeking to balance the energies of the sun and the moon. When the nadis are cleared and energies are balanced, prana can flow more fluently.

Let's try one round together. Sit in a comfortable seated position, with your head, neck, and trunk aligned. Breathe into each nostril separately in order to see which one is flowing more smoothly. Chances are, you'll have an active nostril and a passive nostril. Begin your practice on your active side. Establish your diaphragmatic breath.

Bring the right hand to the nose. Fold the index finger and middle finger so that the right thumb can be used to close the right nostril and the right ring finger can be used to close the left nostril. Inhale through both nostrils.

Close the passive nostril, and exhale completely through the active nostril.

Inhale through the active nostril slowly and completely. At the end of the inhalation, close the active nostril, then slowly and completely exhale and inhale through the passive nostril.

Repeat this cycle of exhaling and inhaling 2 more times for a total of 6 breaths.

At the end of the final inhalation through the passive nostril, exhale through both nostrils and take 3 deep breaths; this completes 1 round.

In summary, for 1 round of nadi shodhana do the following:

1. Exhale active.
2. Inhale active.
3. Exhale passive.
4. Inhale passive.
5. Exhale active.
6. Inhale active.
7. Exhale passive.
8. Inhale passive.
9. Exhale active.
10. Inhale active.
11. Exhale passive.
12. Inhale passive.
13. Exhale through both nostrils and take 3 deep breaths.

Practice a few rounds of nadi shodhana at the end of an asana to restore equilibrium between the two nadis and compensate for any imbalances inadvertently caused during practice.

## Asanas for Deepening

Each nostril relates to different physiological aspects of your being. After practicing a series of the following deep, stimulating backbends, check to see whether the right nostril is active.

○ *Bridge.*  ○ *Camel.*
○ *Cobra.*

Do the same for the following passive-hold poses, checking to see whether the left nostril is active.

○ *Standing forward bend.*  ○ *Squat variation.*
○ *Seated forward bend.*  ○ *Child's pose.*

Finally, note the nostril flow at the end of class. Aim to have a smooth and open air flow through both nostrils so that sushumna (the central main nadi that runs along the spine and ends at the crown chakra) is active.

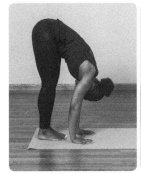
Bridge

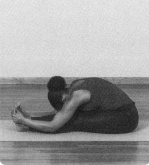
Cobra

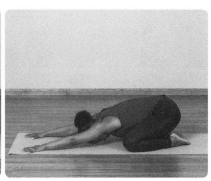
Camel

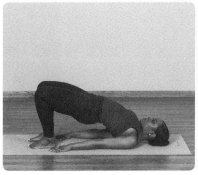
Standing forward bend

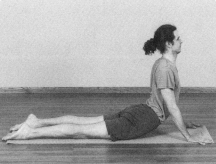
Seated forward bend

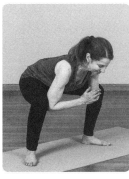
Squat variation

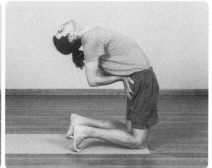
Child's pose

## Motivation Off the Mat

Practice nadi shodhana anytime you need to calm the emotions. Try it first thing in the morning and you'll feel its balancing effects for the rest of the day.

Use nadi shodhana as a light in the midst of a storm. A student of mine reported excusing herself from a heated business meeting to practice several rounds of nadi shodhana in the restroom. She came back feeling refreshed and sufficiently self-reliant to tackle the remainder of the meeting.

To alleviate insomnia, practice nadi shodhana starting with the left (moon) nostril.

## WISE WORDS

> Once you affirm that you're exactly where you want to be, you'll be amazed at how much energy is suddenly within you.
>
> Listen to the sound of your breath. Feel it in every cell. Imagine that the breath is stretching you.
>
> The more awakened the pranic field, the more energetic you feel.

## Teacher Tip

If you want to add an additional round of nadi shodhana, take 3 to 5 breaths after the active-side round, and begin 6 complete breaths on the passive side.

# OPENING THE LEFT CHANNEL

## Intention

To learn to activate the right brain by opening the left nostril.

## Lesson

Have you ever come to class feeling completely agitated or unclear?

When you begin your practice in a relaxed state, it activates the right hemisphere of the brain—the yin side that controls complex memories, internal energy, and holistic thinking. The right side of the brain then integrates more readily with the left hemisphere—the yang side of the brain that manages rational thinking, external energies, and heat-inducing activities like digestion.

There are two main channels of energy—the ida, (left) and pingala (right)—that weave lifeforce through the chakras, the wheels of subtle energy that are housed in the spinal column. Each of these energy channels ends in either the left or right nostril. When the breath—and prana—are carried predominately through the left nostril, the body remains calm and the mind will be quiet. This is an ideal setting to practice gentle asana and meditation.

Today we'll begin our practice by opening the left nostril, which is responsible for activating the right brain. Lie down on your right side, resting your right ear against the inner upper arm. Stay here until the left nostril clears.

Each breath is like an ocean wave, swelling and receding in perfect rhythm. Concentrate on this vital flow of nourishing air into and out of the body. Visualize a slow rolling ocean wave as you breathe completely and effortlessly.

## Motivation Off the Mat

For a simple practice to alleviate anxiety arising in the body or mind, close off the right nostril with the right thumb and breathe out of the left nostril, taking 6 complete breaths. Next, move your thumb away from the right nostril and breathe out of both nostrils for 3 complete breaths. Repeat the practice until the left nostril is active.

## WISE WORDS

The first step in releasing stress is to recognize when you're *feeling* it.

Every time you see a red light or long line, instead of allowing yourself to feel burned by impatience, use your time to practice breathing in and breathing out. Smile. This wait is out of your control.

## Teacher Tip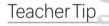

Fill the entire room with your radiance, and create a safe yoga space for inspiration.

# 3

# Asana

*You are a seeker. Delight in the mastery of your hands and your feet, of your words and your thoughts.*

—Buddha

Asana, the third limb along the royal path, is a powerful, practical, and ingenious physical practice. By engaging your internal intelligence in asana, the body reaches deep layers of consciousness that help to advance your own physical, mental, and spiritual healing progress.

Open your mind to the creativity within each posture. For instance, if you experience a new sensation in triangle pose when you turn your upper arm in, out, or over the head, share it with your students. The deeper you delve into the process of self-study and self-discovery, the more inspiring and alive your practice and teaching will be.

# STEPPING STONE VINYASA

The stepping stone vinyasa is a reminder that asana isn't the goal of yoga; it's merely a means to get there, a form of transportation to find the stillness of the mind. Ride the motivational wave as you guide the way through the path of movement.

Take 3 to 5 breaths in each pose before transitioning to the next one.

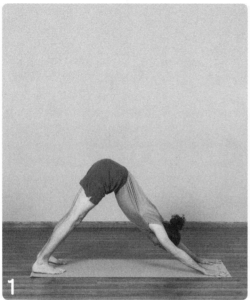

Downward dog

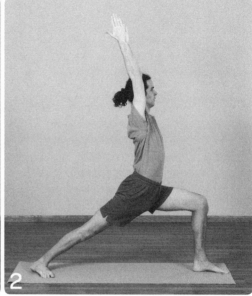

Warrior I

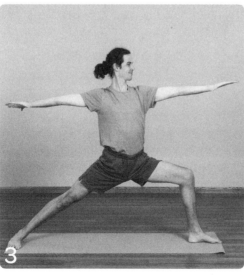

Warrior II with palms up

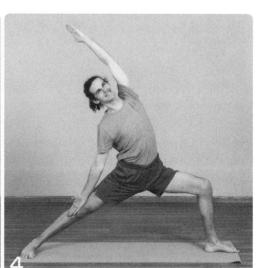

Reverse warrior

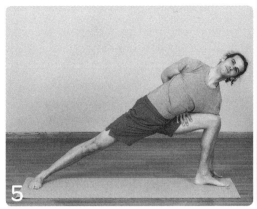

5

Side angle with top arm in half bind

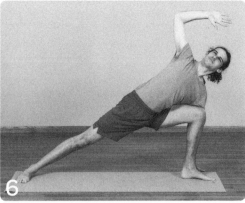

6

Side angle, circling top arm clockwise and counterclockwise

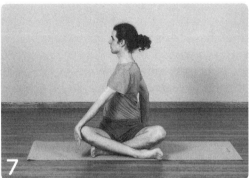

7

Seated twist

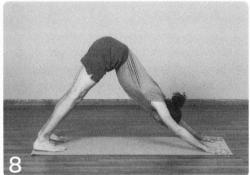

8

Turn to downward dog and repeat the sequence on the opposite side.

# FEET

## Intention

To feel the body's foundation by plugging into the earth's energy.

## Lesson

[Begin class in mountain pose.] Do you know how important your feet are? The average person takes 6,000 steps a day. That's a lot of miles over the years. The feet are your foundation and your connection to the earth. If the foundation is weak, problems will show up in the rest of the body; the lower legs, the back, and even the shoulders can be traced to issues in the feet.

In all of the standing poses, the feet—the part of the body that touches the ground—form the foundation of the posture. If the foundation of a house is out of alignment, the walls will be contorted and disrupt the entire framework. In asana practice, if the feet are misaligned or the body weight is off center, it's difficult to strike a tall, spacious, and centered pose. Your body is like the house; if your foundation is off-balance, you can disrupt the entire framework.

Your weight should be evenly distributed between the outer and inner foot, and between the heel and ball of the foot. Here, we practice samastitihi which means "equal standing." This balance gives your body ideal postural alignment that translates to strong, expansive standing postures as well as other poses in which your feet are engaged.

Close your eyes. As you stand, become aware of the four corners of each foot—the base of the big toe, the base of the little toe, the inner heel, and the outer heel. In a firm, well-balanced foundation, the arch feels lifted and light while the inner heel and base of the big toe stay grounded. Take a moment to feel your foundation, and make any adjustments necessary.

Let's use this foundation consciousness as we begin our asana practice.

## Asanas for Deepening

- *Mountain pose.* Spread your toes, and hug the soles of your feet to the earth. Let the weight of your body snuggle downward into the ground. As the weight of the body moves downward, the earth's inner energetic force rises up to the crown of the head.

- *Warrior I, warrior II, and triangle.* In all standing poses, note the positioning of the feet. Feel the current rising from the ground, through the soles of the feet, traveling up to the pelvic floor.

- *Tree.* In one-legged balance poses, much of the work is accomplished prior to the foot being lifted off the ground. Begin in mountain pose, establishing the balanced action of both sides of your body. Imagine a root extending from each of the four corners of the standing foot, growing into the earth. From that root system, visualize the pranic pathways traveling through the leg to the pelvic floor, and from the pelvic floor through the spine, up to the crown of the head. Then lift the opposite leg and place the foot on the standing leg.

- *Toe seat.* Sitting on curled toes provides a stimulating stretch for the soles of the feet.

- *Butterfly.* According to ancient teachings, the feet are symbols of humility and peace. Bringing the head, the seat of the ego, and the feet together cultivates your humble and introspective potential. Bend forward, aiming the third eye toward the toes.

- *Tennis ball massage.* This simple massage is remarkably effective for tired feet and sensitive soles (and souls!). While standing, roll a tennis ball under the sole of your foot to stimulate circulation and the energy within the meridian points.

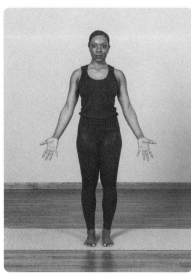

Mountain

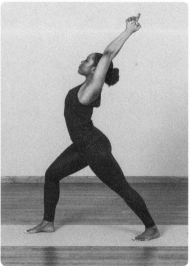

Warrior I

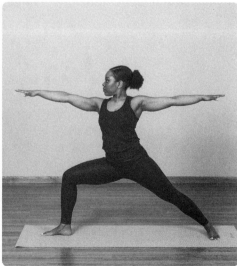

Warrior II

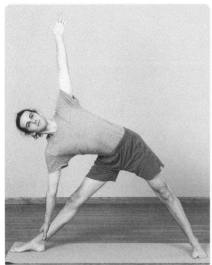

Triangle

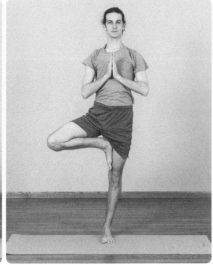

Tree

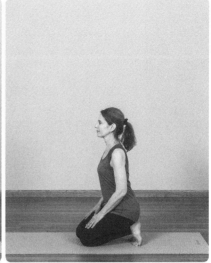

Toe seat

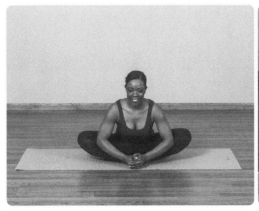

Butterfly

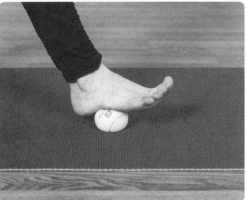

Tennis ball massage

## Motivation Off the Mat

Take your shoes off and let your feet breathe. Walk barefoot, spreading your toes frequently.

Wear comfortable shoes. Avoid shoe styles like high heels, which take their toll on your spine by pushing the hips and lower back out of alignment, putting excess pressure on the balls of the feet and knees.

Try using plastic or gel toe separators. They free the toes from getting too close to each other and help prevent mild corns and relieve bunion pain.

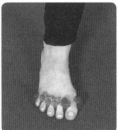

Yoga toe separators

To keep the soles in tip-top shape, massage the feet several times a week. Foot massage helps maintain healthy joints and muscles, improves circulation, and alleviates edema (swelling of the legs and feet caused by fluid retention).

- With your fingers between your toes, circle your ankles 8 to 10 times in each direction, then flex and extend the balls of your feet 8 to 10 times.
- Massage the balls of your feet, toes, arches, heels, and tops of the feet.
- Stamp your feet on the ground as if you were trying to put out a small fire. Feel the tingling response rise up through each leg.

Practice breathing easily in all standing poses, securing your foundation before moving on to the next posture.

Feel the grounding strength awakening through the feet, rising up the legs, and settling into the pelvic floor. From there, create space in the pose by spreading the pelvic floor energy through the rest of the body up to the heart and throat, out to the fingertips.

Ignite and extend the balls of the feet forward, and spread the toes. Use your feet to take up lots of space. Plug in, and power up!

## Teacher Tip

For a soothing effect on your sore feet, put a pair of plastic or gel yoga toe separators in the freezer before use.

# FORWARD BENDS

## Intention

To develop a quiet and patient mind through the settling effects of forward bends.

## Lesson

Forward bends are quieting and settling, and they bring your attention inward, making them compelling counterposes to the more vigorous backbends. Because they're a robust antidote to mild anxiety, they're also used to develop one's patience and humility.

Forward bends are also excellent for relieving mild back pain. They stretch and lengthen the spine, the muscles of the lower back, the pelvis, and the legs. The upper back, kidneys, and adrenal glands are stretched and stimulated as well.

The influences of the mind are observed throughout an entire practice, but forward bends—primarily sustained forward bends—teach us that the integration of yoga requires more mental than physical effort.

Forward bends test our patience to come back to the present. When you hold a forward bend with your eyes closed, become aware of the melodramas and stories in your mind's eye. See if you can wait out those little mind performances until they drop away completely, while your focus rests on your breath and the gentle release into the pose.

[Be sure to balance the forward-bend sequences with backbends and twists.]

## Asanas for Deepening

○ *Seated forward bend.* This posterior stretch is said to be the ideal pose for examining the ebb and flow of the mind. Rather than taking the pose to the edge and folding to your limit all at once, practice patience by first emphasizing the length of the front torso hinging at the hip creases, slowly bending forward, taking the pose deeper with breath. Discover all you can from the inside out.

○ *Standing forward bend.* Try several variations of this pose to explore new sensations in the back, hamstrings, and shoulders. For example, try palms to the ground with legs straight, knees bent, or hands on a block *(photo a)*; hands to the back of the ankles, shoulder blades spread *(photo b)*; and opposite hand to opposite elbow *(photo c)*. Continue letting go again and again using the power of the exhalation.

○ *Child's pose.* Bring the hands next to the feet with your palms up. Hum a soothing exhalation into the mat.

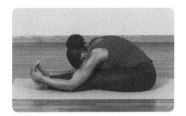

Seated forward bend

## STANDING FORWARD BEND

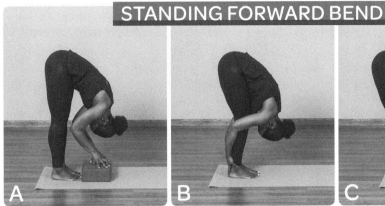

A — Hands on a block

B — Hands to the ankles

C — Opposite hand to opposite elbow

## Motivation Off the Mat

Forward bends teach you about the middle way—the rejection of extremes. Whether you're deciding what to eat for lunch or how to behave toward an unfavorable co-worker, notice the equilibrium and clarity a yogic lifestyle yields as you practice the philosophy of balance.

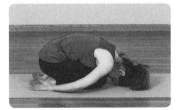

Child's pose

## WISE WORDS

The seated forward bend is often called "the stretch of the west;" the ancient ritual of the yogi facing the sunrise (east) during practice means that the back of the body faces west.

Recognizing what's true for your body can be challenging if your desire is to be in a place that you aren't ready for. Remind yourself to think organically about the pose.

Explore any negative mental patterns you're bringing to the asana, such as an urge to push or a tendency to let the mind wander.

## Teacher Tip

Forward bends calm the brain and invigorate the nervous system. Practice a 2-minute standing forward bend before class to awaken and clear the mind.

# BACKBENDS

## Intention

To explore the physiological aspects of backbends.

## Lesson

Yoga is defined as the restraint of the fluctuations of the mind. The practice is intended to reduce these fluctuations in the frontal lobe of the brain, the part that's most involved in conscious thought.

As you progress in your practice, your time on the mat will be spent moving from the familiar to the somewhat obscure, from the front part of the brain to the back of the brain, and from the front of the body—the known—to the back of the body—the unknown.

Today, we're going to bring the awareness of the unknown to our backbends. Think of the opposite of backbends—forward bends. They're quieting, cooling, and settling, while backbends are stimulating, heating, and exciting. The backbend is the yang to the forward bend's yin. Backbending postures bolster a sense of expansion, confidence, and bravery. They open the entire front of the body, including the chest, abdominal organs, pelvic region, and quadriceps.

Yoga is about oneness and integration of body, mind, and spirit. When areas in the body—front, back, or sides—are closed down, it makes us feel more separate and limits energy flow. When we're are low on energy, it limits what we're capable of doing, which can lead to mild depression and fear.

The physical aspects of backbending work counter to these impressions because they improve circulation along the spine, helping relieve depression and other symptoms of feeling closed off from the outer world. Backbends ignite confidence, courageousness, and aliveness.

[Be sure to balance backbends with forward bends, twists, and neutralizing poses such as child's pose.]

## Asanas for Deepening

Before beginning a backbend, first lengthen the pose, then explore the depth. Depth without length creates constriction. To inhibit overstimulation of the sympathetic nervous system (the fight-or-flight response), and create a calmer pose, develop an even and steady breath with the main consideration on completing the exhalation.

Practice a series of warming asanas such as sun salutations, twists, and moderate backbends like sphinx pose to warm up to wheel. Protect the wide muscles of the back from overextending by practicing gentle stretches like knees to the chest, child's pose, happy baby, and reclining twists between poses.

- ○ Lunge
- ○ Crescent lunge
- ○ Cobra, supported *(photo a)* and unsupported *(photo b)*
- ○ Camel
- ○ Upward dog
- ○ Bow *(photo a)* and bow with teacher assist *(photo b)*
- ○ Bridge
- ○ Wheel

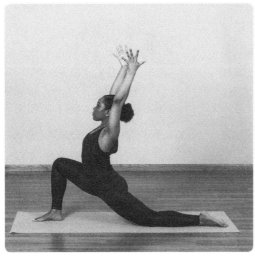

Lunge

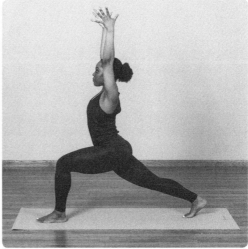

Crescent lunge

## COBRA

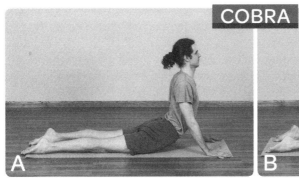

A

Supported cobra

B

Unsupported cobra

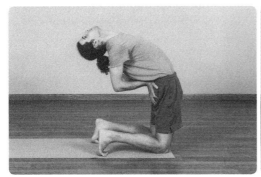

Camel

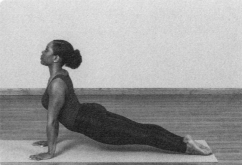

Upward dog

## BOW

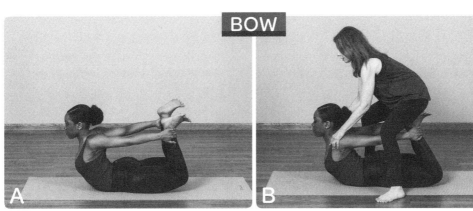

A

Bow

B

Bow with teacher assist

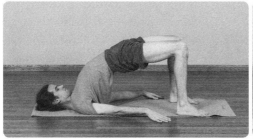

Bridge

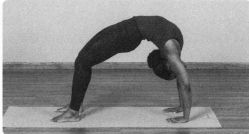

Wheel

## Motivation Off the Mat

Simple backbends such as unsupported cobra and bridge are recommended for anyone with breathing problems. Backbends open the breathing anatomy around the shoulders, collarbone, and chest, eliminating tightness that cramps the rib cage. Once the chest opens, more space is created for the lungs, allowing for deeper breathing and increased oxygen flow.

When you're feeling sluggish, a few breathing bridges (inhale to rise, exhale to release) are an ideal pick-me-up asana sequence.

Backbends help counteract the damage of bad posture by helping to realign the vertebrae while stimulating the sympathetic nervous system.

## WISE WORDS

The power of backbends is subtle, yet immediate. They work directly on the nervous system, assisting relief to ease mild depression.

Think of the backbend as an adventure. It's mysterious, provocative, and stimulating to the senses because it engages a part of the body you can't see.

The posture is a tool that exposes you to more energy and light, making more space to free the spirit.

## Teacher Tip

What's the difference between cobra and upward dog? In cobra, the feet, ankles, thighs, and pelvic triangle are grounded before lifting the front of the spine off the mat. In upward dog, while the knees can remain on the ground, the pubic bone is raised off the mat for a slightly stronger pose.

# TWISTS

## Intention

To observe the cleansing wring-and-release effect of the twist.

## Lesson

The twist is the great asana equalizer. If you're lethargic, it picks you up; if you're stressed, it helps calm you down.

The real virtue of twists is that they compress the body and assist in untying tension. When you release the wringing-out action of the twist, the muscles that were involved in the pose become flooded with nutrients, increased oxygen flow, and fresh blood.

Twists tone and cleanse the organs, strengthen the muscles of the spine and neck, and open the shoulder joints. As the torso rotates, the kidneys and abdominal organs are activated and exercised. This action improves digestion and removes sluggishness. Because the nervous system begins in the spinal cord, every part of the body is given the opportunity to rejuvenate and heal. Twists invite you to become more comfortable in your body and more inspired by your own tenacity.

Let's discover the twist's physical principles by taking a seated twist in easy pose with the pelvis in a neutral position. Bring your awareness to the crown of your head. Open the crown so that the chest, neck, and head are lifted. Elongate and align the spine by pressing the sit bones into the floor. Lift and open your heart center. Bring your left hand to your right knee and your right hand behind you, supporting yourself with your fingertips. Inhale and lift as you lengthen the spine. As you exhale, slowly rotate to the right from the base of the spine up through the low back, waist, shoulder blades, and neck, finally turning your gaze to the right. With each inhalation, continue to lengthen the spine, creating space in the vertebrae; on each exhalation, amplify the twist. [Repeat on opposite side].

[Remember to balance your twist practice with forward bends and backbends.]

## Asanas for Deepening

- ○ *Reclining twist.* The rib cage releases as the feet and knees settle to the earth or a block.

- ○ *Seated twist.* Perform a simple twist *(photo a)* and half spinal twist *(photo b)*.

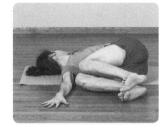
Reclining twist

- ○ *Standing twist.* Step your feet slightly wider than hip-distance apart. Allow your arms to extend straight out, like the letter T. Move side to side, twisting at the waist and allowing the arms to swing with you, bending the knees gradually; reach farther on each repetition. Connect your breath to the twists from right to left; inhale when you twist right, exhale when you twist left.

- ○ *Eagle.* Eagle pose distributes the benefits of twist to the legs and the arms.

- ○ *Revolved triangle.* Squeezing the inner thighs toward each other, while keeping the lower vertebrae near the pelvic floor stable, gently twist up the spine continuing the inner movement up to the crown of the head. Extend upwards through the top arm.

- ○ *High lunge prayer twist.* Move the elbow to outside the opposite knee, and place your palms together in prayer at your sternum.

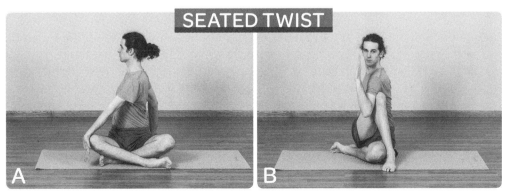

### SEATED TWIST

A — Simple twist

B — Half spinal twist

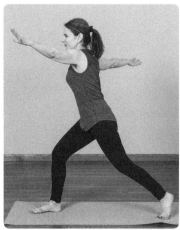
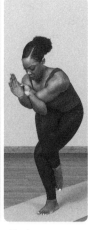
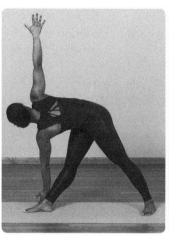
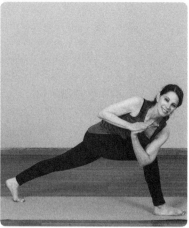

| Standing twist | Eagle | Revolved triangle | High lunge prayer twist |

## Motivation Off the Mat

When you're seated for long periods of time, take several twist breaks in your chair. Move the knees to the right side of the seat and the hands to the armrests on the right side. Reach upwards through the crown as you inhale. As you exhale, gently twist to the right. Repeat the twist on the left side.

## WISE WORDS

Twists keep *avidya*—spiritual tunnel vision—out of your life. By staying present with everything around you and behind you, your inner vision remains clear and unobstructed by illusion.

Twists keep you mindful and present during life's inevitable changes.

Before you begin the twisting movement, lengthen the torso by pressing downward and rooting into your foundation while reaching upward toward the sky. Feel the spine come to life.

# HEADSTANDS

## Intention

To welcome the benefits of the king of asanas.

## Lesson

The headstand is known as the king of asanas. It has legendary benefits, including increased vitality, improved concentration, and enhanced glandular functioning.

Accomplishing headstand though, can be quite demanding. Some students have trouble with it because they don't have enough strength and flexibility in the shoulders and hamstrings, or they have weak lower backs and abdominal muscles. Fortunately, a number of preparatory poses and variations of the headstand address these issues.

A third hurdle, which may be the most overlooked, is that headstand requires overcoming the fear of turning upside down and, with it, the possibility of falling. For anyone in this category, use the wall for support.

Contraindications for practicing headstand include high blood pressure, heart problems, cervical spine injuries, detached retina, glaucoma, osteoporosis, neck and shoulder injuries, excess weight, pregnancy, and menstruation. If you have one of these conditions, it's best to avoid putting any pressure on the top of the head or the cervical spine. Instead of headstand or shoulderstand, (which is a preparatory pose for headstand) please practice legs to the wall pose.

Let's begin class with some postures that lay the groundwork for the king of all asanas.

## Asanas for Deepening

Some schools of yoga counter headstand with mountain pose, while others follow with child's pose to alleviate any dizziness. Trust your inner teacher, and stay connected with what feels best for you.

Practice these preparatory postures before demonstrating headstand.

- *Reclining hamstring stretch*. This posture stretches and warms the hamstrings.

- *Lunge series*. Try low lunge with the back knee on the ground *(photo a)*, high lunge *(photo b)*, and dragon pose with the elbows on the ground near the inside of the front foot *(photo c)*.

- *Locust*. Locust develops the low-back muscles to stabilize the low back.

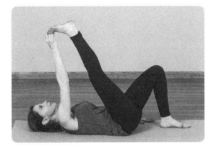

Reclining hamstring stretch

- *Fire series*. Practice a series of postures to strengthen the navel center, digestive system, and the low-back muscles. Include yoga cycling *(photo a)*, scissor stretch *(photo b)*, and double-leg lifts *(photo c)*.

- *Shoulder openers*. Loosen the shoulder area with eagle arms *(photo a)*, cow face arms *(photo b)*, and arm swings *(photos c and d)*.

- *Dolphin*. The movement of the dolphin develops stamina and stability in the shoulders as it strengthens the abdomen and back muscles, and primes the forearms to support the weight of the body.

- *Bridge pose*. The bridge and its variations expand the upper chest and elongate the spine. Press the feet into the earth, lift the thighs, and expand the heart.

- *Shoulderstand*. Take shoulderstand with the elbows and forearms supporting the lower back to prepare the neck, upper back, and shoulders.

## LUNGE SERIES

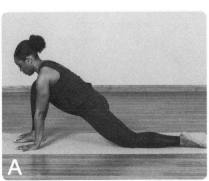

A

Low lunge

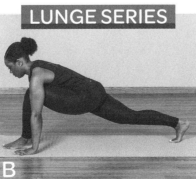

B

High lunge

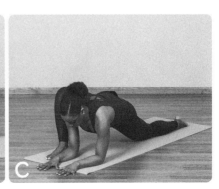

C

Dragon

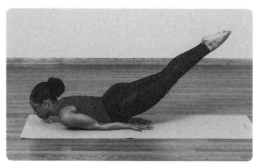

Locust

## FIRE SERIES

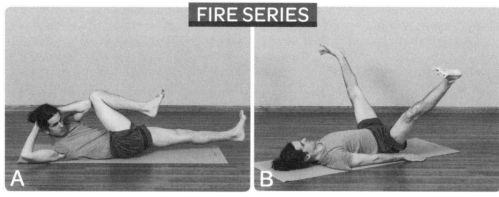

Yoga cycling

Scissor stretch

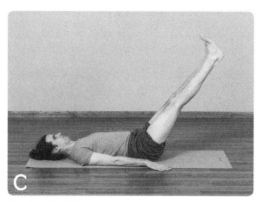

Double-leg lifts

## SHOULDER OPENERS

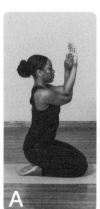

Eagle arms

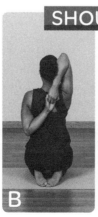

Cow face arms

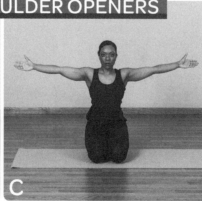

Arm swings with arms open

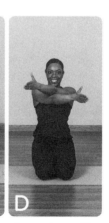

Arm swings with arms closed

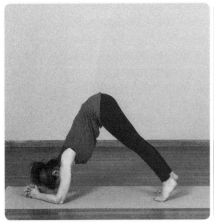
Dolphin

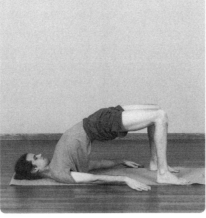
Bridge

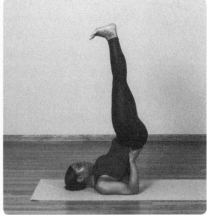
Shoulderstand

The headstand requires a slow start and demands a considerable amount of core and shoulder strength. In fact, in the early stages of learning headstand, try practicing the lift while using the wall for support. To begin, come into the dolphin pose, walk the feet toward your head, and raise the knees to the chest while collecting your balance *(photo a)*. Then, straighten your legs, lifting the soles of the feet up to the sky *(photo b)*. Protect your neck; keep the weight of the pose on your forearms rather than on the crown of the head. Allow your ujjayi breath to flow deeply. To exit the pose, bend the knees to the chest, and release the feet to the ground. Rest in child's pose. Once you build strength and proficiency in the headstand, try the tripod variations *(photos c and d)* as you step into mastery of headstand.

## HEADSTAND

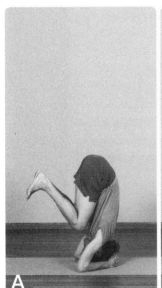

A

Halfway up

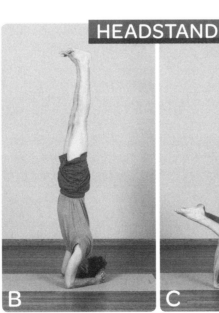

B

Full headstand

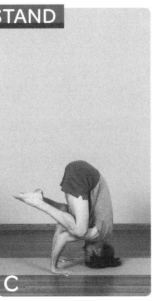

C

Tripod with knees on upper arms

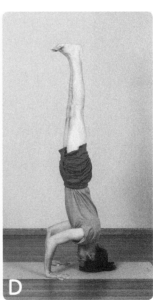

D

Full tripod headstand

## Motivation Off the Mat

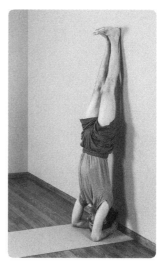

Headstand stimulates the crown chakra, the connection to divine spirit.

Notice the confidence and inner strength that are revealed when headstand is accomplished.

When you practice headstand, the immune system is given an automatic boost. The lymph system moves through the body only when you move, unless you reverse the flow by inverting the body.

Headstand at the wall

## WISE WORDS

If your balance shifts as you raise your legs up into headstand, stop moving until you gain equilibrium.

Moment-to-moment awareness is the secret to balance.

Deepen your headstand by adding ujjayi breath. Ujjayi is effortless in inversions because the throat is already compressed.

## Teacher Tip

Achieving headstand takes exceptional courage and composure. Practice breaking through the fear so that you can benefit by the life-altering exhilaration of turning your life upside down.

# ASANA AND ACCEPTANCE

## Intention

To explore Patanjali's definition of asana, and accepting your place in asana as in life.

## Lesson

In Patanjali's *Yoga Sutras*, asana is defined as a pose that's both steady and comfortable. In this sense, the interpretation is to be fully present, exclusively alive to the now experience.

Learning to be present and participate in something that's both steady and comfortable means freeing yourself from any thought or sensation that allows a resting place for suffering, including self-criticism, future worries, or living with unsettled emotional wounds. When you live in the present, you're practicing yoga and living abundantly.

There are times in practice when many of us respond from a place of unnecessary judgment and criticism, thinking things like *I can't do this posture* or, *Everyone else is more flexible than I am*. Today's practice is to silence your inner critic. When you catch yourself criticizing something or someone, notice the judgment, then check to see if it's coming from your emotions, your past experiences, your body, or your breath. Then, exhale your inner critic's voice out into the stratosphere.

If you're forcing asana or other parts of your life, ask yourself *Is this the true spirit of yoga*? When things are steady and comfortable, there's no forcing, only progress.

## Asanas for Deepening

Teach postures that you (and your class) find challenging, such as half moon with the foot hold (candy cane), firefly, or yoganidrasana (yoga sleep pose). The practice is not to *perfect* these poses but to feel the potential ease and comfort that's possible anywhere in any asana when you practice acceptance. Warm the muscles with sun salutations, quadriceps stretches, and hip openers.

○ *Half moon.* If you're unable to reach the ankle or foot in the candy cane variation, use a strap around the arch as a connector from your hand to your foot.

○ *Compass pose.* The compass points your focus in the right direction as it warms the shoulders, hips, and hamstrings. For a less challenging variation, try leg cradles.

○ *Firefly.* Have fun and be playful in this pose. Ground the heels of your hands and fingertips to the earth, and practice lifting one leg up at a time. Light up like the firefly!

○ *Yoganidrasana.* For this unusual pose, try lifting one leg at a time behind the arm or shoulder, planting the opposite foot on the ground. Chip away at an outdated attitude of *I can't do it* by breathing the mantra *I can.*

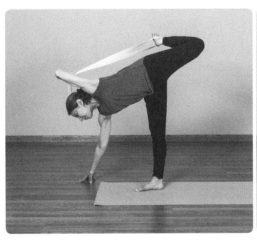
Half moon with candy cane using strap

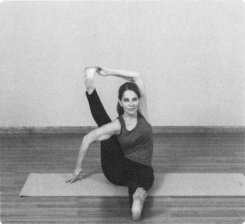
Compass pose

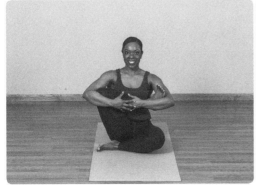
Leg cradle

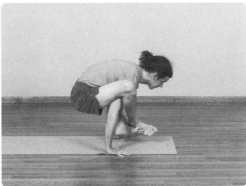
Firefly

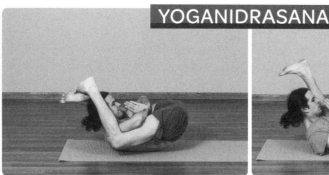
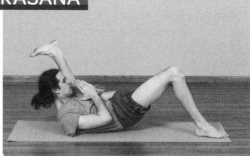

## YOGANIDRASANA

Yoganidrasana

Yoganidrasana with one leg

## Motivation Off the Mat

Take a bird's-eye look at your life. Do you see areas that you'd like to change or eliminate entirely, places that don't feel steady and comfortable? Can you make adjustments in your mind-set as you practice and adjust your asana? Allow these areas in your life to flow through you so you can accept them rather than agonize over them.

Feel yourself becoming sensitized and responsive. Be passionate about the choices you make, tuning into your heightened perception of being alive.

When something or someone is of your control, accept it by changing your attitude.

## WISE WORDS

Don't concern yourself with what anyone thinks about you. The problem with craving acceptance is that it puts the base of power outside of yourself.

Accept where you are in this moment without striving, without comparing, and without judgment. Go where it feels the most desirable, where your energy flows best. You have the ability to sense this. Trust it.

Everyone has a different idea of what the words *steady* and *comfortable* mean. What do these words mean to you today?

If there's a place in your body or an aspect of your emotions that needs extra attention, invite your benevolent loving spirit to embrace those areas with joy and compassion. Don't allow remorse or shame to occupy any space in your being.

## Teacher Tip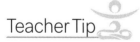

Live your life without an inner critic, and abandon the *I'm not good enough* chatter in your head. Accept where you are in your journey.

# ASANA AND PEACE

## Intention

To learn how yoga practice has a positive impact on peace.

## Lesson

Most yogis benefit from a nonviolent, benevolent spirit. The practice introduces a tranquil frame of mind; it asks you to become more sensitive to yourself as it heightens your compassion toward your fellow human beings.

As you become more awakened, you move away from forcing and controlling events, and you move toward letting the universe take care of your daily dilemmas. You give up attempting to control situations that aren't yours to control. These changes influence the consciousness and actions of every person you meet. The sensitivity you develop on your yoga mat touches everyone in your personal universe. They, in turn, influence everyone in *their* universe, and the ripple effect continues.

You soon begin to notice that you can shift the direction of the world.

## Asanas for Deepening

○ *Parrot.* This pose symbolizes neutrality, one who takes action without analysis, repeating what others say without attachment.

○ *Clam.* Experience the wonder of the body breathing autonomously. Who is in control of this breathing? It happens 24 hours a day, every day, for your entire life, without conscious effort. As you follow the breath up and down the spine, breathe awareness into your back muscles.

○ *Peaceful warrior flow.* Move from warrior II *(photo 1)* to warrior I *(photo 2)* to warrior III *(photo 3)*. Be bold. Feel the fortitude, firmness, and determination it takes to practice being the warrior. Dare to confront the difficulties of life head on with a peaceful intent to face internal conflicts.

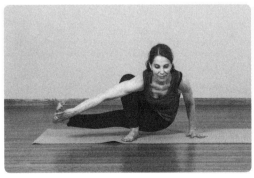

Parrot

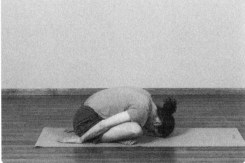

Clam

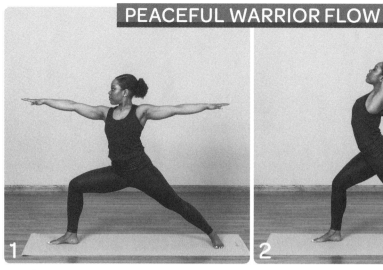
## PEACEFUL WARRIOR FLOW

1 Warrior II

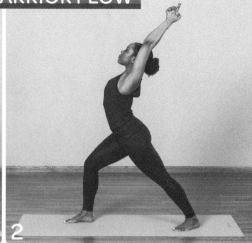

2 Warrior I

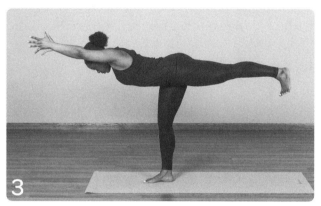

3 Warrior III

## Motivation Off the Mat

The moment you use force in a situation, you lose awareness of your emotions and the truth of the circumstance. This happens during times of impatience and desperation, and it creates struggle and discomfort in your consciousness. Breathe thoroughly, and look for peace in every occasion.

## WISE WORDS

Forcing the body past the point of resistance is an act of self-aggression, the opposite of practicing peace. Allow your practice to unfold organically without pain.

Be the one to spread peace wherever you go.

The surest way to be happier is to do all you can to improve the lives of others.

# SEQUENCING A CLASS

A healthy, logical yoga sequence opens with simple warm-ups, progressively moving to more challenging postures, then gradually cooling down by returning to less challenging poses to prepare for relaxation.

Despite what style or level of yoga you teach, always practice your sequence to ensure the postures you've selected impart your intention, both physically and emotionally.

## BEGINNER SEQUENCE

The poses indicated within each category of postures are suggestions only. Please select and modify postures based on the length, level, and intention of the class.

### Centering

Begin class by setting the intention. Students can be seated, standing, or in a reclining position. Create a space to invite presence and awareness of breath and body, focusing attention inward.

### Warming

Supine stretches, such as the following:

*Knees to chest*

*Hip openers*

*Reclining twists*

*Breathing bridge*

### Transition Poses

*Seated side stretch*

*Easy pose twist*

*Cat–cow*

*Modified side plank*

*Thread the needle*

*Low lunge*

*Downward dog*

*Standing forward bend*

*Mountain*

### Sun Salutations

The postures in sun salutations stretch and strengthen all major muscle groups. See chapter 4 for a full description of sun salutations.

### Standing Poses

*Warrior I*

*Warrior II*

*Reverse warrior*

*Side angle*

*Triangle*

*Crescent lunge*

*Balance poses: tree, eagle, half moon*

## Seated Poses

*Hero*

*Full or half lotus*

*Butterfly*

## Navel Center Work – Series

*Boat*

*Yoga bicycles*

*Leg lifts*

## Backbends – Series

*Cobra*

*Locust*

*Bow*

## Twists

*Seated twist*

## Seated Forward Bends – Series

*Posterior stretch*

*Head to knee*

*Wide-leg forward bend*

## Inversions

Depending on the level of your class, pick one, two, or three of the poses below.

*Inverted action pose*
*(supported shoulderstand)*

*Plow*

*Fish*

## Relaxation

*Savasana*

## Pranayama Practice

*Alternate-nostril breathing*

# Salutations in Motion

*If anything is worth doing, do it with all your heart.*
—Buddha

The yoga salutation is interpreted as vinyasa, a series of asanas linked with the breath. In the context of this chapter, the salutation refers to a movement of gratitude toward the self, those you love, the blessings you have in your life, and finally, the earth and sun's life-giving properties. By acknowledging the connection of mind and body, the salutation becomes a method for demonstrating your appreciation for your own existence.

A salutation has unlimited potential. Create your own salutation, blessing, or movement in the form of honoring your students, children, parents, home, the food you eat, and the roof over your head. By honoring your space with movement and intention, these practices celebrate the wondrous attributes of all living things in the world. Make it real; take it personally. Bring your movement and breath into your heart and share it.

# SURYA NAMASKARA (SUN SALUTATION)

## Intention

To awaken to the physical and spiritual benefits of the sun.

## Lesson

Surya namaskara (sun salutation) is the graceful sequence of postures executed as a continuous, flowing motion. Each posture, linked by the breath, counterbalances the one before it, stretching the body and elongating the spine forward and backward. These movements alternately expand and contract the chest to regulate breathing.

Sun salutation is one of the most popular vinyasas practiced in yoga class, and according to yoga philosophy texts, it was created as an invocation to honor the life-giving energies of the sun. To many practitioners, sun salutation is performed as a prayer to commemorate one's inner light. It shows devotion to the external sun, the creative lifeforce of the universe that yogis believe radiates both inside and outside the body.

Sun salutation begins with a focus on gratitude; the inner eye is turned toward the spiritual heart. Filling the heart with awareness and appreciation for what the sun provides, internally, externally, and symbolically transforms these postures from mere exercises into an act of devotion toward all aspects of nature.

To practice the sun salutation with an attitude of gratitude, visualize the sun rising and setting day after day for millions of years. See it lighting, beautifying, and warming the environment, while supplying the necessary elements to grow food. Connect with this visualization by feeling the heat in and around your body. Before we begin our first round of salutations, imagine drawing that sun energy into your heart, and let it radiate within you.

## Asanas for Deepening

○ *Sun loops.* Lifting the arms to the sun, open yourself to greet and receive the fortitude of the universe.

1. Bring the hands to the heart in anjali mudra (prayer position).
2. Inhaling, reach the arms up and over the head, rising up on tiptoes as if to reach to the sky.
3. Exhaling, lower the heels to the ground, burst your arms wide apart with palms up, then at shoulder height, turn the palms down, moving the hands toward the thighs, returning to anjali mudra.
4. Perform with a swift, heat-generating movement. After doing 3 to 5 sun loops, pause to feel the circuits of heat around your body, gradually resting your attention in the heart center.

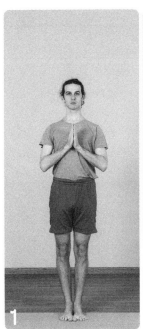
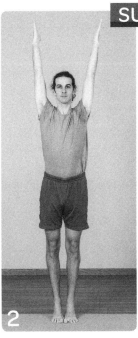
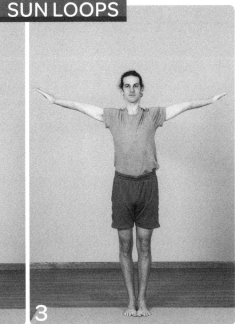
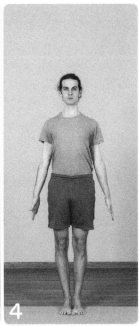

**1** Hands to heart in anjali mudra

**2** Arms reach overhead, lift to tiptoes

**3** Arms burst apart

**4** Arms move toward thighs

*Surya namaskara.* The sun salutation stretches and strengthens every major muscle group in the body. Move through the sequence in a continuous, flowing motion leading with the breath.

1. Stand in mountain pose with hands to prayer.
2. Inhaling, reach the arms overhead.
3. Exhaling, lower the torso to standing forward bend.
4. Inhaling, step the left leg back to lunge.
5. Exhaling, to plank.
6. Continuing to exhale, lower the plank to chaturanga or supported plank with knees to the ground.

7. Inhaling, lift your chest to cobra.
8. Exhale to downward dog.
9. Inhaling, step the right foot forward to lunge.
10. Exhale to a standing forward bend.
11. Inhale to mountain pose with the arms overhead.
12. Exhaling, join the hands and lower them to prayer.

Repeat, leading on the opposite side.

## SURYA NAMASKARA

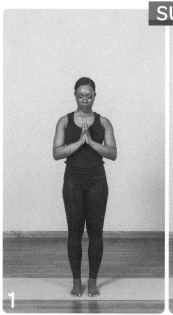

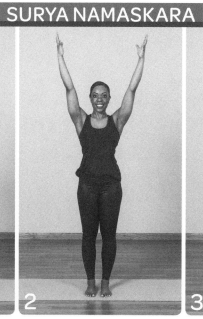

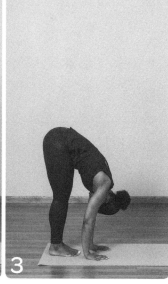

1 Mountain, hands to prayer

2 Mountain, arms overhead

3 Standing forward bend

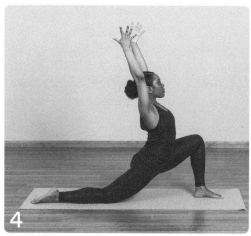

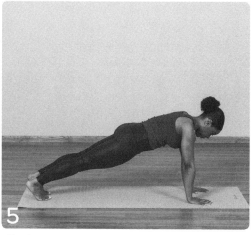

4 Lunge

5 Plank

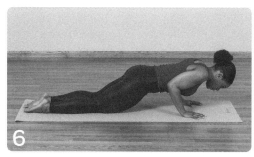

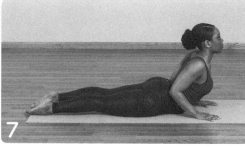

6 Chaturanga (supported plank)

7 Cobra

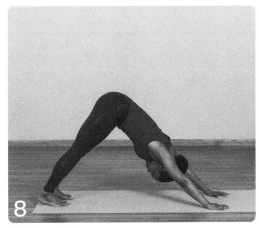

Downward dog

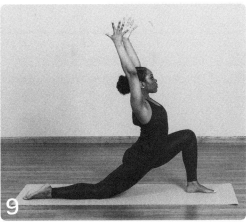

Lunge (opposite leg)

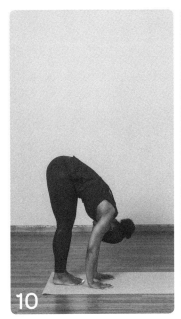

Standing forward bend

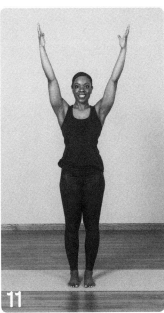

Mountain, arms overhead

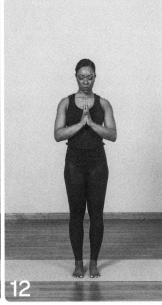

Mountain, hands to prayer

## Motivation Off the Mat

At sunrise, thank the sun for its life-giving powers and be grateful for this new day.

At sunset, thank the sun for another sacred day.

The sun is constant and always there to light and warm the earth, even on cloudy days.

Go outdoors every day to soak up the sun's energy and activate production of vitamin D.

The outer sun is a representation of your inner sun; it corresponds to the spiritual heart. Let it shine.

The ancient yogis describe the heart as the only place in the subtle body that knows the truth. The ritual of practicing sun salutations unleashes the truth of the deeper Self.

The Sanskrit word *surya* means "sun." The word *namaskara* is the Hindi word for *namaste*, from the root *nam*, meaning "to bow."

## Teacher Tip

Remember to love and respect yourself first before anyone else. Your devotion is an inspiration to your students.

# CHANDRA NAMASKARA (MOON SALUTATION)

## Intention

To arouse the cool, female energy of the moon.

## Lesson

Chandra namaskara (moon salutation) is the sun salutation's equalizer. While the sun salutation heats the body using male-orientated and external energies and emphasizes pingala (the right nostril), the moon salutation acknowledges the cooling, lunar, internal female energies associated with ida (the left nostril).

Moving through the two salutations in one practice helps fulfill the ideology of hatha yoga—the integration of ha (sun) and tha (moon) to balance the opposing factors of your conscious and unconscious patterns.

The phases of the moon represent the growth, maturation, and death cycle that all things in nature experience. Each phase of the lunar cycle has its own personality, and each is expressed within the human body. The waxing phase (from new moon to full moon) represents the growth stage. The waning phase (from full moon to new moon) correlates to the seeding, flowering, and dying stages within your consciousness.

Moon salutations cultivate a calming, rejuvenating quality and are thought to be most beneficial when the moon is visible. We'll begin with several rounds of sun salutations to heat the body and activate external forces. Next, we'll follow with moon salutations to balance the energies of ha and tha.

## Asanas for Deepening

To establish harmony within the body when experiencing too much solar energy or during intense or anxious moods, practice the restorative postures of reclined bound butterfly and supported open angle. Use blankets or bolsters beneath the torso to release cooling energies and open the lower belly and pelvic floor. Lead with an even breath.

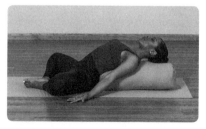

Reclined bound butterfly

○ *Chandra namaskara.* The moon salutation cools and calms the nervous system. Visualize the moon on a clear night sky shining brightly overhead. Repeat the salutation to lead on both sides, holding each posture for 3 to 5 breaths.

1. Stand in mountain, palms in prayer.
2. Side moon. Interlace the fingers, pointing the index fingers up in steeple. Lean to one side, then to the other.
3. Temple.
4. Five-pointed star.
5. Triangle.
6. Pyramid. Lower the hands toward the ground.
7. Step to a lunge, lowering the back knee to the ground.
8. Extended-leg squat. From lunge, walk the hands to the center. Take the front knee into squat, and lengthen the back leg to the side.
9. Squat.
10. Extended-leg squat. Extend the opposite leg.
11. Step to a lunge on the opposite side. Release the back knee to the ground.
12. Pyramid on opposite side.
13. Triangle to opposite side.
14. Five-pointed star.
15. Temple.
16. Side moon lean to one side, then the other.
17. Stand in mountain.

## CHANDRA NAMASKARA

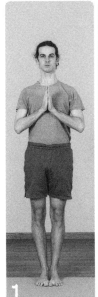

1

Mountain

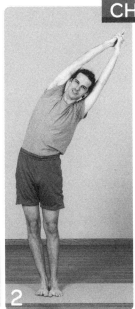

2

Side moon

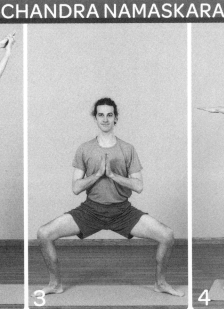

3

Temple

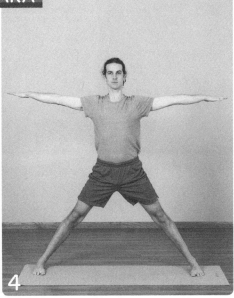

4

Five-pointed star

*(continued)*

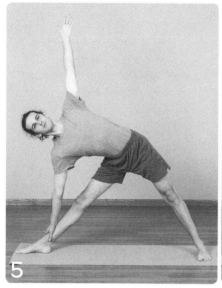

5

Triangle

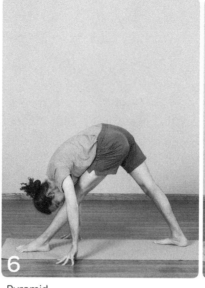

6

Pyramid

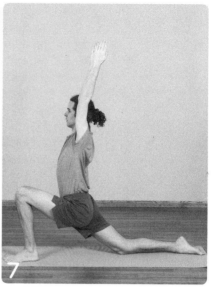

7

Lunge

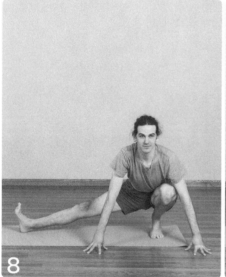

8

Extended-leg squat

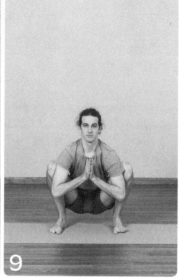

9

Squat

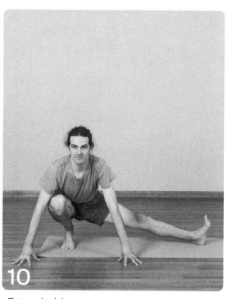

10

Extended-leg squat

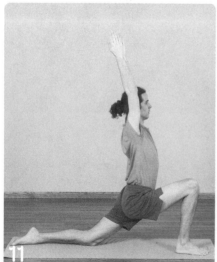

11

Lunge on opposite side

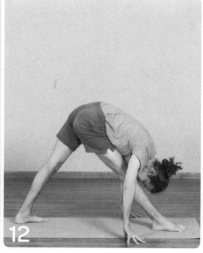

12

Pyramid

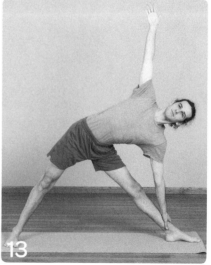

13

Triangle

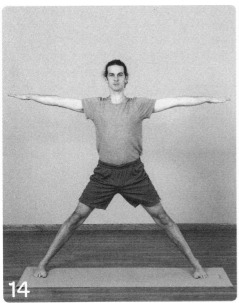

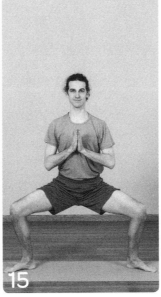

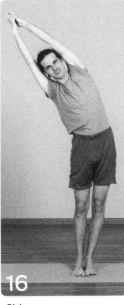

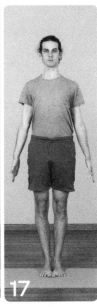

| **14** | **15** | **16** | **17** |

Five-pointed star          Temple        Side moon      Mountain

○ *Pranayama practice: Chandra shodhana.* To open the lunar energies, close the right nostril with the right thumb and breathe from the left nostril. Begin with 1 round of 6 complete breaths. Chandra shodhana is often practiced to defuse stress, anxiety, and mood swings associated with hypertension. (For instructions on alternate-nostril breathing, see Nadi Shodhana in chapter 2.)

○ *Chandra mantra (chant to the moon).* Chant *Aum som somaye namah aum* meaning "Atman (universal spirit), your moon fills me with passion. I call out to you with love, my Atman."

In yoga philosophy, the moon is the master of the human mind. Chanting the chandra mantra is said to enhance the mind's potential.

## Motivation Off the Mat

Full-moon days are called "days of opportunity." If you want to manifest something into your life, the best time to take action is between the new moon and the full moon. The new moon is a time to take advantage of the energies of the high tides and begin a new project, career, or relationship.

## WISE WORDS

Just as the tides of the ocean are affected by the phases of the moon, so are the waters (the tides) within the body.

The full moon represents the awakened mind. The ancient yogis believed that the lunar phase present on the day you were born sets the tone for your soul's evolution during this lifetime.

## Teacher Tip

When teaching on full moon days, allow the class to unfold intuitively. Create the sequences and themes that benefit your students, not yourself. If you are not sure what your students need, ask them.

# STAR SALUTATION

## Intention

To meet the "king of salutations" and experience the tenacity of the galaxy.

## Lesson

A star is a celestial body that's visible from the earth at night. Stars that are grouped together form galaxies that make up the universe. The nearest star to Earth is the sun, the main source of energy on this planet. Star salutation, which honors the entire galaxy, is befittingly called the "king of salutations."

As we practice star salutation, notice how many of the movements expand the body into the shape of a pentagram. From the physical perspective, you're stretching in all directions, using your arms, legs, and head as the tips of the star. Spiritually, the pentagram is associated with mystery and magic, yet it's the simplest form of a star shape. It can be drawn with a single line. For yogis, this symbolizes the endless energy patterns within us.

Star salutation offers a tremendous side stretch and strengthens the torso muscles. Unlike the basic sun salutation, star salutation adds a twist so that you can explore the solar system circulating within you. Feel your individual power, and remember that every miniscule drop you create in this universal ocean has a ripple effect on everyone around you.

Now, stretch your internal and external universe by learning the star salutation, the king of salutations.

## Asanas for Deepening

○ *Star salutation.* Be a star and shine prana into every point in your body. Think of the head, arms, and legs as points of the star. Hold the postures for a minimum of 3 complete breaths; more experienced students can hold longer. Repeat the sequence on the opposite side.

1. Mountain. Take three centering breaths, remembering your purpose in the universe today.
2. Mountain. Lift the arms up toward the biggest, brightest star in our galaxy, the sun.
3. Forward bend. Reach toward the earth.
4. Downward dog.
5. Upward dog.
6. Downward dog.
7. Five-pointed star. Lengthen, open, and energize the whole body.
8. Temple. Lift the ribs off the pelvis, and imagine someone pushing down on your thighs, taking your posture deeper. Lift up on your toes to get taller. Bend the knees deeper, fold at the hips, and bow to the earth. Feel the connection between the cosmos around you and the earth beneath you.
9. Triangle. Visualize triangle as a star tipped to the side.
10. Revolved triangle. Transition into revolved triangle from triangle without coming to stand.
11. Half moon. Merge the standing foot with the earth as you flex the top foot and move it upward toward the sky.

12. Warrior III. Shine and breathe into your five star points—the legs, the arms, and the crown of the head.

13. Five-pointed star.

14. Forward bend.

15. Mountain. Take 3 centering breaths before beginning on the opposite side.

## STAR SALUTATION

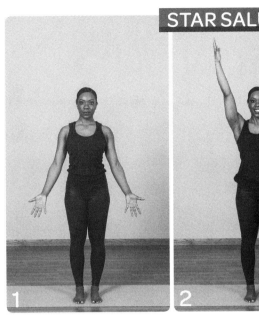

Mountain

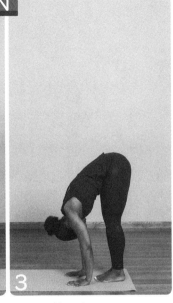

Mountain (arms lifted)

Forward bend

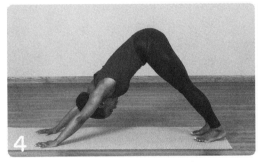

Downward dog

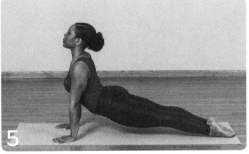

Upward dog

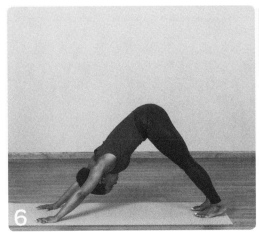

Downward dog

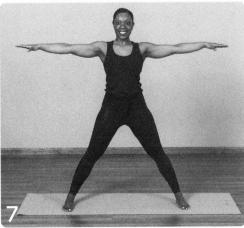

Five-pointed star

*(continued)*

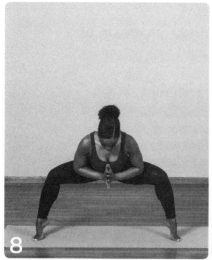

8

Temple

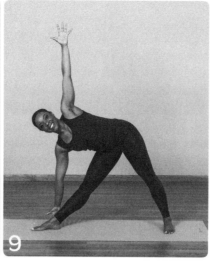

9

Triangle

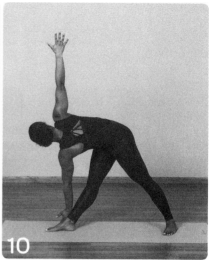

10

Revolved triangle

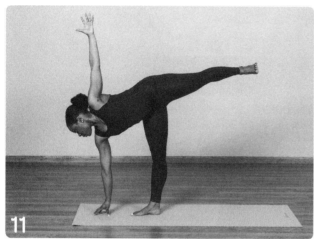

11

Half moon

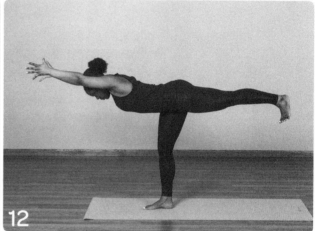

12

Warrior III

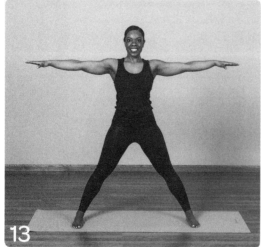

13

Five-pointed star

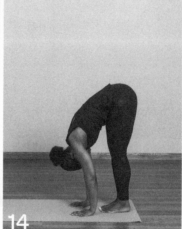

14

Forward bend

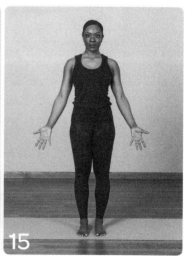

15

Mountain

## Motivation off the Mat

Imagine the head, arms, and legs as five points of a star, and the heart as its center. Feel your lifeforce radiate through you. The more you practice this visualization, the sharper you become at sensing your shining self.

When stars accumulate, they become a galaxy. Who in your life is part of your galaxy?

## WISE WORDS

As you expand the body, every cell expands and becomes porous.

Connect from the core of your being to the core of the universe.

Visualize everyone in the class forming a small but influential galaxy of like-minded fields of energy.

## Teacher Tip

Embrace your radiant star mentors. Remember that you're a shining star to others, including your students.

# EARTH SALUTATION

## Intention

To experience feeling grounded by taking the class outdoors.

## Lesson

Coping with the challenges, sensations, and sensitivities of the human body is an opportunity to learn more about it. If you feel scattered or spacey, you can call on Mother Earth to root you, to use her potent, grounding energy of the mountains, trees, and fields. Human beings are tied to the earth, but yogis are constantly unfolding, reaching up to the sky in an effort to both lengthen the spine and feel their connection between heaven and earth. The process of yoga practice begins with feeling your foundation; when you're connected to Mother Earth, you can open yourself to all of nature's possibilities.

Let's witness that feeling today by taking the practice outside. Our physical awareness begins at the feet, carrying the earth energy up the legs, into the pelvis, and traveling up the spine. If wind, sounds, insects, and birds distract you, know that it's Mother Nature's way of drawing your focus back to the earth.

## Asanas for Deepening

○ *Earth salutation.* Feel the ground beneath the feet. This practice may be taught on grass or sand, with or without the use of yoga mats.

1. Child's pose. Extend through the arms and touch the earth.
2. Downward dog. Inhale and exhale as you rise up on the toes.
3. Candlestick.
4. Mountain.
5. Tree.
6. Standing splits.
7. Crescent lunge.
8. Extended forward bend, twist.
9. Mountain.
10. Candlestick.
11. Child's pose

## EARTH SALUTATION

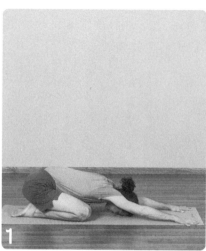
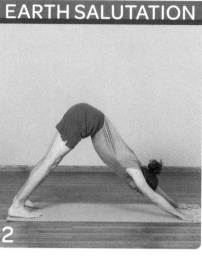
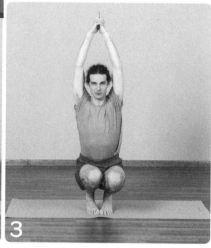
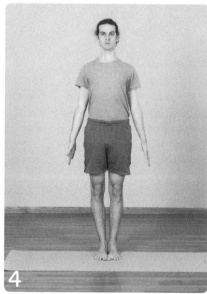
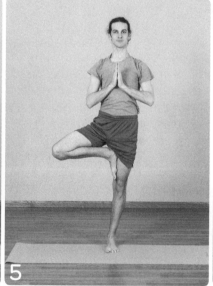
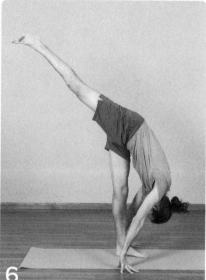

Child's pose

Downward dog

Candlestick

Mountain

Tree

Standing splits

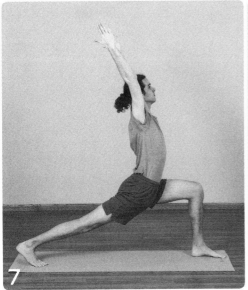

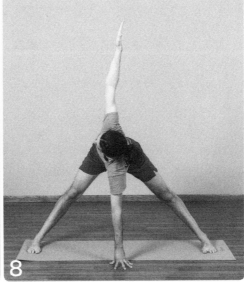

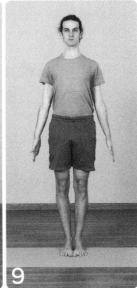

7 Crescent lunge

8 Extended forward bend, twist

9 Mountain

## Motivation Off the Mat

Celebrate Earth Day on April 22 with a walk through nature.

Take a walking meditation, syncing each step with your breath.

Spend a day at the beach building sand castles, feeling the sand and water on your feet. Listen to the waves, catch the breeze, and turn your senses outward. Bury your toes and practice tree, triangle, and lunges in the sand or water, digging your feet into the ocean's floor.

Practice impermanence. Build your sand castle close to the water, and watch the surf carry it away.

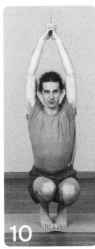

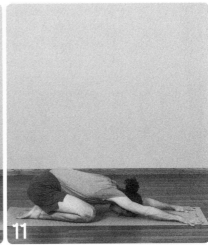

10 Candlestick

11 Child's pose

## WISE WORDS

Use the earth salutation when you're feeling scattered and unable to concentrate. Visualize the grounding effects of Mother Earth.

In winter, when the ground is frozen, the earth is in a spiritual slumber until the birth of spring.

During the spring and summer months, notice the vitality and potential of the earth's rebirth and fortitude beneath you. Trees sprout new growth, flowers bloom, and the light of each day grows longer.

## Teacher Tip

An outdoor practice on a warm summer day may sound wonderful, but be warned: It could draw unwanted attention. Select a private area, a place where you won't have random spectators observing or walking through your class.

# SALUTATION TO THE SELF

## Intention

To honor your inner light.

## Lesson

Honoring yourself and your inner light is an act of self-love. When your heart is full of compassion, empathy, and gratitude for yourself, you can share it with the rest of your world.

The path of honoring yourself begins with self-acceptance. You might fear being judged for your choices, your character, or how you look. In reality, you're the only one entitled to judge yourself. In his infinite wisdom, Buddha said, "No one is more deserving of your love than you." Why not fall in love with yourself, accept who you are, and see what happens?

Today we'll practice the salutation to self. Stay awakened in your body, feeling the sensations of the skin, bones, and muscles. Take a deep breath, and feel the feet on the floor. Notice the way your rib cage moves as you breathe, and how you're attuned emotionally at this moment. Remember that outer joy is an extension of the love we have for ourselves. Forget about the things you wish you were and weren't, and honor yourself for who you are right now.

Let's begin with a moment of gratitude. Think of all the ways your body and spirit have served you along your journey, and thank yourself accordingly.

## Asanas for Deepening

○ *Self salutation.* Express each asana in your soul and the correlating vibrations of appreciation for your body. Take the time to fully inhabit your amazing self.

1. Mountain with arms folded.
2. Warrior I.
3. Warrior II.
4. Reverse warrior.
5. Humble warrior.
6. Resting pigeon.
7. Downward dog.
8. Rabbit pose with the hands interlaced behind the back and weight on the crown of the head.
9. Hug-asana, pausing in humble adoration of the self.

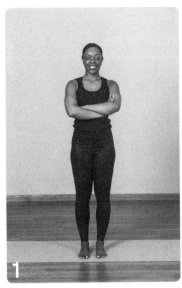

**1** Mountain

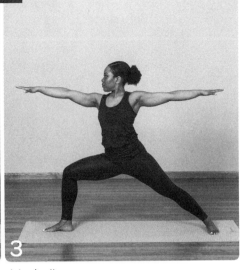

**2** Warrior I

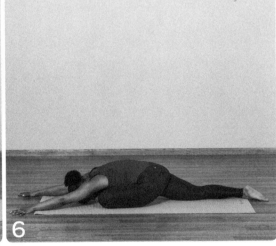

**3** Warrior II

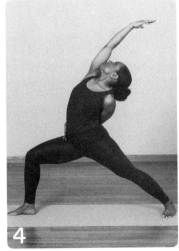

**4** Reverse warrior

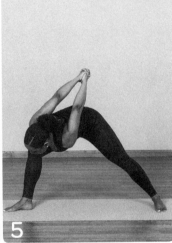

**5** Humble warrior

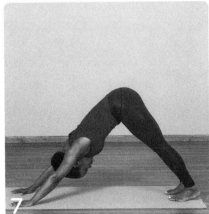

**6** Resting pigeon

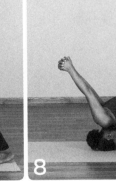

**7** Downward dog

**8** Rabbit pose

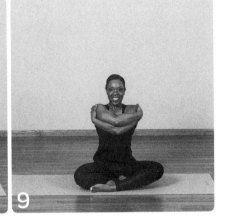

**9** Hug-asana

○ *Breath of Joy.* The breath of joy awakens the whole system, increasing oxygen levels in the bloodstream, stimulating the sympathetic nervous system, and circulating more prana to help you rock your day!

1. Place your feet shoulder-width apart, knees slightly bent. Inhale one-third of the breath, filling up the bottom of the lungs, while lifting the arms out wide to shoulder height, palms facing up.
2. Inhale the next third of the breath, filling two-thirds of your lung capacity, while lifting the arms higher; raise the upper arms toward the ears.
3. Inhale the last third, completely filling the lungs while lifting the arms to the sky, palms facing each other.
4. Take one robust, open-mouthed exhalation to the sound of *ha* while bending forward, hinging at the hips, swinging the arms along the sides and up behind you.

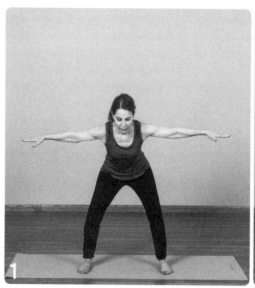

Inhale (one-third of the breath)

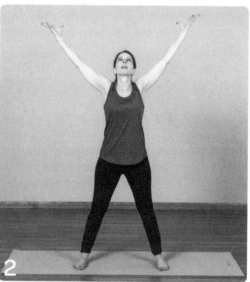

Inhale (two-thirds of the breath)

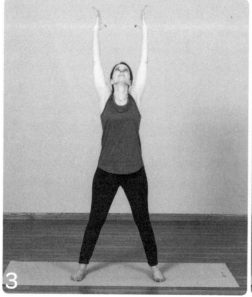

Inhale (last third of the breath)

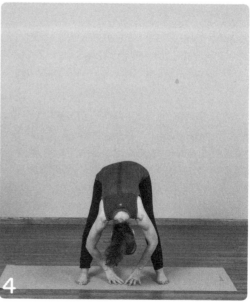

Exhale *ha*, folding at the hips

## Motivation Off the Mat

Listen to your speech, including your inner thoughts. Do you criticize your body or spirit more often than you imagined? Can you enjoy a compliment, or do you immediately disagree with the praise given to you? If you catch yourself criticizing your body or actions in any way, send yourself loving, compassionate messages about how special a being you are. When someone throws light your way, say "Thank you."

Learn to enjoy being by yourself. If you rarely get a chance to be alone, set aside a time once a week to enjoy your own company and be your own best friend.

Participate in activities that lift your spirits—dancing, making pottery, flying a kite, cooking—anything you love. Feel the joy in your body when you do something that feels emotionally invigorating.

## WISE WORDS

Self–acceptance ends all forms of emotional pain, and leads to a lifelong love affair with yourself.

The body is a miracle, and you're inside of it. You are the miracle!

Love and cherish your body. As long as your precious vehicle is healthy, let go of doubts and self-criticisms about how it looks.

To be the most compassionate and loving beings we can be, we must first be compassionate to ourselves.

*Your task is not to seek for love but merely to seek and find all barriers within yourself that you have built against it.*

—Rumi

## Teacher Tip

During relaxation, instruct your students to focus on and nurture one thing they truly love about themselves.

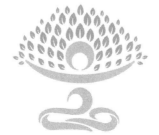

# 5

# Prana

*Drop by drop is the water pot filled. Likewise, the wise man, gathering it little by little, fills himself with good.*

—Buddha

The term *prana* means "lifeforce." It refers to anything that animates life, including any living thing in the universe. The complexities of the pranic journey can be simplified with the understanding that the lifeforce that moves through you also moves through every*one* and every*thing*—the trees, the squirrels in the tree, and the forest floor around the tree. The visceral comprehension of prana can alter a student's yoga class experience forever.

Every being is a pranically connected wave in the ocean of life.

# WAVE VINYASA

The wave vinyasa adds power and sensitivity to your practice. Relish in the inherent joy of your yoga discipline. Add the ujjayi breath, close your eyes as you move, and ride the wave of life.

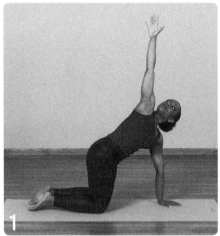

Table twist

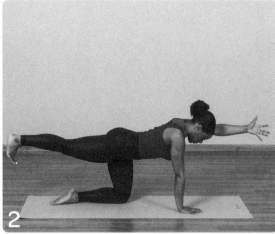

Table balance

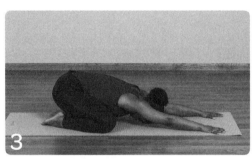

Child's pose to table (exhaling to child's pose and inhaling to table)

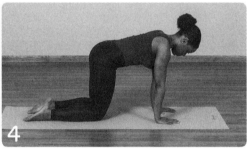

Table

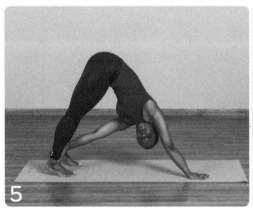

Downward dog twist

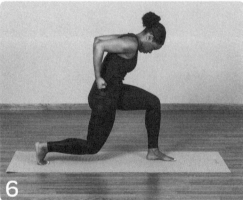

Moon dip lunge (bending back knee on exhalation)

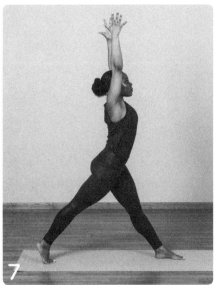
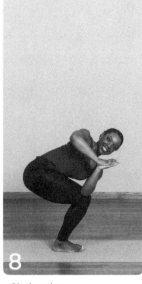
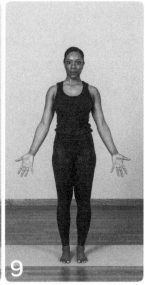

7 Moon dip lunge (straightening legs on inhalation)

8 Chair twist

9 Mountain

# HOLDING ON TO PRANA

## Intention

To cultivate pranic balance.

## Lesson

To thoroughly appreciate the holistic practice of yoga, it's important to recognize prana, the energy that inhabits every living thing. *Prana* is a Sanskrit word that means "lifeforce." It signifies the energy that flows through the nadis, the body's subtle energy channels.

The most significant way to bring lifeforce into the body is through the breath. So, it is imperative that here on the mat, you stay watchful of every breath you take.

We also receive prana from food, sleep, and positive emotions such as love, gratitude, and happiness. If your emotions are disturbed or the foods you eat are inadequate, prana can be scattered, eventually depleting your lifeforce. To be strong and healthy, it's essential to learn how to contain and direct prana.

That often means stepping away from negative or draining situations, a discipline that's vital for holding on to prana. In asana practice, we watch for distractions and notice when the mind wanders. This focus develops the ability to retain enough lifeforce to stay balanced and in the moment.

In today's practice, observe when the mind wanders, and how long it takes to come back to the moment. This is how you begin to sharpen and control your thoughts. Physically, we discover areas where prana is stuck. Then, through mindfulness, focus on what you've been giving too much physical or emotional energy. An unnecessary drain of energy can leave you empty so that you have nothing left for yourself.

When you discover this connection, you'll have aroused your awareness—the first step in experiencing crystal clear thinking, understanding your purpose, and taking action to make substantial changes.

## Asanas for Deepening

Practice uniting the body, mind, and spirit in celebration of the vitality of the pranic energy within you, the basic stimulus that sets all living things into motion.

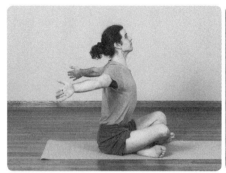

Easy pose heart lift

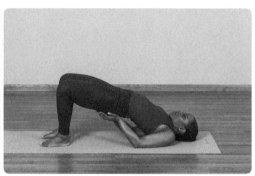

Reclining eagle-leg twist

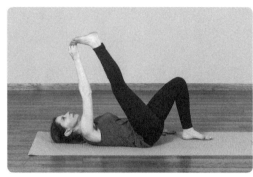

Reclining hamstring stretch

Bridge with hand support

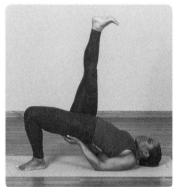

Bridge with one leg extended

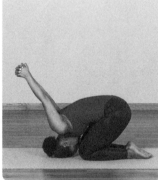

Rabbit pose

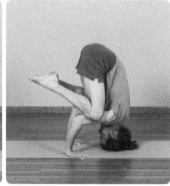

Tripod

## Prana Shower Breath

When you're at an event or place that you don't want to be, note the way your body instinctively prepares. If you're like most people, you take a breath, hold it for a moment, and then, with a deep sigh, think, *Okay, let me get this over with*. You may not even be aware of it, but when you hold the breath before speaking or acting, you're organically harnessing pranic energy to help you accomplish the unpleasant task at hand.

**How to Do It**

1. Sit with your head, neck, and trunk in alignment. Inhale through your nose opening your eyes wide, and imagine yourself drawing in light energy through your ears, face, and the top of your head. Take in as much air as you can.

2. When your lungs are full, hold your prana-filled breath. Close your eyes, and bring your awareness to the point between your eyebrows. Visualize the energy you inhaled forming a ball of bright light at the center of your forehead. Hold the breath for as long as it's comfortable.

3. Exhale slowly, feeling the light disperse into an invigorating shower of energy throughout your system. Repeat the breath cycle in this manner up to 10 times.

## Motivation Off the Mat

Release negative attitudes and energies from the high-maintenance people that drain your prana. At one time, they may have had important reasons for being in your life, but now, respect yourself enough to let them go. It's better to be alone than to be in toxic company.

## WISE WORDS

If you're filled with toxins, tensions, and closed-down body parts, you don't have room for prana to flow.

A purposeful attitude has the power to transform the experience of life itself. Live with intention.

Prana follows thought.

If you knew how powerful your thoughts were, you wouldn't think another negative thought again.

## Teacher Tip

As you stand before your students, remember what brought you here. You're the person who made the life-transforming decision to teach yoga because you're in love with the practice, you believe in the philosophy, and more than anything else, it ignites your being to share that joy.

# FEELING THE FLAME

## Intention

To access prana through thought.

## Lesson

Today we'll practice a technique called feeling the flame, which delivers a definitive sensation of prana. This exercise explores the emotions that bring pranic awareness of breath into the nadis, the subtle energy channels.

Begin by lying on your back. Close your eyes, and recall the physical excitement of a genuinely happy experience. It could be falling in love, the birth of a child, or a fabulous vacation—anything you want.

Visualize the event in your mind's eye. Inhaling the experience, spread your arms from the heart center slowly out to the sides. Imagine your breath as an expanding flame that moves your arms effortlessly up toward your head. As your inner flame expands, this feeling of elation expands with it.

Let the flames of joy spread from your heart center, reaching out to the tips of your fingers, up to your head. As you exhale, move the arms downward, back to your sides, feeling the joy travel into your legs and feet. Flowing slowly and rhythmically, take 3 to 5 breaths, filling the body with breath awareness, light energy, and true happiness.

## Asanas for Deepening

As with any asana practice, pause to establish pranic intention before beginning.

- *Pyramid.* Examine the pranic energy flow from the pelvic floor.
- *Warrior I, hands behind the head.* Sense your inner warrior penetrating into the earth beneath you from the strong back heel foundation, opening the throat center, and expanding through the arms. Stand your ground.
- *Gate.* Attempt to close and lock the pose's "gate" to any unwanted negative energies in your life by reaching the top arm toward the straight leg or foot.
- *Seated forward bend.* Reach for your legs, ankles, or toes as if you were reaching for someone or something you love.

## Motivation Off the Mat

Thoughts are the seeds of the mind. Tap into the emotional power of prana by accessing an instant vacation or fantasy through creative visualization. Close your eyes, and see yourself on a sandy beach, in a cabin in the woods, or getting the job you've always wanted. Energy nourishes intention.

## WISE WORDS

During asana, focus on how you're directing your prana rather than the physical aspect of your muscles and bones. What happens to the breath when a posture is easy for you? What about when a posture is difficult?

Your thoughts are living things and whatever you feed will grow. If you want more light and prana in your life, plant healthy thoughts.

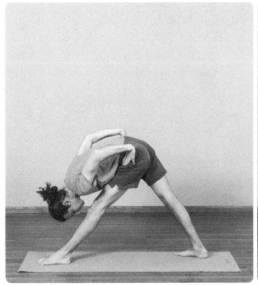

Pyramid

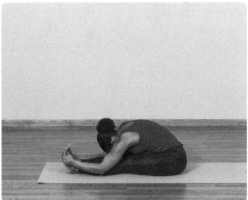

Warrior I, hands behind the head

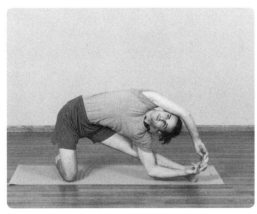

Gate

Seated forward bend

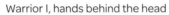

## Teacher Tip

It's impossible to be liked by every student who attends your classes. The need to be liked by everyone is an ego-driven illusion that will distract you from your authentic voice. Believe in yourself without seeking anyone else's approval, and your true light and truth will always shine.

# PRANA AND THE FOCUSED MIND

## Intention

To demonstrate how the mind affects prana.

## Lesson

Prana is the vital energy of the universe. Just as the ocean is represented in a single drop, the human body exists by the same prana that sustains every living thing.

Prana can be increased and decreased at will, or moved to where we need it most. The process of learning postures, breathing techniques, and practicing meditation gives you the tools to control and move your own prana.

Dealing with adverse circumstances like stress can deplete your lifeforce. For instance, take worry. When you're worried about 10 different things, it's possible that prana could drain out of you in 10 different directions. Or, if you're angry with someone or something, you may be giving away your precious prana to the *thought* of that person or situation. The loss of prana is draining to your consciousness and toxic to your system.

Learning to detach from negative situations is vital for keeping your prana flowing. When you work with pranic intelligence, you learn to manage stress and negative conditions to form and maintain a watchful mind.

## Asanas for Deepening

Asana practice gives you a system for identifying when, where, and how you're losing or blocking energy. As you move through your postures, notice where you're tight, weak, distracted, or uncomfortable.

- *Half moon.* Move energy up to the pelvis and out through the limbs, focusing on the supporting leg.
- *Boat balance.* Root through the sit bones, locating the balance from the floor to the toes.
- *Pigeon.* Magnify the sensations and pranic ripples that run through the hip, back, and groin in the backbend *(photo a)*, twisting *(photo b)*, and resting *(photo c)* variations.

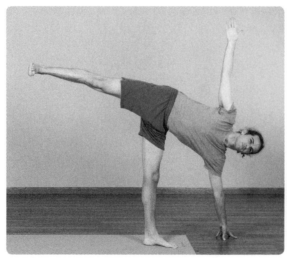

Half moon

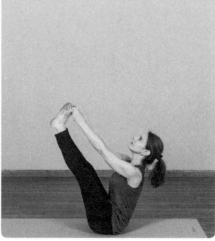

Boat balance

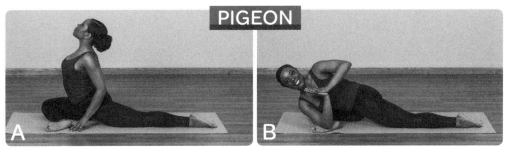

**PIGEON**

Pigeon with backbend

Pigeon, twisting

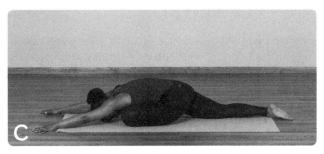

Pigeon, resting

## Motivation Off the Mat

Protect your prana! Distance yourself from toxic energy, situations, and people. Anyone in your personal universe—coworkers, relatives, even friends—can be an energy drain.

Practice bhastrika (bellows breath) for a quick boost of energy. Perform 3 rounds of 11 breaths, drawing air in and out of the lungs rapidly while maintaining a complete breath. Bhastrika builds mastery of the energy flow in the body, energizing every cell and awakening the serpent power of kundalini, the dormant energy at the base of the spine.

## WISE WORDS

It's impossible to tune into asana and be absorbed in a personal drama at the same time.

After releasing tighter, binding postures such as a seated twist, pause to observe the newly created flow of energy through the spine. Take time to notice prana.

## Teacher Tip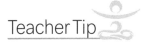

Observe your life experiences with a fresh perspective. Share your wisdom and life lessons with your students to help them on their journey.

# STORING PRANA

## Intention

To identify the body's energy storehouse.

## Lesson

Most people begin the practice of yoga to experience its physical advantages. With continued practice they discover its esoteric benefits, many of which come from yoga's pranic powers.

Prana is interwoven within the philosophy of hatha yoga and can be learned and acclimated through various yoga practices. To illustrate this point, consider that in ordinary breathing, you absorb prana. However, through controlled and regulated breathing exercises, you can elicit a much greater supply of prana to be stored and used when you need it most. Think of it as stockpiling prana, just as a storage battery can store electricity.

Today we'll work with a breathing exercise that stores prana in the solar plexus, the body's central prana storehouse, and the place that relays strength and energy to all parts of the body. Let's start with the pranic boost breath.

Please lie down on your back. Bring your hands to the solar plexus and breathe evenly. Visualize how each inhalation draws in a massive amount of vital energy from the universal supply. This prana is taken in by the nervous system and stored in the solar plexus.

On each exhalation, note how each breath shines energy to all parts of the body. Imagine how this vital energy is distributed to every muscle, bone, organ, vein, and cell, from the top of your head to the soles of your feet. Feel it invigorating, stimulating, and recharging every nerve center as it sends power and strength through your layers of consciousness. Envision pranic light as a great white light rushing in like waves entering through the lungs and flowing into the solar plexus. On exhalation, see your body light up, and savor the lifeforce streaming to all parts of the body, out to the fingertips and down to the toes.

## Asanas for Deepening

- *Agni sara with fanning.* Agni sara increases the flame of the solar plexus and distributes lifeforce through the body. It helps support the abdominal muscles, intestines, ovaries, fallopian tubes, uterus, spleen, gall bladder, kidneys, diaphragm, and lower back muscles. From a standing position, bend forward and rest the hands just above the knees. Exhale completely and pull your belly in and back toward the spine *(photo a)*. Continue to hold the breath out as you let the belly drop *(photo b)* and pull it in and back again, let it drop, and pull it in again. Repeat this process until you need to inhale. Practice 3 rounds, then stand in mountain and welcome the heat wave within the body.

- *Boat.* Extend the arms to encourage strength in the solar plexus. Engage the lower abdomen and lift up through the lumbar spine.

- *Cat stretch variation.* As you exhale, pull up on the navel center like a pranic pump; as you inhale, release into table pose and sense the new energy running through the back and limbs.

## AGNI SARA WITH FANNING

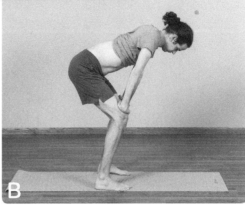

**A** Exhale the breath

**B** Inhale, release the navel center

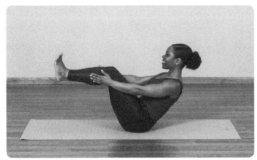

Boat

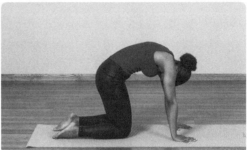

Cat stretch variation

## Motivation Off the Mat

Smile and rejoice in a calm body and heart center.

The pranic boost breath recharges and lifts the spirit, and can be an effective method to top off your lifeforce before applying energy-healing techniques.

Use intention. Do you want to stretch the hamstrings, calm an anxious mind, or make a decision? As you consciously inhale, allow the universe's energy to spread throughout the body. Make a mental picture of what you want to produce.

## WISE WORDS

Nature is never at rest. From the smallest blade of grass to the world's largest ocean, to your own body, everything is alive with pranic vibration.

When you're charged with prana, you have the ability to transfer that energy to others.

## Teacher Tip

A relaxed body is vital for storing prana. Give your students the gift of time to relax.

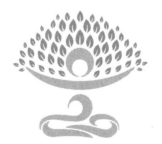

# 6

# Pranayama

*No one saves us but ourselves. No one can and no one may. We ourselves must walk the path.*

—Buddha

Hatha yoga is designed to help clear the body's subtle energy channels so that prana can flow freely toward more spiritual endeavors.

Pranayama is the fourth limb of the eight-limbed path of raja yoga, and considered the last of the external limbs. Although the advanced breathing exercises of pranayama are sometimes taught separately from postures, asana practice helps prepare the body for these exercises by reducing body tension, opening up the breathing anatomy, and prompting awareness to the flow of breath.

Asana, united with a practice of pranayama and rightful living, directly supports the aspirant's journey to enlightenment. On this glorious path of liberation, be sure to visit all the transformational stops along the road.

## Intention

To encounter the science and practice of pranayama.

## Lesson

Pranayama is the fourth limb of the eight-limbed royal path as taught by Patanjali.

The word *pranayama* is a combination of *prana*, "lifeforce," and *yama*, "control." The practice of pranayama is the use of breathing practices that bring lifeforce under control. Pranayama can also be interpreted as prana + *ayama*, a Sanskrit word which means "to expand" the vital lifeforce throughout the body.

Pranayama is an instrument that helps control the thought waves of the mind. When you have control of your breath and prana, you have control of the mind.

A regular pranayama practice nourishes the body's subtle energy channels and prevents their decay. It also helps increase lung capacity. Each day, people take about 23,000 breaths and use 4,500 gallons (17,034 liters) of air. With regular pranayama practice, you can deepen the breath and utilize up to 6,000 gallons (22,712 liters) of air a day.

Today, after relaxation, we'll enjoy a pranayama practice using anuloma krama, a segmented inhalation that fills the torso with prana and expands lung capacity.

## Asanas for Deepening

The asana practices that prepare the body for pranayama stretch and strengthen the supporting anatomy around the lungs and diaphragm.

○ *Thread the needle.* Begin in table pose. Thread the right arm behind the left arm, lowering the right shoulder blade to the ground. Twist the rib cage to the left. Repeat the movement on the opposite side.

○ *Twisting triangle.* Take a wide stance with feet facing forward. Place one hand on the ankle, ground, or on a block in between the feet, binding the opposite arm. Twist your rib cage toward the side of the bound arm. Repeat the posture on the opposite side.

○ *Camel.* Elongate and widen the front of the body from the quadriceps to the throat, gently pressing the spine forward.

○ *Shoulderstand.* The position of the pose increases circulation around the neck and chest, providing relief for bronchitis, asthma, breathlessness, and throat ailments.

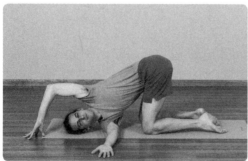

Thread the needle

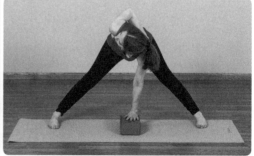

Twisting triangle

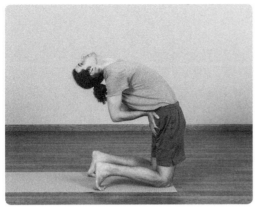
Camel

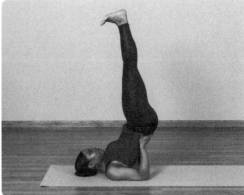
Shoulderstand

○ **Anuloma krama.** After relaxation, use this segmented inhalation routine to activate the mind, increase focus, and expand the capacity of the lungs.

1. Exhale deeply and fully.
2. Inhale the first third of the breath in 2 to 4 seconds, expanding from the pelvic floor to navel center. Pause.
3. Inhale the second third of the breath in 2 to 4 seconds, expanding from the navel center to heart center. Pause.
4. Inhale the last third of the breath in 2 to 4 seconds, expanding from the sternum to throat center. Pause.
5. Exhale slowly and fully from the throat center to the pelvic floor.
6. Repeat the breathing sequence for 5 more breaths.
7. As you inhale, visualize your torso as a tall glass filling with water until it's filled to the top. Exhale, pouring out all the water, before filling again.

## Motivation Off the Mat

Who do you want to be? The choice is up to you. You can choose to be uptight and hardened, or a relaxed, adaptable, enlightened being.

## WISE WORDS

Maintain the mind's receptivity and sense of observation.

Listen to the vibrations of your exhalation and inhalation.

Open your pores and breathe through your skin.

Inhalation is the process of drawing universal energy into the body, bringing the cosmic breath into contact with the individual breath. Exhalation is the removal of toxins from the body, providing more space for prana to expand.

## Teacher Tip

Breathe loudly and purposefully to set an example for your class. Fill the entire room with your presence, and ignite the space with inspiration and motivation. Eliminate your own distractions, false beliefs, fears, and comparisons.

# BENEFITS OF PRANAYAMA

## Intention

To learn the physical, mental, and spiritual attributes of pranayama practice.

## Lesson

Pranayama is the current that removes impurities from the body, mind, intellect, and ego. The practice increases lung capacity, benefitting every system in the body. During normal inhalation, an average person takes in about 30.5 cubic inches (500 cubic centimeters) of air; that volume is about three times the size of a tennis ball. A deep inhalation will allow you to take in about six times as much.

The practice of pranayama has countless benefits.

- Purifies the nadis, protects the internal organs and cells, and neutralizes lactic acid, which causes fatigue.
- Relaxes the respiratory muscles of the neck.
- Softens the facial muscles. When the face is relaxed, the muscles release their grip on the organs of perception—the eyes, ears, nose, tongue, and skin, reducing tension in the brain.
- Improves concentration, clarity, and confidence.
- Improves digestion, vitality, perception, and memory.

After relaxation we'll practice nadi shodhana and kapalabhati, the shining skull breath.

## Asanas for Deepening

○ *Chest beating.* To loosen the "armor" and closed off emotional layers around the heart center and the lungs, make fists with the hands and gently tap on the upper chest, shoulders, rib cage, and side ribs. Experience the heart beating inside the chest.

○ *Cat-cow.* Savor the movement of the breath through the spine.

○ *Side angle with upper-arm rotations.* Reach from your rooted toes and heels, through the intercostal muscles, up to the active fingertips, as you circle the top arm clockwise and counterclockwise.

○ *Rag doll.* From standing, round forward, dropping the head as you reach toward the ground. Let the arms hang. Feel the torso swell and lift with each inhalation.

○ *Backbend series.* Access and expand the breathing passages in the front of the body with cobra *(photo a)*, locust *(photo b)*, and bow *(photo c)*.

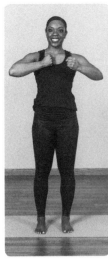
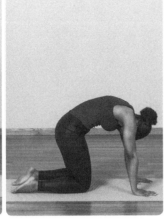
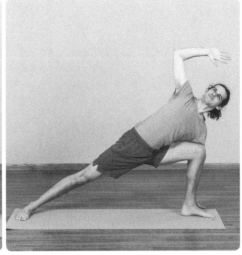
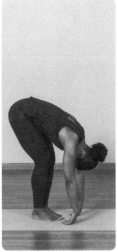

| | | | |
|---|---|---|---|
| Chest beating | Cat-cow | Side angle with upper-arm rotations | Rag doll |

**BACKBEND SERIES**

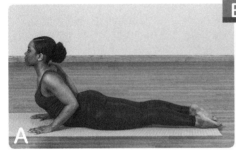
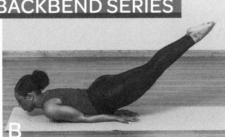
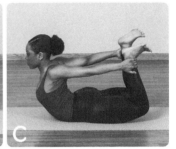

Cobra | Locust | Bow

## Pranayama Practice After Relaxation

*Nadi shodhana.* Take 2 rounds of nadi shodhana (see chapter 2 for practice instructions). Before starting the first round, check to see which nostril is active and which one is passive. Begin on the active side.

*Kapalabhati.* Kapalabhati, the shining skull breath is an invigorating and purifying pranayama that cleanses the nasal passages and lungs, stimulates the brain, and energizes the body. To practice, take a natural inhalation and follow it with a deep, rapid exhalation, pressing the diaphragm in and up. Repeat 20 times.

> **Kapalabhati is contraindicated for individuals with high or low blood pressure, heart disease, hernia, gastric ulcer, epilepsy, vertigo, migraine headaches, detached retina, glaucoma, history of stroke, and for anyone who has undergone recent abdominal surgery. If you become dizzy or nauseous, stop the practice and return to normal diaphragmatic breathing.**

*Nadi shodhana.* Take 2 rounds of nadi shodhana beginning with the passive side.

## Motivation Off the Mat

Changing your energy state can be as simple as noticing how you're breathing. If you're feeling tired or dull, a longer inhalation will energize you; if you need to calm down, a longer exhalation can relax you.

## WISE WORDS

Give your day purpose. What will empower you today?

In yoga philosophy, consistent pranayama practice is essential to attaining mastery over the mind's modifications.

Yogis are empowered with the wisdom and tools to remove anything that stifles consciousness and creates suffering.

Invite your mind to breathe into every part of the body.

## Teacher Tip

Discourage mindlessness by encouraging safety. Watch your students, and talk them through their practice.

# WORKING WITH *HA* AND *THA*

## Intention

To balance the lunar and solar manifestations of the body and mind.

## Lesson

The core practices of hatha yoga are created to balance ha and tha, the solar and lunar currents that represent the dual nature of man—the sun and the moon, male and female, hot and cold, light and dark, mental and physical, right and left. This balance includes working with the two major nadis that manage our experience of the world—ida (the current that ends in the left nostril) and pingala (the current that ends in the right nostril).

When we become aware of nostril dominance, as in the practice of nadi shodhana, we notice that one nostril often flows more freely than the other. When both nostrils are equally open, the central current, sushumna, the most important nadi in the body, is active. The sushumna channel is the pathway where awakened energy rises from the core to the crown chakra, creating a state of balanced energy. The open sushumna pathway is called the way to liberation.

Today we'll begin our class by working with ida and pingala. Get into a comfortable seated position with your head, neck, and trunk aligned. Soften the belly, and feel it naturally move with the breath. To check which nostril is most active, close off your right nostril with your right thumb and take a complete breath out of your left nostril; then close off your left nostril by bringing your right ring finger to the left nostril, and take a complete breath out of the right. Next, bring your attention to the sensation of breath in the active nostril. Focus on the breath as if it's flowing only through the active side. If thoughts outside of this practice come into your mind, acknowledge them, then tell them they're not welcome here, and let them go.

Now, move your attention to the passive nostril. Feel the touch of breath in there without letting the mind wander. Keep your attention on this side longer than on the active side, noticing whether your focused intention opens the passive nostril.

Finally, direct your breath into both nostrils. Inhale from the nostrils to the crown of the head. Exhale from the crown to the nostrils. Relax the mind as you breathe back and forth between these two points.

## Asanas for Deepening

Multiply the benefits of your practice by using the full attention of your mind, body, and spirit.

- *Squat.* Get close to the ground in the squat position as you practice 11 bhastrika breaths. When the pranic field has been cleared, savor the subtle shift in energy.

- *Lotus/half lotus.* The lotus pose helps to free congested areas in the hips, back, groin, and buttocks. Encourage the shoulder blades to slide down the back while holding the pose.

- *Palm tree.* Bring balance to the breath by exhaling into the intercostal muscles of the rib cage; on the inhale feel the lungs fill with air, on the exhale stretch further. Take 3-5 complete breaths on each side.

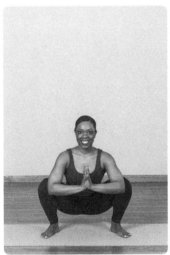
Squat

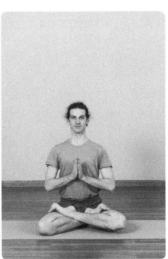
Lotus

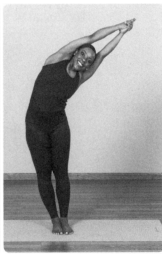
Palm tree

- ***Alternate-nostril breathing with retention.*** This vigorous practice alternates the flow of breath from the right to the left nostril. Before starting, practice 3 rounds (6 complete breaths per round; 3 breaths per nostril) of nadi shodhana followed by 11 bhastrika breaths.

   1. Sit in an upright position.
   2. Bring the forearms to the belly.
   3. Exhale, fold forward over the arms, reaching the third eye toward the floor.
   4. Inhale deeply, and retain the breath as long as is comfortable, returning to an upright, seated position.

5. Exhale, bringing the chin toward the chest. Inhale, lift the head. Close the active nostril. Exhale forcefully through the passive nostril.

6. Inhale through both nostrils, close the passive nostril, and exhale forcefully through the active side. Repeat this exercise until both nostrils are flowing freely.

> **Don't practice these techniques if you have high blood pressure or chronic problems in the eyes, nasal passages, or ears. If you feel dizzy or lightheaded, stop and return to normal diaphragmatic breathing.**

## Motivation Off the Mat

Pay attention to your breathing for the next several days, noticing nostril dominance and how it relates to your environment and energy level.

Note the muscular energy in your body, and observe your emotional states throughout your day.

Sustaining a balanced ha and tha can be a helpful approach to bring harmony to your day. For instance, if you need to quiet your mind while doing computer work, try opening the left nostril by closing the right nostril and breathing through the left until the breath flows smoothly. Or, try a few rounds of nadi shodhana with emphasis on the left channel to activate the right brain. Alternatively, if you need to present a new idea at work, keep a social engagement, or balance external left-brain energy, activate the right nostril by closing the left and breathing through the right.

## WISE WORDS

The point between ha and tha is the place of balance and harmony.

Tension restricts the flow of lifeforce.

Positive results from asana practice can only be perceived when there's an absence of tension.

When you've reached your edge, don't go beyond it. Instead, pause to feel the extremes—the hot and the cold, the good and the bad, the sharp and the soft. Attempt to find your middle ground between ha and tha.

## Teacher Tip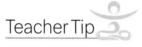

Like balancing ha and tha, watch the ebb and flow of your lesson plan. Teach the fierceness of the strong power asanas juxtaposed with the laid-back, relaxed stretches. Get comfortable with the awkward places that feel too hot or too settled, discovering the middle way between extremes.

# BOOSTING THE IMMUNE SYSTEM

## Intention

To integrate asana with pranayama practices to strengthen the immune system.

## Lesson

Most people get a cold or the flu once or twice a year. But if you're frequently sick, it could be a sign of an exhausted or compromised immune system.

The chakra most related to the immune system is manipura chakra, located at the navel center. This chakra is linked to the adrenal glands, and often gets overworked during times of extreme stress. When the adrenals are overworked, the immune system can weaken.

To boost the immune system, today's practice includes asanas that work the manipura chakra along with agni sara pranayama and two-to-one breathing. Outside of class, to help the flow of food and toxins through the intestines, be sure to drink 8 to 10 glasses of water a day, and eat a diet rich in fiber. Include vitamin C and zinc in your daily supplements, and get at least 7 hours of sleep to rejuvenate the mind and the body.

## Asanas for Deepening

*Immune system booster.* This routine strengthens the manipura chakra and improves the immune system. Follow this practice with 5 to 10 minutes of relaxation.

- *Sun salutation.* Perform the sun salutation (see chapter 4) 2 to 4 times to warm the body.
- *Agni sara.* Practice 3 rounds of agni sara (see chapter 5), pausing between each round for 1 complete breath.
- *Fire series.* Include 1 to 6 variations depending on the class level.
- *Bow.* Balance agni (fire) by practicing bow up to 3 times, holding the pose for 5 breaths. Follow with child's pose.
- *Seated forward bend.* Eliminate accumulated toxins and improve circulation in the digestive tract by holding the pose at the deepest extension for 5 breaths, returning to center, and repeating 5 times. Welcome a deep exhalation each time you fold into the pose.
- *Seated twist.* Seated twists trigger the squeezing and rinsing process of the large muscles along the spine, and stimulate the organs of elimination and digestion which help energize metabolism.
- *Shoulderstand.* The "queen of asana" soothes the nerves, helps relieve hypertension and insomnia, and stimulates the thyroid gland. Sustain the pose for at least 5 breaths.
- *Two-to-one breathing.* Maintain a 2-minute practice. (See chapter 2).
- *Savasana.* Invite relaxation into your body. Allow your pores to open and the body to breathe.

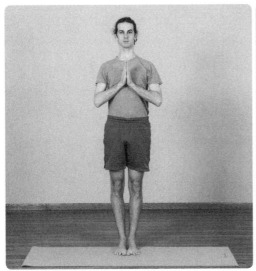

Sun salutation

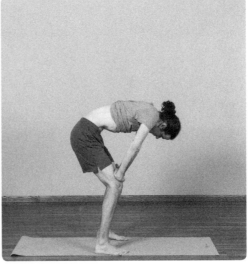

Agni sara, belly lifted

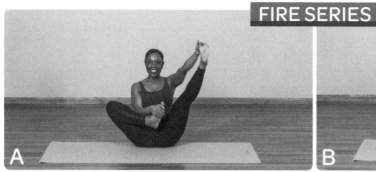

A

Butterfly lift

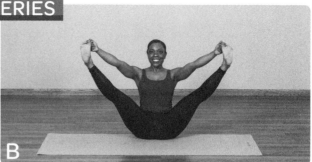

B

Butterfly balance

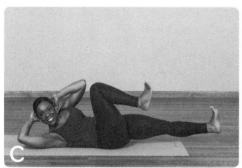

C

Yogic bicycles

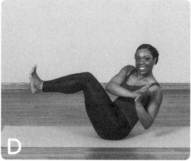

D

Boat twist

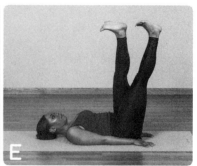

E

Supine scissors

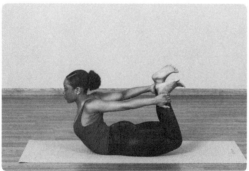

Bow

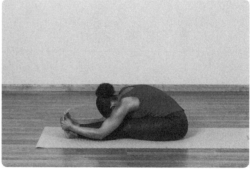

Seated forward bend

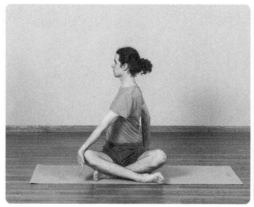

Seated twist

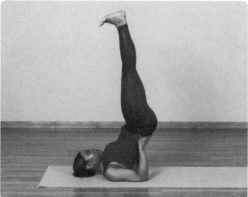

Shoulderstand

## Motivation Off the Mat

During cold weather, most people spend 90 percent of their time indoors, inhaling filtered air and other people's germs. To stimulate your brain and get your blood flowing, get outside at least once a day on cold days, taking time to go for a brisk walk or stretch.

Absorb the sun. The sun gives us our primary source of vitamin D. A lack of vitamin D can exacerbate autoimmune disorders and inhibit healthy functioning of the thyroid gland. Try to soak up at least 10 to 20 minutes of sun exposure 3 to 4 times a week to support brain chemistry and the endocrine system.

Sleep. Getting a full night's sleep is the most underrated health habit and healing tool we have at our disposal. The body needs time to heal, cleanse, and rejuvenate from the day's activities. Sleep is linked to balanced hormone levels (including the stress hormone cortisol), weight management, and clear thinking.

## WISE WORDS

Increased oxygen in your body gives the immune system more ammunition to fight off germs—yet another reason to breathe with awareness!

Practice being present, riding (rather than fighting) the rhythm of your life. When you're content, you're far less likely to become run down and sick.

## Teacher Tip

Hold space for your students by creating a safe, welcoming environment. Smile, say hello, and take time to talk to your students before and after class. People come to yoga to feel better; empower them to do that.

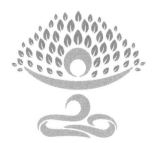

# 7

# Motivation

*There are only two mistakes one can make along the road to truth; not going all the way, and not starting.*

—Buddha

Yoga is a pure holistic life philosophy. It's complete, foolproof, and has stood the test of time. The practice of motivational yoga teaches us to face our fears, vulnerabilities, and inner enemies in order to live a more enriched life. Your transformative words, practices, and teachings are critical connectors to help ensure that happens for your students.

Moreover, no matter what you need to enhance your own spirit, there's a motivational yoga practice that will empower your decisions, strategies, and results. The lessons in this chapter outline distinctive action-oriented assignments to help you live your best life so that you can inspire your students to do so too.

# MOTIVATION IN MOTION

Yoga's meritorious effects on your physiology provide the motivation to practice every day, but these improvements are just the beginning. A regular practice creates a more disciplined mind that reflects on everything you do.

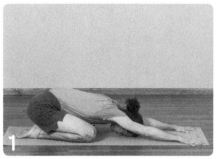

1

Child's pose

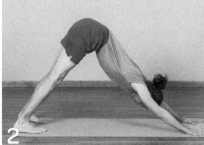

2

Downward dog

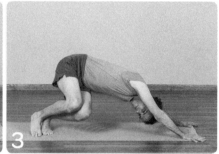

3

Downward dog twist

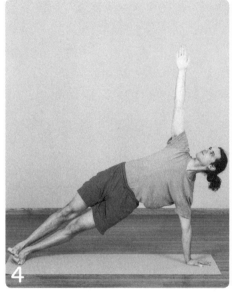

4

Side plank

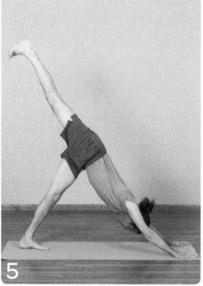

5

Downward dog split

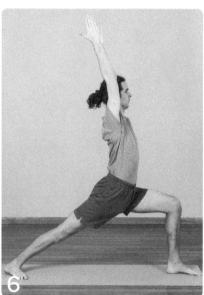

6

Warrior I with open arms

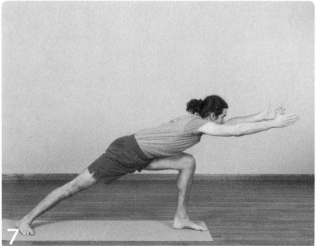

7

Warrior I with forward reach

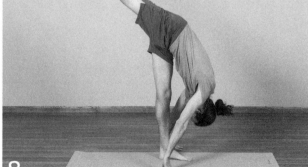

8

Standing split

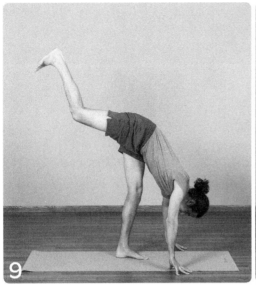

9 — Kick bombs (exhale and lift the knee to the chest, inhale and extend the leg to kick back)

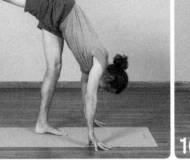

10 — Mountain

# MOVING FORWARD

## Intention

To take control of your energy state.

## Lesson

On any given day, the choices you make can be significantly altered when you live in an active state of energy. Your energy state is your current identity, what you're feeling right now is who you are. If you feel tired, your identity at this moment may be lethargic. If you feel sad, your identity may be withdrawn. Recognizing that fact, you can improve your mindset simply by changing your physiology.

Check in with yourself. How do you feel? Get very clear about how it. Can you put a name to the feeling? A low, fearful, or angry mood can ruin your day and turn people *off*, just as your bright, high-energy positive self will turn people *on*. When you have the ability to improve your mood and shift the direction of your energy and emotional state, your entire physiology—even the expression on your face and the light in your eyes changes. Researchers who study life experiences and the effects on body chemistry know this: When you *feel* different, you *are* different.

Today's practice is dedicated to cultivating your exquisite field of energy. Changing your mood will change your destiny.

## Asanas for Deepening

These practices increase blood flow, move you out of your comfort zone, and get the blood pumping to give you the power to transform your consciousness.

○ *Mountain.* Notice how your feet face forward to symbolize taking one step at a time in a progressive direction.

- *Lunge switch.* Focus on your strong legs as you strengthen your lunge by switching legs with a single jump.
- *Downward dog–upward dog.* Begin in downward dog *(photo a)*, and inhale to upward dog *(photo b)*. Repeat the sequence 5 times.
- *Crescent lunge twist.* Extend the arms out to the side, and move the front thigh bone parallel to the ground.
- *High lunge twist.* Bring the opposite elbow to the outside of the knee for a twist.
- *Universal temple.* As you exhale, round the upper back, pull the chin to the chest, and wrap the arms in a self-love hug *(photo a)*. As you inhale, lift the torso, arch the spine, and reach up through the heart center while opening the arms to send your loving energy to all that need it *(photo b)*.

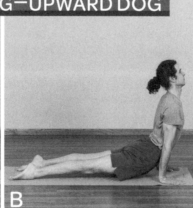

Mountain

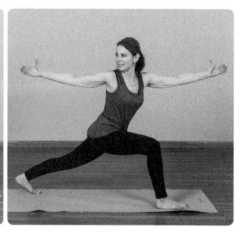

Lunge switch

**DOWNWARD DOG–UPWARD DOG**

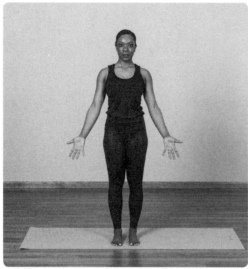

A

Downward dog

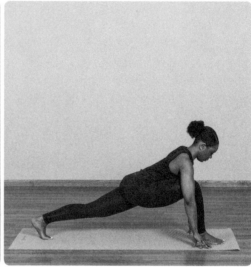

B

Upward dog

Crescent lunge twist with arms open to the sides

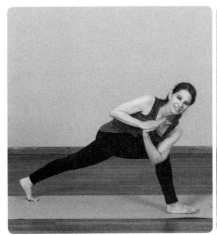

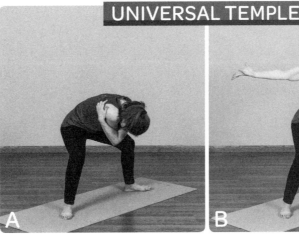
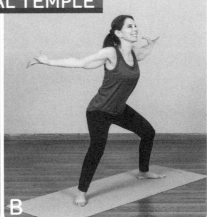

**UNIVERSAL TEMPLE**

High lunge twist | Universal temple, exhaling | Universal temple, inhaling

## Motivation Off the Mat

Be mindful of the emotional changes triggered by other people's actions or words. Visualize a shield of light energy protecting you from unfavorable influences; don't let negative people ruin your day. To stimulate positive lifeforce around you, embody the kind of energy you want to attract.

If a word or phrase is meaningful to you, acronyms such as the following can help you remember the mindfulness of motivation.

**AMF**
- Always
- Moving
- Forward

**NOW**
- No
- Opportunity
- Wasted

**IM DEEP (I'm deep)**
- Inspiration
- Motivation
- Dedication
- Education
- Exploration
- Perspiration

## WISE WORDS

If you don't like where you are, move; the choice to change is yours.

Don't be the reason you don't succeed.

Yoga is like power fuel for life.

Keep it simple, do the practice, and applaud your daily transformations.

*Only the wisest and stupidest of men never change.*

—Confucius

## Teacher Tip

Motivate yourself first before attempting to motivate others. Watch your attitude; it's the first thing people notice about you. Take action, read books, experiment, travel, and never stop learning. Be an inspiration for someone today.

# MORNING GRATITUDE MEDITATION

## Intention

To feel grateful for your life.

## Lesson

If you want to get motivated and destroy fear and anxiety, learn to live in gratitude. Don't just put yourself on autopilot and say "thank you;" really mean it when you say it, and sense it in the heart center. Gratitude is a transformative practice because it leads to contentment and appreciation for what you *have,* not for what you *don't* have.

When the mind gets used to thinking negatively, it's easy to stay there and get comfortable; this dark place can feel like "home." In time, it can weigh heavy on us, and we don't even realize there's another way to be. Sadly, we forget that there's a truly bright side to life.

Thankfully, with practice, gratitude can become first nature. Let's begin our attitude of gratitude now.

Close your eyes, and acknowledge all the good things in your life. [Pause] Are you able to sit on the ground without discomfort? Be grateful. Allow your body to feel relaxed and open. Feel how day after day, year after year, you've cared for yourself. Sense a rush of gratitude for yourself and the people and things that have supported you in this care. Get specific as you envision your family, friends, neighbors, co-workers, pets, your home, your job, your education, and your health. Use your inhalations to concentrate on what you're grateful for; use your exhalations to imagine the energy of your gratitude circulating through your body out into the world.

> *Bring your hand to your heart center, and silently repeat the following:*
> *With gratitude, I honor the people, animals, places, and things that have blessed my life.*
> *I am grateful for my health and safety.*
> *I am grateful for my loving family, friends, and the good people who have touched my life.*
> *I am grateful for my education.*
> *I am grateful for my strength of character.*
> *I am grateful for the blessings of this life that I lead.*

## Asana for Deepening

Embark on a path toward cultivating gratitude by dedicating your practice to someone you love. A gratitude practice is a reminder of how lucky we are to have loved ones in our lives. Within each pose, bring that person to mind while taking 5 to 8 ujjayi breaths, enjoying the body's expansion of lifeforce.

- *Mountain.* Honor your stoic mountain strength, and scan the body as you stand tall. Feel the power of the floor supporting every action as you shine your heart open.
- *Warrior II.* Protect the people you love with the strength of the warrior. With arms wide, create a wall of safety and refuge.
- *Humble warrior.* Bow to the earth, holding gratitude and humility in your heart. Silently send a loved one your healing thoughts.

- *Pigeon.* Meet the physical blocks in your body by sending the breath into the hips and forgiving those you love.
- *Downward dog split.* Lift the top knee and hip toward the sky. As you stretch the pelvic center open, imagine your heart center sending love out into the world.
- *Wild thing.* Who are you wild for? Dedicate this exuberant heart-opening pose to the great love in your life.
- *Supported savasana.* Slide a bolster lengthwise beneath your spine. Position the sit bones on the ground while the back body, neck, and head are supported with the bolster. Open the chest as you let the mind's eye scan every body part, thanking it for its service.

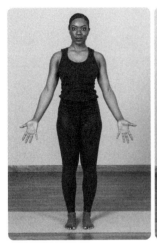
Mountain

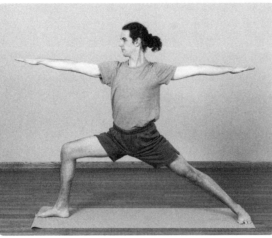
Warrior II

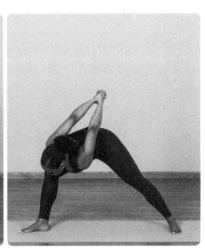
Humble warrior

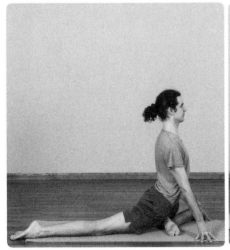
Pigeon

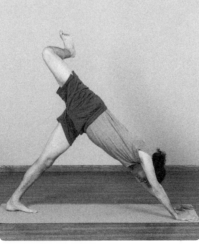
Downward dog split

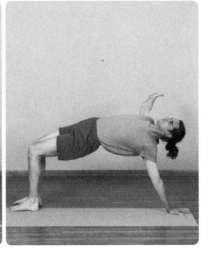
Wild thing

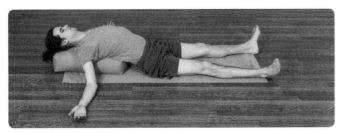
Supported savasana

## Motivation Off the Mat

Keep a daily gratitude journal. Include the small, everyday details of your life and the situations you may have taken for granted, like finding the perfect parking space. Once you start to write down the things you're thankful for, you'll notice when they happen.

Look at yourself every day, staying in constant gratitude of your body and mind.

Everyone wants to be appreciated. Tell your significant other how much joy they bring you and how important they are in your life. Practice this communication often, giving compliments and getting specific about what you appreciate. Gratitude communication can exponentially increase a couple's love connection.

Practice loving kindness meditation while visualizing someone that you appreciate, such as your child, a parent, your spouse, a teacher, or friend. Send this person gratitude and love as you breathe through your heart center. Envision the whole person with unconditional love. Let yourself well up with sentiment. When you feel some degree of natural gratitude for the true happiness of this loved one, extend the practice to another person you care about, then another, and another.

## WISE WORDS

You don't need a reason to feel good, but remember, there are plenty of them.

Be grateful for the doors that didn't open.

When you feel fear or sadness tell yourself, *This is one small uncomfortable moment. I came this far in life, and I will get through this.*

Focusing on your weaknesses will distract you from your purpose. Focus on your strengths, and you'll be more productive in your journey.

While others may complain about the size of their butts and bellies, their wrinkles, thinning hair, or varicose veins, be thankful that you can breathe, move, and stretch. And when your body lets you down (which it eventually will), remember that you *never* took it for granted.

*You have no cause for anything but gratitude and joy.*

—Buddha

## Teacher Tip

Dedicate your class to someone who inspires you. Use that visceral energy to move gracefully, paying attention to all the valuable lessons that person has taught you.

# ENERGY IS YOUR IDENTITY

## Intention

To recognize how energy levels influence life.

## Lesson

Your current energy state is a connector to help you move forward in life. Or *not*. How does your energy level feel right now?

Imagine you're going to a job interview, trying to convince someone to hire you. What's your energy like then? If you're not enthusiastic, if you're not sharp, if you're having an off day, or worse, if you don't believe in yourself, it's nearly impossible to influence anyone to do anything.

Energy is the key to success. The higher your energy level, the more efficiently your body will run, and the more efficiently your body runs, the better you'll feel inside of it.

Every positive result takes mindful effort and consistency. If you want to make progress in your job or improve communication with your partner, you have to take the appropriate steps toward that goal. As a yogi, your energy comes from daily observances like nurturing your emotional, physical, and spiritual self. This is more than coming to a yoga class a few times a week. The discipline of the practices will pull you in the direction you want to go, but the work begins with you.

To start the process, don't think too hard. Just start. Ask yourself, *What's one simple thing I can do today to take a step toward a goal in my life?*

Now, let's get energized to take action and responsibility for our life choices with a discipline called the Morning Trio. The Trio is made up of the three practices that, when combined, will stimulate the mind and physiology to get your psyche in a positive place. It's like starting your morning motor.

First, sit with your eyes closed and connect to your desire to live your best life. Get clear about what that looks like. Where are you? What are you doing? Who are you with? See and feel the entire place. Feel the courage of the warrior energy, and connect with your confidence. Your energy field will begin to shift with this thought. Motivation comes from within.

Next, stand with your feet wide apart. Inhale to a count of 4, raising the arms above your head while rising up on the toes, embracing your vision. Then, exhale to a count of 4, lowering the arms to your sides, bending the knees, and bringing the heels to the ground, sending your vision out to the universe. Repeat this movement and thought 5 times.

Finally, use an affirmation that inspires you. You have to say it like you mean it, so pick a thought, a word, or a short sentence that lights you up. You should feel the exhilaration of these words. Like a mantra, your affirmation is a tool of the mind. Chant out loud, and use your body to express the conviction that's deep in your soul. March in place, wave the hands, and use your body to concentrate on your outcome. Outside of class, you can use any expression you'd like, but today, because we're doing this together, we'll use the affirmation *I hold the key to my destiny.* Speak with certainty and intensity. Speak what you want to become.

## Asanas for Deepening

○ *Warrior I.* What is it about the movement and placement of the legs and arms in warrior I that fills you with pride and bravery? How do you breathe when you feel this pride? What other postures evoke a courageous response within you?

○ *Crescent lunge.* Empower your strong torso to lift up high, feeling the toes dig into the earth while your arms reach to the stars.

○ *Humble warrior.* Take a graceful bow in gratitude for all the people who have supported you in your journey. How do you describe this feeling in the body?

○ *Firefly.* Throw some unexpected physical adventure into your lesson by introducing variations of firefly, wheel, splits, or headstand. No one has to be a contortionist to work *toward* an advanced posture. The adventure is in the endeavor, acknowledging the intensity of a challenging movement.

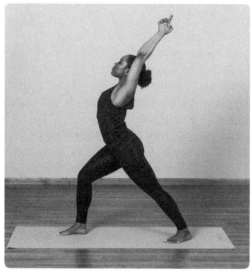

Warrior I

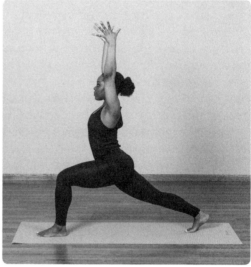

Crescent lunge

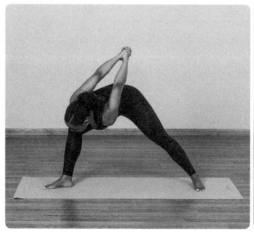

Humble warrior

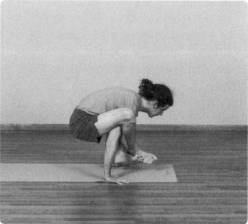

Firefly

## Motivation Off the Mat

Walk strong. First shake out your whole body to loosen up and get your circulation flowing. Taking longer strides, walk with authority, feeling yourself in complete control of your movement.

Time is your most precocious commodity. You can't buy more of it, and once it's gone, it's gone forever. Use each moment of your day judiciously.

## WISE WORDS

Your conscious energy begins when you say it does; prana follows thought.

Your greatest value is the effect you have on others.

## Teacher Tip

As you tell your students to be present, to drop their thoughts of past or future, remind yourself to do the same. Be your most mindful self when you teach.

After practicing the Morning Trio, ask your students to walk around the room and introduce themselves to one another. Instruct them to shine their bright spirits while greeting each other with affection.

# TRANSFORMATION

## Intention

To reveal that change can happen in an instant.

## Lesson

Most of us don't follow through on the things we truly want. We think it takes too much preparation, knowledge, time, and resources. The truth is that to transform your life, even right this minute, you simply have to decide to do it. Once you make that decision and commit to it, your mind will find the way to make it happen.

Yoga helps us define our emotional groundwork when we don't always know who we are or what we're capable of. We often think we're going to do this thing we always wanted to do, but instead, we find a way to self-sabotage the whole idea. Suddenly out of fear and doubt, we decide we're not good enough to meet our goals. We stop when something feels too demanding, or we tell ourselves it's just not the right time for change.

Yoga philosophy teaches us how to have an open mind, spirit, body, and a long-term commitment to living a meaningful life; one that will pay residual effects for years to come. When do you start to take the steps to realize your goals in life? Right now. You just have to begin.

*Today's class is about transformation. We can transform at any time, as long as we make the decision to do so. As you inhale, allow your heart center to lift, feeling fully grateful for everything you have in your life. Now close your eyes; keep the back long, wide, and open, and lift the crown of the head toward the sky. Feel what's inside of you now. Be truthful with the answer that you tell yourself. Are you joyful, anxious, impatient, sad, or curious? Without judgment, simply observe the sensation of that emotion.*

*Next, think of everything that's good in your life. Think of all that you are grateful for, such as your health, your parents, siblings, children, your relationships, your job, your home, your pets, your favorite music, places you like—whatever comes up. Feel it as a massive embrace of devotion and tenderness. Take it all in, and absorb its life-boosting strength.*

*Now, with this inner strength generated by all the beauty in your life, think about what you'd like to manifest. What would be the best part of attaining that goal? Put aside how to do it, which the logical mind will do; put aside the naysayers, and see yourself already doing it—living your purpose and your dreams. Feel as if it already exists; own it. Enjoy the pleasure and progress of attaining that level of accomplishment and purpose. Your mind will build certainty around this future vision and help you attract the resources to achieve it. Remember that everything you create in your life exists first as a thought, feeling, or desire.*

## Asanas for Deepening

Building belief in your purpose takes practice. It's like building a muscle; you've got to use it or lose it.

- *Child's pose.* Bow to your life and all its blessings.
- *Wide-leg standing forward bend with hands interlaced.* As you move into this pose, dip into your soul. Lead with the crown of the head, connecting to your divine self. Open your heart and, squeezing the shoulder blades together, expose the purpose of your life to Mother Earth.
- *Self-love hug.* Be your own inspiration. You can do anything you set your mind to.
- *Shoulder rolls.* Shrug your shoulders up toward your ears, and roll them back and down, continuing to circle in this direction for a few rounds; then switch directions. Feel the surge of possibility tingling throughout the upper torso.
- *Tree.* Above all else, stand tall. Catch yourself when you fall. And when you do fall, get back up and try again.
- *Temple toes.* Roll onto the balls of your feet with hands in prayer. Feel the ebb and flow of balance, the strength fluctuating in your legs, and challenge yourself to be present and in charge of your evolution.
- *Dolphin.* Press the forearms firmly to the ground and lift the chest. Bring the crown of the head toward the floor, lift the hips, close the eyes, and hold the image of your perfect future self in your mind's eye, the space between the eyebrows.
- *Cobra.* Use the cobra pose to help you overcome obstacles that are keeping you from moving (or slithering!) forward. Meet your fears head on so that you can move past them. Feel your chest fill with air as you rise up against the pull of gravity.
- *Supine moxie breath.* Interlace the fingers behind the head to open the shoulders and collar bones. On an exhalation, move the knees to the chest, curling the back by rolling the tailbone slightly off the mat while lifting the upper body, aiming the elbows toward the knees (photo a). On an inhalation, stretch the legs out parallel to the ground, and return the upper back to the mat (photo b). Repeat this movement

5 to 10 times using a forceful, audible "ha" on the exhale. This rigorous heat-inducing movement invokes the fire element in the solar plexus by creating the moxie to embrace your personal power and transform.

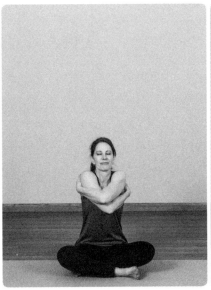

Child's pose

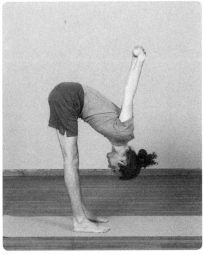

Wide-leg standing forward bend with hands interlaced

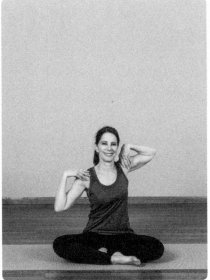

Self-love hug

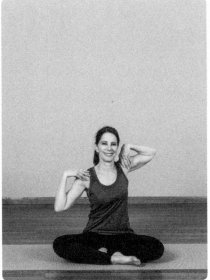

Shoulder rolls

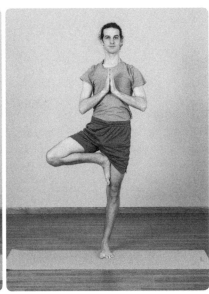

Tree

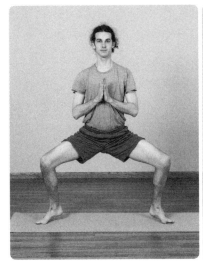

Temple toes

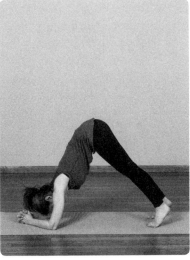

Dolphin

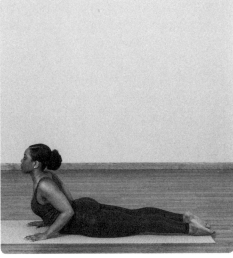

Cobra

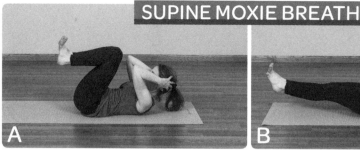

**SUPINE MOXIE BREATH**

A — Supine moxie breath—exhale

B — Supine moxie breath—inhale

## Motivation Off the Mat

Nothing is permanent, including self-motivation. Commit to your transformation practice on a daily basis. Make it part of your morning routine, like brushing your teeth.

Keep your distance from people who say you can't attain your goals. Don't give up your personal power to someone else; other people aren't living your life.

Every morning when you wake up, see and feel your path opening before you. Then, release any negative thinking, self-doubt, or destructive relationships that no longer serve you.

## WISE WORDS

Practice poses that induce heat. Fire is the element of change and transformation. Qualities associated with fire include determination, drive, commitment, passion, and intensity.

Only you are responsible for your success, health, and the decisions you make.

Think about how it would feel to attain your goal, rather than the steps to get there or the pain of the process.

Live your life as if your dreams have already come true.

## Teacher Tip

While in dolphin pose, offer this fun fact: In Greek mythology, the dolphin symbolizes rebirth and renewal. Throughout the process of one's own transformation, the symbol of the dolphin provides the bravery, persistence, and strength to endure tumultuous waters.

# REFRAMING

## Intention

To train the brain to reframe its thoughts.

## Lesson

Here's a parable about the persistent battle of good and evil within all of us:

*A grandmother tells her grandson, "Inside of each of us live two wolves that are always ready to fight each other. One is a good wolf; he's kind, generous, and brave. The other is a bad wolf; he's greedy, mean, and angry."*

*The grandson thinks about it for a moment and says, "Which one wins?"*

*The grandmother replies, "The one you feed."*

Knowing which wolf *you* feed is a crucial step toward having control over your emotions. Thoughts are like seeds. Whatever thought gets fed—negative or positive—is the one that will grow. Both exist only in our minds; while positive thoughts can reap blessed rewards and encourage a life of joy, negative thoughts can manifest as anger, self-inflicted pain or self-sabotage.

The concept of reframing negative thinking involves identifying unhealthy thoughts and replacing them with healthy ones. One way to do this is to recognize that you assign your own meaning to every situation and event. Even when something seemingly negative happens, it's only negative because of the way you decide to look at it.

When you counter a limiting belief by reframing a thought or opinion, you break down the negative system, reducing its chances of stifling your happiness. Reframing is easy to do. First, observe the negative thought, then replace it by putting the thought in a positive context.

During today's practice, challenge your assumptions and negative thoughts, and notice which wolf you're feeding.

## Asanas for Deepening

Use your asana practice to look at yourself. For example, one of my students struggled with doing twists because of limitations related to her weight. She reframed her struggle after realizing that the twist was never going to happen if she kept thinking, *I hate myself. I hate my body.* Instead, she focused on her long, healthy spine and the beauty of having a body that's free of pain. Eventually, she accomplished a stress-free twist.

○ *Standing forward bend.* Imagine you have a little trap door on the crown of your head, and when bending forward, it opens. Empty out your past and future. Be in the now.

○ *Downward dog.* Because downward dog reverses your body's blood flow, use it to reverse an angry spirit or low day.

○ *Bow.* Like most backbends, the bow releases endorphins and increases the body's ability to take in more air. Feel how the pose brings joy into your body.

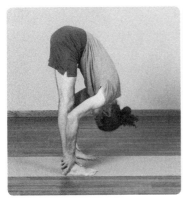

Standing forward bend

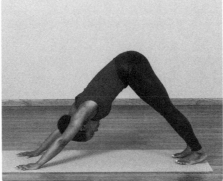

Downward dog

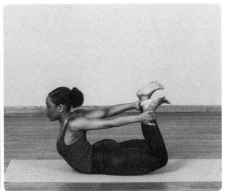

Bow

○ *Fish.* Open the chest and heart center to alleviate feelings of anxiety and help unlock the cage of trapped emotions.

○ *Moon dips.* From crescent lunge, on the exhalation dip (bend) the back knee into a pool of possibility, making fists with the hands while bringing the elbows close to the side body, and chant, "Yes!" *(photo a)*. As you inhale, straighten both legs and reach your hands toward the sky *(photo b)*. The sky's the limit!

○ *Backbend on a stool.* Unless you have stools in your yoga practice space, you'll have to save this one for your home practice. Carefully lean backward over a bar stool as you free the throat center, releasing the neck, and lift the heart organically. Note how the mind automatically reframes the room, which in relation to you is turned upside down. What's it like to walk on the ceiling?

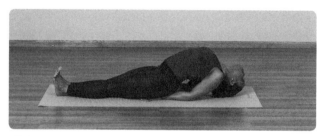

Fish

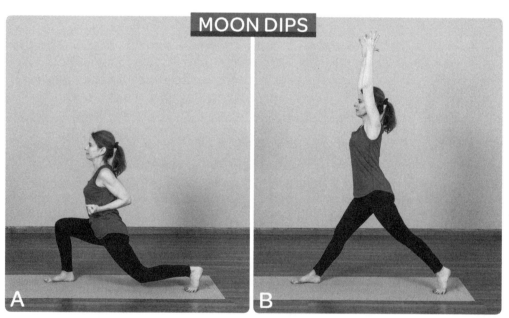

MOON DIPS

A

Moon dips, exhaling

B

Moon dips, inhaling

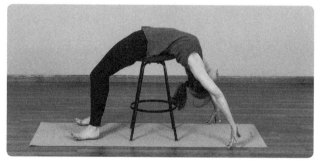

Backbend on a stool

## Motivation Off the Mat

Observe when and where your negative thoughts arise. Then, reframe the meaning you give to each thought. One way to notice these patterns is to keep a thought journal. Any time you have a pessimistic thought, write it down in the journal. The practice will help stop these thoughts from spreading, while it directs your attention toward your most common problem areas or limiting beliefs.

Describe your situation as accurately as possible. A negative mind loves to see things worse than they are. Using the reframing technique, see your reality as it is, as if you were reporting on a news item. See the entire experience, including all the negative and positive factors, but without subjective distortions.

## WISE WORDS

When you find excuses for not moving forward, reframe your excuses. Make a shift in an instant by changing your attitude. Use the affirmation *Nothing is stopping me from achieving my goals.*

Fear and uncertainty will impede your ability get into the postures. Yogis practice asana to come into contact with these emotions and discover what it takes to let it go or make peace with them.

Focus on what you *can* do rather than what you *can't* do. Celebrate the *can.*

## Teacher Tip

Encourage students to focus on their positive aspects before starting their physical practice. What do they like about themselves? What are they proud of? Prevent any destructive focus before it starts.

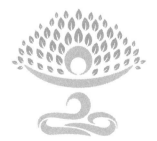

# Yamas

*To enjoy good health, to bring true happiness to one's family, to bring peace to all, one must first discipline and control one's own mind. If a man can control his mind he can find the way to Enlightenment, and all wisdom and virtue will naturally come to him.*

—Buddha

As codified by the Hindu sage Patanjali, the yamas, the first limb of raja yoga's eight-limbed path, are comprised of five moral disciplines and restraints. Once you explore them, you'll discover how to apply them to your life. For now, consider each sacred value as it relates to work, play, emotions, social interaction, and the yoga you take to the mat. So much more potent than a physical discipline, yoga's ancient philosophy is as relevant today as it was thousands of years ago.

**Yamas: Moral Disciplines and Restraints**

*Ahimsa*—Nonharming, nonviolence. Be kind to yourself and to all creation. Refrain from physical violence as well as criticism and judgment. Do not take or covet what belongs to someone else, whether it's credit for an idea or a physical object.

*Satya*—Truthfulness. Avoid all falsehoods and fabrication.

*Asteya*—Nonstealing. Do not take or covet what belongs to someone else, whether it's credit for someone's idea or a physical object.

*Brahmacharya*—Moderation. Avoid excess in all areas of life.

*Aparigraha*—Nonpossessiveness. Abstain from greediness, hoarding, or possessing beyond one's needs.

## Teacher Tip

Hand out a printed copy of the yamas and niyamas to your students.

# YAMA 1: AHIMSA

## Intention

To learn how to live a nonviolent life.

## Lesson

The five yamas, the first step on the eight-fold path of raja yoga, are restraints for cultivating happiness in our inner and outer worlds. The first yama, ahimsa, sets the groundwork for all the others. Ahimsa is the practice of nonviolence. Yoga philosophy teaches that the highest virtue is to do no harm.

Violence isn't limited to killing or hurting another person or animal. It can take many other forms, such as selfishness, anger, or negative words. To paraphrase an ancient Taoist proverb, *If there is to be peace in the world, there must be peace between neighbors. If there is to be peace between neighbors, there must be peace in your heart.* The practice of ahimsa begins within.

Consider the subtlest examples, such as self-criticism, to the most obvious manifestations, such as physical abuse, bullying, and war. Today's practice focuses on ahimsa in action and the dedication to patience, compassion, and love. Let's set our intention on inviting peace, stillness and nonviolence into our bodies and spirits through the focus of ahimsa. Do no harm.

## Asanas for Deepening

Be kind to yourself. Listen to your edges. Find balance by working with challenge and effort, without pushing toward injury or pain. Smile. Take pleasure in the transitions as well as the postures.

○ *Standing yoga mudra.* As you bend forward with your hands clasped behind your back, let the weight of the arms organically open the back. Feel the ribs sliding off the pelvis as the hamstrings awaken, stretching to their edges. Release the weight of the world from the shoulders.

○ *Warrior I.* Place the hands in prayer position, thumbs to the heart center. Use the pose to meditate on the beauty of strength and peace from within.

Standing yoga mudra

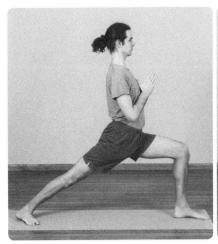

Warrior I

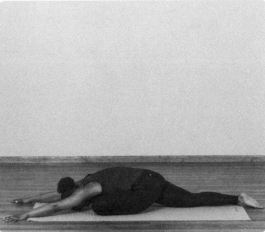

Resting pigeon

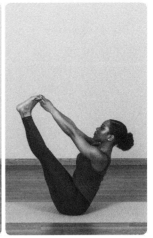

Boat balance

○ *Resting pigeon.* Relax, breathe, and witness pigeon's organic openings.

○ *Boat balance.* Hold the spine long and lifted, hook the big toes with the first two fingers, and gently press your feet away from your pelvis, slowly straightening the knees, feeling the stretch of the hamstrings. If you fall over, calmly persevere.

## Motivation Off the Mat

Notice when you unintentionally do harm to yourself. Be alert to self-criticism, angry words, lack of self-confidence, even sleep and work imbalances. Once you become mindful to self-harm, forgive and nurture yourself, knowing that ahimsa can be your guiding light of self-love.

Avoid harm to your peaceful self by turning off the news. The news creates an overloaded feeling of negative energy and displeasure with the world. Recognize that so much of what we see and hear from the media is out of our control.

## WISE WORDS

Ahimsa is the deep awareness of actions and thoughts, the same insight practiced in asana.

Ahimsa can be most challenging when you apply it to yourself.

A careful and restrained use of force is sometimes necessary for preventing even greater violence. It's said that in one of his past lives, Buddha killed a man who was planning to murder 500 others.

Asana practice is a forceful tool for liberating harmful emotions locked in the body's tissues.

## Teacher Tip

Forcing a posture works against ahimsa. If a student can't get into a pose, show variations or offer child's pose.

## Intention

To explore the meaning of truth.

## Lesson

In the *Yoga Sutras,* satya (truthfulness) is the second yama on the yogic path.

How do we begin to define truth? We each have our own version of truth and what it means to us. For instance, if three people witness a car accident, each person may have a different account of the same scene—not because someone is lying, but because we all have our own subjective truths based on how we remember that reality.

The guiding principle in adhering to satya is to remove the "veil" of self-deception. When the veil is removed, the meaning of satya is also interpreted as avoidance of distortion, embellishment, or any type of falsehood.

The simple truth is, there *is* no simple truth. Truth is more than avoiding telling lies. Truth begins when you look within. Do you put your own worries, anxieties, and fears into conversations that you have with others? Or do you listen without judgment, without attaching to past conversations? How truthful are you with yourself? Do you often exaggerate just to get your point across?

Consider how the yamas guide you in your life. Take a look at the first yama, nonharming. What happens when your friend buys what she describes as the "perfect dress" and asks you whether you like it? If you don't, do you tell her your truth? Yoga philosophy suggests that if truthfulness brings more harm than good, the choice is to remain silent. Your first obligation in adhering to the yamas is to do no harm.

Today, notice the truth in your practice. Do you tell yourself that you can't do a pose even if you've never tried it, or that a posture doesn't cause pain when in fact it does? Open your awareness to see things as they are.

Apply satya, working with honesty and integrity in every movement. Listen carefully to the inner voice, and see how truthfulness is a remarkable tool for liberating your energies.

## Asanas for Deepening

To explore honesty in your practice, ask yourself meaningful questions as you move in and out of the poses. *Is the truth that your mind is wandering? Is the truth that you feel anxiety in a pose?* Notice how prana is enhanced or cut off by a conscious shift in mental attitude. Continue to look inward to learn more about yourself.

- *Tree.* Relax into holding your balance as you observe the interplay between the outer body and the will to stand tall.
- *Splits with blocks.* The hamstrings don't lie. They challenge you to stay alert to the spark of give and take within every breath. Show the hamstrings some respect, and they'll reward you with openness and light in the back body.
- *Hero.* The hero tells the truth about your skeletal system, including your ankles, feet, knees, thighs, and pelvic bones. How are your muscles responding? Feel your weight sink toward the floor.
- *Head to knee.* Be mindful of pushing to a place where you think you should be but aren't there yet.

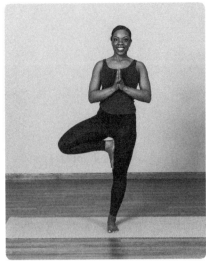

Tree

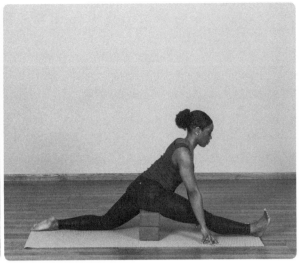

Splits with blocks

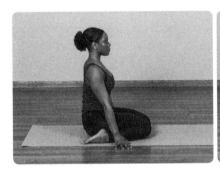

Hero

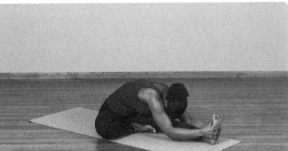

Head to knee

## Motivation Off the Mat

Sharpen your listening skills. Can other people's words obscure our own truth?

True listening means engaging in other people's words without projecting or adding your own opinions. When my children were quite young, an older friend told me to cherish every moment with them; they would soon grow up, move out, and start their own families. Was she suggesting that I was a bad, unappreciative mother, asleep at the maternal wheel? Or was I misinterpreting her words with my defenses? When I listened with satya, I took my own projections out of the conversation and genuinely listened to what my friend was saying. As one who had walked this road, she was simply telling me to embrace this time of my life.

## WISE WORDS

When body and mind are in sync, truth rises to the top.

Take time to listen for inner truth.

As awareness expands, perception becomes clearer and you come closer to the truth, seeing life as it is in each moment.

## Intention

To absorb the concept of nonstealing.

## Lesson

The third yogic observance is asteya (nonstealing). Asteya means we should neither steal, nor have the intention to steal any object, speech, or thought belonging to another person. In fact, asteya is an extension of ahimsa, because theft is a type of violence against another.

The concept of asteya comes in many forms. Let me give you an example that you may not have thought of as stealing.

> *Emily was a copywriter in a marketing firm. She worked with Brian, an art director, to create advertising campaigns and promotions. One Monday morning, as Emily shuffled past her coworkers and into her office, she overhead the office clamor: "We were robbed over the weekend!" "What did they take?" "How did they break in?" Abuzz with the news, the staff was shocked and frightened. As Emily sat at her desk to take a quick inventory of her belongings, Brian rushed into her office and jokingly screamed, "They stole all my ideas!"*

Although Brian's remark made light of the tense situation, this is one accurate depiction of how asteya works in our lives. The philosophy of asteya goes beyond simply not taking objects that aren't yours. It also refers to not taking credit for the actions of others, not accepting too much change from a cashier, or not being late and thus stealing time from the person who's waiting for you.

Look for ways that asteya relates to your asana practice. In yoga class, people often compare themselves to others; they want what others have, whether it's their flexibility, strength, body shape, or an advanced forward bend.

Sometimes, when the body can't perform the so-called finished pose, people might strain or injure themselves, violating the first yama (nonharming) as well as the second yama (truthfulness).

As a result, the pattern of how the yamas build on one another, creating a foundation for life, begins to emerge.

## Asanas for Deepening

Work on postures that are challenging, if not downright impossible for you. Treasure the fact that you can bend forward, although you may need to bend your knees. Be honest with yourself, and honor your boundaries.

Let go of the craving to do a picture perfect pose, making each variation of the posture your own. Use props where needed.

- ○ *Headstand.* When doing the headstand, do a preparation lift at the wall or a half headstand at the wall.
- ○ *High lunge with bound arm balance.* Use a strap if the hands don't connect.
- ○ *Bound lotus.* Use a strap if the hands don't reach and connect to the toes.

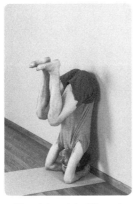

Headstand, half head-
stand at the wall

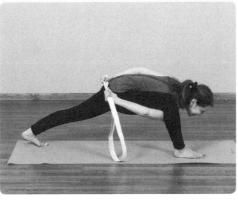

High lunge with bound arm balance

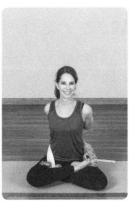

Bound lotus

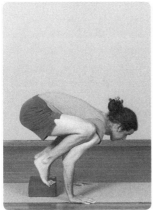

Crow

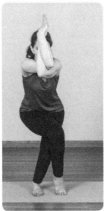

Eagle

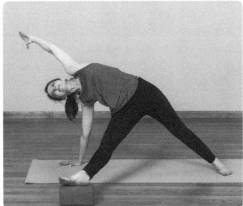

Lifted fallen triangle

- *Crow.* Practice with both feet on a block, lifting one foot at a time, before "flying" your crow.
- *Eagle.* If eagle challenges your balance, keep the toes of the top leg on the ground.
- *Lifted fallen triangle.* Place the foot of the extended leg on a block to capture the lifted feeling.

## Motivation Off the Mat

You may be stealing without even knowing it. Do you use office supplies for personal use? Do you use more natural resources than you need? Do you take too many napkins or sugar packets when you dine out?

Appreciate the things you have. When you look outside yourself for more, you neglect the riches that you already have. Foster a sense of abundance in your life.

## WISE WORDS

Be aware of taking up too much of someone's time or patience.

Cultivate a sense of completeness and self-sufficiency; let go of cravings.

*You wander from room to room in search for the pearls that are already around your neck.*

—Rumi

## Intention

To interpret the age-old advice, *Everything in moderation*.

## Lesson

Imagine reaching for your third piece of candy and hearing a voice in your head say, "Everything in moderation." You've already had two pieces, so you decide not to have a third. That's the key principle of the fourth yama, brahmacharya, which means "moderation."

Brahmacharya can also be interpreted as a way to stop wasting one's energies. In other words, when you live in moderation, your energy won't be wasted on things that don't serve your higher good. This idea includes avoiding pleasures that feel wonderful for a short period of time but are ultimately fleeting, such as the high from drugs and alcohol. Instead, this yama encourages us to move toward discovering the sustaining peace and happiness that are already within us.

Many of us don't know how to achieve consistent moderation in our lives, so we fall into the cycle of excess and deprivation. Yoga philosophy suggests that if you're going to indulge, recognize it, then do it mindfully and joyfully. On the flip side, ignoring moderation will throw you off balance, adversely affecting your physical and mental health.

On the mat, brahmacharya can teach you a new approach to asana. In today's practice, take each pose as if you've never done it before—with a fresh, open mind and receptive body. Use beginner's mind; you have nothing to compare the pose to if it's new to you. Listen and trust the voice within that seeks balance, harmony, and peace in every movement. As you let go of the bonds of past pleasures and pains, you'll discover hidden abilities, new energies, and playfulness in your practice.

## Asanas for Deepening

Brahmacharya is dedication to the perception, understanding, and awareness of the divinity within.

With the mind of a neophyte, practice deeply and honestly without spending too much mental or physical energy on one pose or another. Coordinate holding postures with moving through them, leading with the breath. Tune in to ask what your body needs today. Be sure to incorporate poses that you normally resist.

- *Sun salutation.* Salute the sun with respect for its healing energies and your own divine lifeforce.
- *Chaturanga.* Practice chaturanga with knees up or down, holding for up to 10 breaths, stopping before you get fatigued.
- *Camel.* Root yourself into the present moment through the shins and feet, lifting through the heart, while maintaining equinity between the inhale and exhale.
- *Revolved triangle.* Before reaching toward the ground in twist, note the stillness before the movement. Focus on your inner balance.
- *Cow face.* Simultaneously stretch the top and bottom of both sides of the body. Use a strap if the hands don't reach each other. Sit in the full posture for 5 to 10 breaths focusing on balancing your spiritual self.

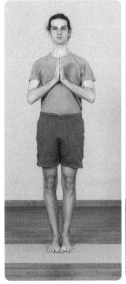

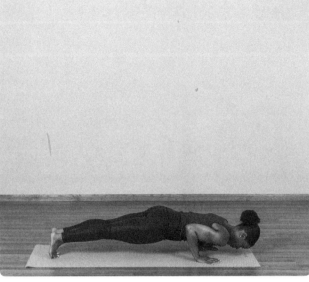

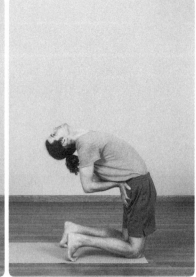

Sun salutation    Chaturanga                                    Camel

## Motivation Off the Mat

Practice moderation by meeting each moment with a fresh attitude. Experience the fullness and magic of each moment while going to work, hugging a loved one, or taking a deep breath.

If you decide to indulge (taking that third piece of candy or cocktail, sleeping too long or too little, or surround-yourself with toxic people), reframe the temptation by remembering the energetic benefits and goals of *Everything in moderation.*

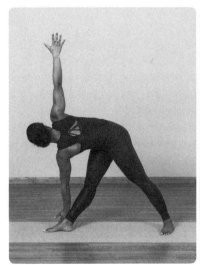

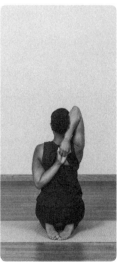

Revolved triangle                Cow face

## WISE WORDS

Think about the things you overdo—food, drink, caffeine, sleep, work, play, exercise, shopping, feeling sorry for yourself—the list goes on and on. Is it possible to do any of these things in moderation?

If you want candy, have candy! Rather than feel guilty, enjoy it. Let the candy melt in your mouth, and find pleasure and appreciation in the sweetness, flavors, and texture.

When your inner and outer lives are balanced, the mind becomes calm, natural serenity flows, and you feel content with life.

## Intention

To recognize greed within yourself.

## Lesson

Aparigraha (nonpossessiveness) is the fifth yama on the yogic path. From a yogic perspective, possessiveness and greed are signs of a vacant search for happiness.

The desire to buy or accept more than you need clouds the mind and prevents you from understanding the joys and deeper motivations for a fulfilled life.

What's necessary for you to be healthy, happy, and gratified? Ask yourself if you really need all the clothes, toys, books, or trinkets in your home. How much of it is no longer useful and has become clutter? Can you see how easy it is to lose perspective of what's truly important in life, especially if all you want is *more*?

Greed also extends beyond things to people, including your loved ones. You can have an unhealthy, controlling attachment to people such as your children, parents, spouse, and friends.

You can also be possessive with your thoughts. People tend to hold onto ideas, principles, and precise methods of doing things, becoming set in their ways. This state of inflexibility can transfer to the body's muscles and tissues. The practice of aparigraha is to learn to let go of harmful attachments to possessions, people, thoughts, and actions.

Possessiveness also shows up in asana practice. Some yogis are attached to old tensions or injuries, doing a perfect pose, or to putting their mat in the same spot in the room.

Your challenge today is to detach emotionally from the posture, from the outcome, from what you think you are—and let go of the way you want it to be. Then, let the possibilities flourish. Detach.

## Asanas for Deepening

Emotional attachment to strains and injuries can block the natural flow of circulation in the muscles. When you feel tight, use breath awareness to create balance and space.

Let go of your expectations of how your body *should* perform or how a pose *should* be practiced or taught. Stay available and receptive to the deeper experiences of yoga. Each time you practice asana, you begin anew.

- *Savasana.* Let go of the senses and thoughts to be free to be who you really are. Encourage total detachment.
- *Rag doll.* Hang effortlessly with the knees bent, and tune in to the vibrations arising in the spine with every breath.
- *Standing forward bend.* Surrender any effort; this pose requires you to simply listen and remain present with the variety of sensations along the spine and down the legs.
- *Seated forward bend.* The seated forward bend is calming for the system when the body is able to rest. Let your mind and breath release any conscious aggression within the pose.
- *Pigeon.* Relinquish your weight to the ground, allowing the pelvic area to spread.

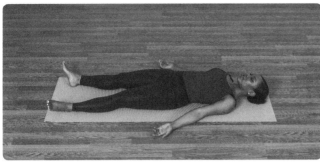
Savasana

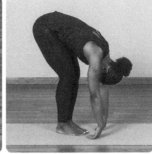
Rag doll

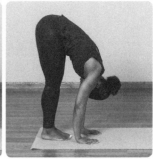
Standing forward bend

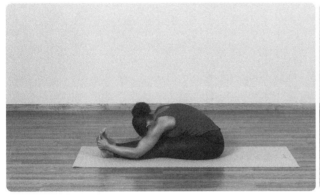
Seated forward bend

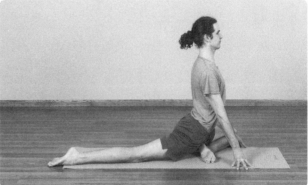
Pigeon

## Motivation Off the Mat

Do you have too much stuff? If it's not useful or beautiful, donate it or throw it out.

Are you so attached to your partner or child that you constantly worry about them? Are you envious of your neighbors? What happens when you don't get what you want?

When you let go of the mental blueprint of the way you think your life *should* be, you can evolve organically instead of willfully.

When you feel jealous, a common impediment to aparigraha, shift to the awareness of gratitude for all that you *already* have.

## WISE WORDS

The yogi trained in the art of greedlessness is generous with time, possessions, and warmth.

Never cling to a person, place, or thing in the hope that it will bring you happiness. Clinging brings you more clinging, and with it, an endless cycle of want.

The possessions you acquire will never completely fulfill you.

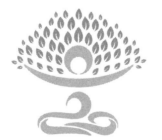

# Niyamas

*To walk safely through the maze of human life, one needs the light of wisdom and the guidance of virtue.*

—Buddha

The niyamas, the second limb of the eight-limbed path, offer practical advice for leading a healthy, happy life through five observances that encourage a natural state of joy and clarity. Not intended as strict or static rules, these guidelines are designed to be fluid, adapting as you adapt and ever-changing as you are.

**Niyamas: Observances**

*Saucha*—Purity. Keep the mind, heart, and body pure.

*Santosha*—Contentment. Accept life as it comes; be satisfied with what is.

*Tapas*—Determined effort. The consistency of discipline to bring about any kind of change.

*Svadhyaya*—Self-study. Study self, scriptures, and the internal states of consciousness.

*Ishvara pranidhana*—Surrender to the divine. Live with awareness of a divine presence. Surrender ego-driven activities to divine energy.

# NIYAMA FLOW

As you flow, empty and surrender the clutter in the mind, letting go of the discomfort that manifests in the body.

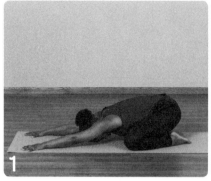

**1** Child's pose

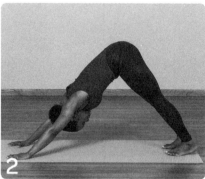

**2** Downward dog

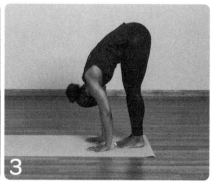

**3** Standing forward bend

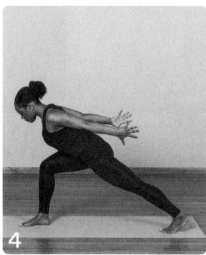

**4** High lunge, floating arms toward the back

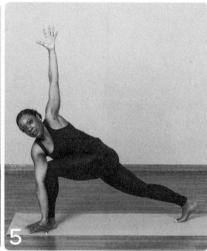

**5** High lunge twist

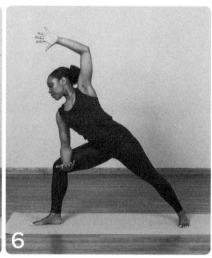

**6** Side angle, rotating the top arm

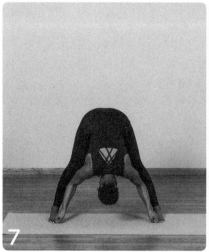

**7** Extended-leg forward bend with big-toe hold

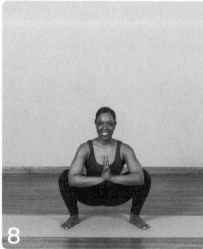

**8** Squat

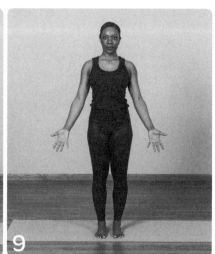

**9** Mountain

# NIYAMA 1: SAUCHA

## Intention

To define saucha of body, mind, and spirit.

## Lesson

In yoga philosophy, there are five niyamas, or observances, that help us navigate our decisions through life. The first niyama is saucha, which means self-purification.

We use saucha as a model for physical health, but it's also a way to cleanse the mind of negative emotions and thoughts.

Body and mind always work in partnership. As the mind moves toward calmness and transparency, it becomes sensitive to toxins and dis-ease in the body. That's why fasting and cleansing techniques alone don't produce self-purification. The mind, full of impurities and mental garbage, must also come clean.

A messy home, office, or car can also reflect your state of mind. When your home is cluttered, we feel smothered by a lack of space. A clean environment provides room to move, breathe, and clear our thoughts.

The focus of today's practice is to cleanse your spirit in order to bring more light and energy to your journey. Engage in pure thinking, directing your thoughts toward the positivity of your practice, the meaning of the postures to your body, and to the concept of saucha.

## Asanas for Deepening

- *Uddiyana bandha (stomach lift).* Massaging and toning the internal organs in the abdominal area relieves constipation, gas, and indigestion.

- *Squat.* Squatting stimulates the digestive tract and releases toxins from the densest parts of the body—the pelvis and legs—both of which are prone to retaining fat and water.

- *Shoulderstand twist.* The change in gravity in shoulderstand helps drain lymph while it stimulates digestion and elimination. Inversions loosen toxins, and they encourage excess mucus to be excreted through the mouth and nose. To add the twist, take shoulderstand and rotate the hips without moving the neck and head.

- *Lion.* Sit on your heels. On exhale, extend the arms, open the mouth wide and stretch the tongue out toward the chin, roaring *AHHHHH!* to cleanse the tongue and remove mucus from the throat. Sit back on the heels on the inhale. Repeat 3 times.

- *Half-hero head-to-knee twist and seated twist.* The squeeze-and-soak action of twisting postures helps clear the abdominal organs; the squeeze forces out waste, while the soaking releases fresh blood, bathing the cells with oxygen and nutrients.

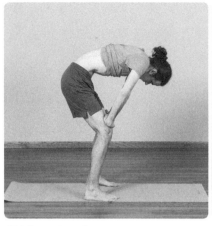

Uddiyana bandha

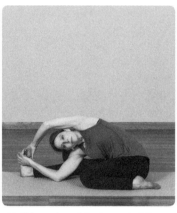

Squat

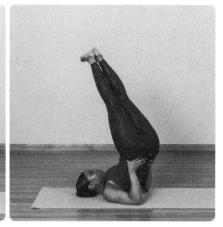

Shoulderstand twist

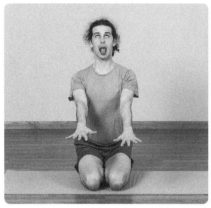

Lion

Half-hero head-to-knee twist

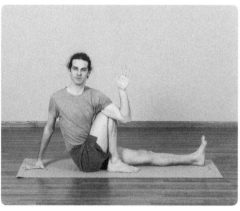

Seated twist

## Motivation Off the Mat

For the mind to be clear, the body and its surroundings—the home, office, practice space, yoga mat—must be kept clean.

Your environment often reflects your state of mind. Don't let dirty dishes, laundry, unread mail, or garbage pile up.

Use neti cleansing to remove mucus and buildup from the sinuses and tissues, and keep the nasal passages clear. Fill a neti pot with a mild, lukewarm saltwater solution, then place the spout of the neti pot to one nostril. Tilt the head to the side opposite that nostril, allowing the saltwater solution to pour through the open nostril. Repeat on the opposite nostril.

Move the bowels once a day. If the system is sluggish, waste stays trapped in your body, along with the tension and slothfulness locked within the tissues. The yogic remedy is to practice deeper, longer-held twists, such as the supine variations before getting out of bed in the morning. Drink 8 to 10 glasses of water a day, avoid white flours, and load up on fresh fruits and vegetables.

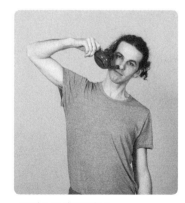

Neti pot cleansing

> The body, breath, and mind have an automatic cleansing process. The breath ebbs and flows, and thoughts constantly enter and leave. On every level, waste is released and replaced with energy and light.

## Teacher Tip

Show respect for yourself and your students by bathing before class, wearing clean clothes, and keeping your mat clean and fresh smelling.

# NIYAMA 2: SANTOSHA

## Intention

To recognize contentment in daily living.

## Lesson

*Santosha* means contentment, and it's the second niyama, or observance in yogic philosophy. Many people tend to think of contentment as the fulfillment of desires, but yoga philosophy teaches that this kind of bliss is short lived. As you learned from the yama aparigraha (nonpossessiveness), desire builds on itself, creating more desire and more cravings. Like a well that can never be filled, greed is a vacant search for happiness. Think about all the happiness beliefs you've told yourself, such as "When I get a new car, I'll be happy." "After I take a vacation, I'll be happy." "Once I'm married, I'll be happy." Was it true? If so, how long did you stay in that state?

The yogi's view of contentment develops from accepting whatever life brings. Contentment is the mindfulness of living in the moment, something we naturally apply to asana.

Here's a parable about two women who seemed to live similar lives:

> There were two women who were very much alike: They were the same age, had similar homes, families, and income levels. They even looked alike. But there was one significant difference. One woman was satisfied with her life, while the other felt empty and frustrated. She wanted more than what she had, and was frequently dissatisfied with her daily activities, finding fault with herself and her family.

As we see from this parable, happiness—the *feeling* of contentment—is a choice. Santosha requires a sense of inner acceptance, which happens when you stop comparing yourself with others. As long as you judge and measure your life by what others have that you don't, you'll never feel content.

In today's asana practice, accept the choices you made that brought you here today. Accept your body, abilities, and limitations as they are right now. Once you decide that what you have is all you need, contentment will find a home in your heart.

## Asanas for Deepening

Personal practice teaches you to accept your body as it is. Surrender any sense of competition among your fellow yogis.

○ *Triangle.* Witness the breath flowing into the awkward spaces. Stay in the pose, and watch your body unfold through time and patience. If a movement feels disagreeable, stay unattached to the outcome and observe whether what you sense is pain, curious sensation, or emotional discomfort. Does santosha arise, even for a moment?

○ *Bridge.* Open the heart, and explore the truth and beauty of the inner and outer worlds. The bridge prevents you from shutting out the reality of your needs, prevailing into the sensation of the present moment.

○ *King dancer.* Experience the cause and effect; and the strength, balance, and flexibility needed to perform the pose. Notice how prana moves inside you, creating more space in your field of energy. Conversely, does the breath struggle, blocking the flow of energy? The choice is yours. Where are you resisting? Smile, feeling the contentment of the beautiful king dancer, Nataraja.

○ *Upward dog–downward dog.* This anti-blues flow is a quick fix for melancholia and the afternoon energy slump. Move from upward dog *(photo a)* to downward dog *(photo b)* with the breath; inhale into upward dog, and exhale to downward dog. Repeat the sequence 6 to 20 times. Rest in child's pose.

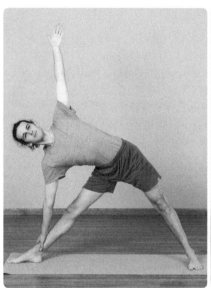

Triangle

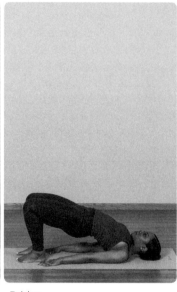

Bridge

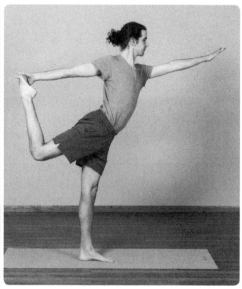

King dancer

**UPWARD DOG—DOWNWARD DOG**

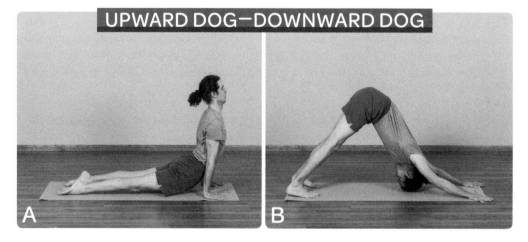

A

B

## Motivation Off the Mat

Contentment practice reveals that you're exactly where you are supposed to be.

Find the time to discover and enjoy the things that make you happy. The simplicity of a walk in the woods, reading a good book, or holding hands with a loved one can awaken a renewed appreciation for the magic in your life.

Live in the present moment without regretting the past or anticipating the future.

Instead of constantly seeking a better body, car, or job, enjoy your perfectly imperfect life.

Before you eat, remember the blessings you have in your life. There are thousands of extraordinary things around you to be grateful for.

## WISE WORDS

Happiness is a way of life.

Nothing is missing. You are complete. You are enough.

Living with santosha frees the mind of the trivialities that rob the spirit of energy. Let go of life's technicalities that are out of your control and look at its larger context with detachment, grace, and acceptance.

# NIYAMA 3: TAPAS

## Intention

To stoke the fiery will to attain goals.

## Lesson

The third niyama or yogic observance is tapas, the willingness and action to reach one's goal. Tapas implies austerity, sacrifice, and discipline; the translation means the "heat" or "fire" which incites transformation. For instance, when someone has an extreme sense of determination, it's referred to as having a "fire in the belly."

According to yoga philosophy, the fire that's created through yoga practice destroys impurities in one's consciousness and leads to control of the body and senses.
To induce lasting change on any level, whether it's to lose weight, master the splits, or attain enlightenment, it's essential to commit to tapas. Putting tapas into practice requires eliminating distractions and obstacles, including negative thinking or naysayers, so that your full attention is on your goal. You might begin by observing the quality of conscious action that you bring to an activity. How often do you dedicate 100 percent of your focus to something?

Discover what drives you to your mat. Tapas in asana opens a new standard of discrimination. Today's practice centers on respecting your goals while working with mindful, determined effort and the fire of will.

## Asanas for Deepening

Put the effort into every pose to get the change you need.

○ *Plank.* Envision a flame at the navel center as you hold plank. Expand the internal fire with your focus and breath.

○ *Elbow plank twist.* Stay high on the toes while slowly dipping the hips side to side, moving toward the knife edge of the foot with each dip. Pause to absorb the body's heat, strength, and power.

○ *Warrior II.* Move your energy from the pelvic floor into the fiery solar plexus, and spread the shoulder blades wide. Breathe, sending determination and action into the whole body.

○ *Fire series.* Point your focus to the navel center, fueling the tapas fire. Include variations of leg lifts such as yoga bicycles, leg circles, single- and double-leg lifts, horizontal and vertical scissors, double-sole kicks, and leg lift twists.

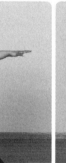

Plank

Elbow plank twist

**FIRE SERIES**

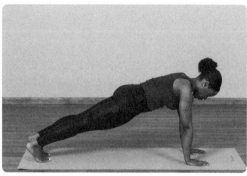

Warrior II

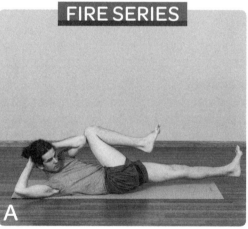

Yoga bicycles

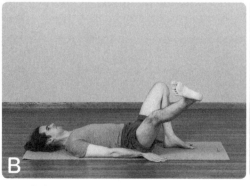

Leg circles

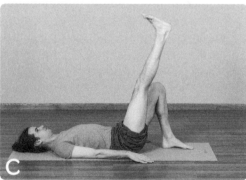

Single-leg lifts

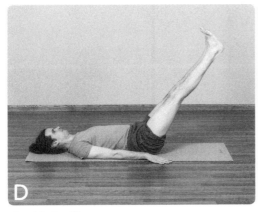

D

Double-leg lifts

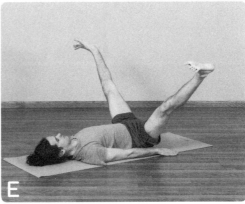

E

Horizontal scissors

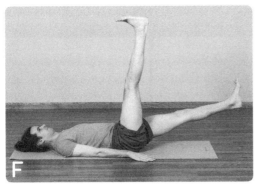

F

Vertical scissors

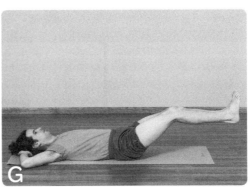

G

Double-sole kicks

## Motivation Off the Mat

Tapas is the *will* to find the way. Every day, will yourself to make one small, positive change. For example, make your bed every morning, drink a full glass of water every afternoon, or take an evening walk.

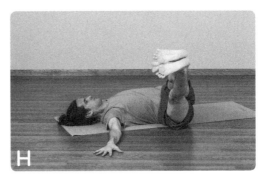

H

Leg lift twists

Don't let daily challenges and disappointments stay within and turn into unhealthy energy. Instead, use the disciplines of tapas to burn them off.

Do something today that your future self will thank you for later.

## WISE WORDS

Tapas is stirred by knowing that life is a miracle, and the desire to make the most of it.

Tapas practice is to purify and destroy anything that holds you down and perpetuates suffering.

Yoga cannot exist without tapas.

## Intention

To encourage the study of self.

## Lesson

Today's class centers on learning more about yourself through the fourth niyama, svadhyaya. The word *svadhyaya* means "the study and observance of oneself." The practice refers to the self through the study of inspiring and sacred texts, books, or teachers, as well as to the skill of self-observation.

Svadhyaya engages the discipline of sayta (truth), which requires total honesty about how you view yourself. Within your yoga practice, svadhyaya asks you to be an observer of the moment-to-moment changes in your body and mind. Self-study is a way of looking within and connecting to your inner truth.

As you practice and move, focus inward to get inside the flow of your experience. Pause between postures to listen and learn from them. Be honest about what you learn and what you don't understand. Be present to pain versus discomfort. It's time to learn something new about yourself.

## Asanas for Deepening

Turn your attention inward and become aware of your breathing. Imagine how the breath creates space in the abstract parts of the body. Observe how prana vibrates, activating every layer of consciousness.

- *Cow face arms.* Does your body have a definitive response to this playful, yet extreme shoulder stretch? Does your upper body feel liberated or locked?
- *Cobra.* Attend to the prana flowing up the front of the spine and down the legs.
- *Crocodile.* Sense the tingling of the back muscles as energy and mood gradually shift.
- *Seated angle.* Take yourself to your edge through astute awareness driven by your physical and mental adjustments. Challenge yourself to stay mindful.
- *Tree.* Observe the ego, that part of you that desires a perfectly balanced tree. Drive awareness to the sole of the standing foot, examining the subtle waves of movement from the edge of the heel to the balls of the toes.

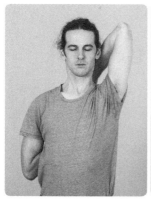
Cow face arms

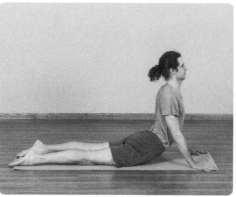
Cobra

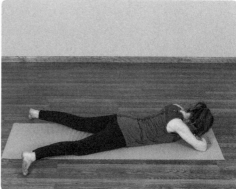
Crocodile

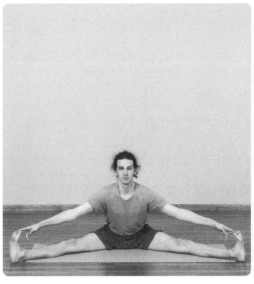

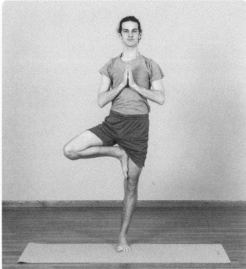

Seated angle                                    Tree

## Motivation Off the Mat

Practice self-study during your day. Every movement is asana, every breath is pranayama, and every thought is meditation.

Each night before going to sleep, ask the question *What did I learn today?*

Observe yourself as though you were watching a video of someone else. Notice the tone of your voice and body language when you speak to family and friends. How does it differ from the way you engage coworkers, customers, or strangers? Does your body feel as if it's wide open and available, or are you shut down and introspective in either situation?

## WISE WORDS

Svadhyaya gives you pause to breathe, relax, feel, and learn. Make it possible to receive and enjoy the spirit of your own exploratory adventure.

Study and practice go hand in hand. Acquire yoga reference books, scriptures, or other inspirational readings that have significance to you such as Patanjali's *Yoga Sutras*, the *Hatha Yoga Pradipika*, and the *Bhagavad Gita* (also see the Recommended Reading List at the end of this book). Determine how the concepts in these books change over time as you grow and change, uncovering the deeper meaning of life.

## Teacher Tip

Remind your class of the choices they have within every pose, offering options for them to consider. As your students attend to their inner worlds, cue them to close their eyes, and don't interrupt by making physical adjustments.

# NIYAMA 5: ISHVARA PRANIDHANA

## Intention

To surrender with faith and devotion to a higher source.

## Lesson

The fifth niyama is ishvara pranidhana. The words *ishvara pranidhana* translate to "surrendering to the divine." This observance asks you to study your relationship to the universe's divine spirit and honor a higher ideal or consciousness.

Yoga philosophy suggests that by uniting your individual self with that of a higher divine principle—be it God, Buddha, Jesus, or Mother Nature—all egotism, trivialities, and selfishness are removed. When you surrender your ego-driven activities to divine spirit, doorways open for positive energy to flow into all areas of your life. With the practice of ishvara pranidhana, every action is taken with significance, every word is spoken with meaning and truth, and every thought is given with clarity.

Ishvara pranidhana redirects energy away from selfish desires as you learn that you're a fragment of something much bigger than your job or body shape. The practice of surrendering to a higher self is in fact a relief from the effort it takes to focus on ego-driven daily dramas.

Today, take your practice within to find the truth of who you are. Offer the fruits of yourself, your work, and your love to a divine force, whatever that may be for you. Notice the difference in your practice when you surrender the ego and free yourself to a concept much bigger than you.

## Asanas for Deepening

Guide the class to become more genuine and receptive to their higher force.

- *Namaste circles.* Inhale and move the arms upward and outward *(photo a)*. Exhale and move the hands to the heart in namaste *(photo b)*. Connect to the universal spirit within the heart center.
- *Tripod.* Place the knees on the forearms. This posture awakens the crown chakra, the connection to divine consciousness, located at the top of the head.
- *Temple.* Bring the hands to namaste. Feel the grounding in the feet and legs. Bring both earth and heaven energy into the heart center.
- *Standing forward bend.* With each forward bend, bow to the power that's guiding you.
- *Supported bridge.* Lift and offer your heart to the universe so that every thought, word, and action is felt as a ripple of love and devotion to the universal spirit.
- *Savasana.* Get quiet, feeling the release of old patterns, traumas, and ideas that clutter the mind.

## NAMASTE CIRCLES

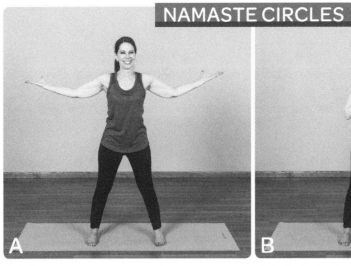

A

Inhaling, move arms up and out

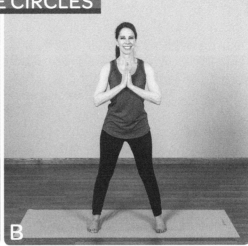

B

Exhaling, bring hands to heart

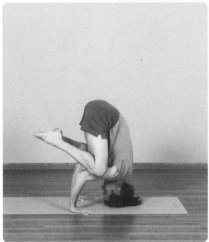

Tripod

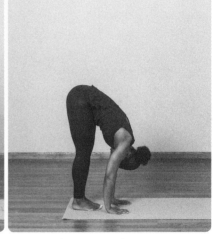

Temple

Standing forward bend

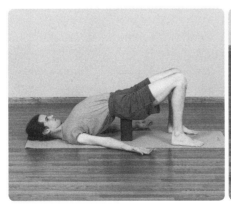

Supported bridge

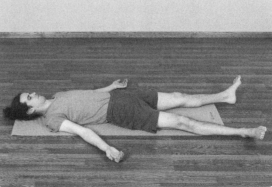

Savasana

## Motivation Off the Mat

Meditate on what you do each day, who you talk to, where your mind goes, and how your body moves. Start your meditation when you awake, and continue as you brush your teeth, eat your breakfast, commute to work, and so on through the rest of your day. How is ishvara pranidhana woven into your daily activities?

Surrender your ego and devote yourself to humanity by volunteering in your community.

## WISE WORDS

The practice of ishvara pranidhana is a way of living with awareness of supreme intelligence.

As you surrender, get quiet and listen for guidance.

When you embrace ishvara pranidhana, your yoga practice becomes a way to stay positive, selfless, and vibrant so that you may contribute to the world at large.

# Chakras

*All things appear and disappear because of the concurrence of causes and conditions. Nothing ever exists entirely alone; everything is in relation to everything else.*

—Buddha

The *chakras* are the body's seven major hubs arranged vertically from the base of the spine to the top of the head, that regulate the flow of subtle energy. The Sanskrit word for wheel, chakra is a spinning vortex of energy. Each chakra is associated with a particular part of the physical body, mental or emotional state, color, element of nature, and sound. Intended to awaken and balance these centers of consciousness and facilitate healing, the lessons in this chapter teach you how to savor the sacred fruit within each chakra.

## Chakras

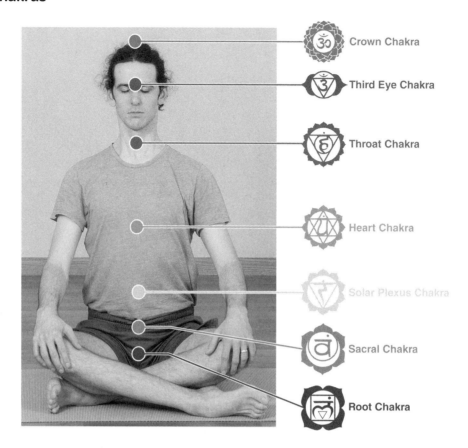

*Root*—Survival; color: red; element: earth; seed sound: *lam*

*Sacral*—Pleasure; color: orange; element: water; seed sound: *vam*

*Solar plexus*—Will; color: yellow; element: sun; seed sound: *ram*

*Heart*—Love; color: green; element: air; seed sound: *yam*

*Throat*—Communication; color: blue; element: sound; seed sound: *ham*

*Third eye*—Intuition; color: indigo; element: light; seed sound: *om*

*Crown*—Divine connection; color: purple; element: thought; seed sound: *om*

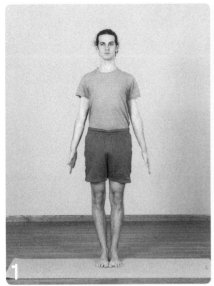

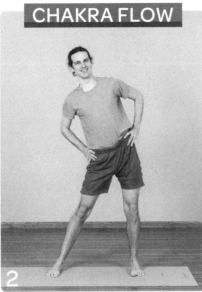

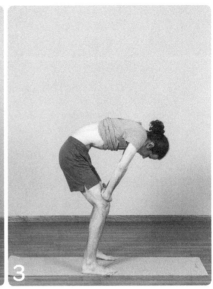

1

Mountain – Root: earth

2

Hip circles – Sacral: water

3

Stomach lift – Solar plexus: sun

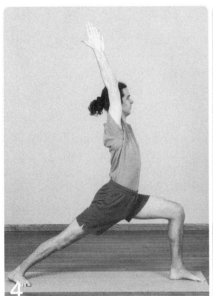

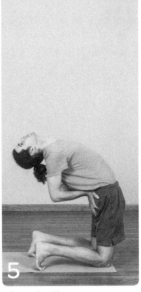

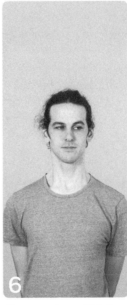

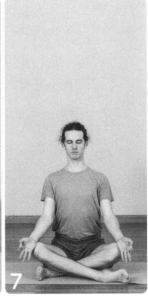

4

Warrior I – Heart: air

5

Camel – Throat: sound

6

Eye exercises – Third eye: light

7

Meditation – Crown: thought

# CHAKRA 1: MULADHARA (ROOT)

## Intention

To activate the root chakra.

## Lesson

The first chakra, *muladhara,* is the root chakra. *Muladhara* means "support" or "foundation." The root chakra is the foundation of all the chakras and guides our survival and self-preservation instinct. It's located at the base of the spine at the pelvic floor, vibrates to the color red, and relates to the grounding element of earth.

When your survival needs are met and the root chakra is balanced, you feel grounded, stable, comfortable in your body, and safe in your environment.

If the root chakra is out of balance, any progress in your life will be made without roots and will lack the stability necessary for long-term growth. When the first chakra is overactive, you feel too grounded in the body—too heavy, too sluggish, and too slow to move. In this state, people tend to overeat and oversleep, and are resistant to change. When the root chakra is deficient of energies, you feel ungrounded and without roots, embodied in insecurity, fear, and anxiety.

Physical imbalances of the root chakra manifest as aches and pains in the legs, feet, and bones, and as problems with the body's elimination system. A person with an overactive first chakra may experience constipation, while someone lacking first chakra energy may have frequent diarrhea.

Our practice today will focus on noticing gravity, feeling safe in the body, and mindfully moving to sense your earthly roots.

## Asanas for Deepening

○ *Foot stomping.* Stomp on the soles of the each foot, sensing the flutter of flow from the earth up the legs.

○ *Tree.* Awaken and strengthen the lower body, rooting the attention downward. Feel yourself supported and connected to the earth as you plant your tree.

○ *Standing forward bend with chant.* Chant the sound *lam,* the seed sound of muladhara, as you exhale down to the earth. Repeat 3 to 6 times chanting *lam* each time you bend forward.

○ *Warrior II.* Reach through the fingertips, extending your subtle body outside of your physical body, while hardily rooting through the feet, supercharging the earth element through this pose.

○ *Triangle.* Feel for spaciousness as you ground your legs and feet, extending the roots up through the body.

○ *Asvini mudra.* Lie in crocodile pose with the legs together. Exhaling, contract the buttocks, pulling the anal sphincter muscles inward. Inhaling, relax completely. Asvini mudra helps strengthen and energize the muscles around the base of the spine and pelvic floor, distributing awareness to the root and directing prana through the sushumna nadi. Repeat the sequence 8 to 10 times.

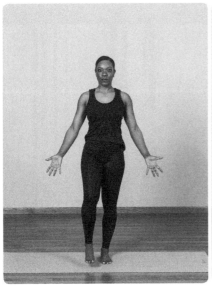
Foot stomping

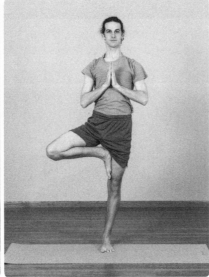
Tree

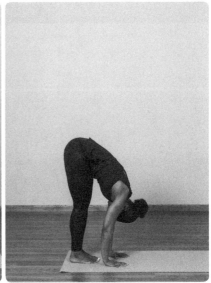
Standing forward bend with chant

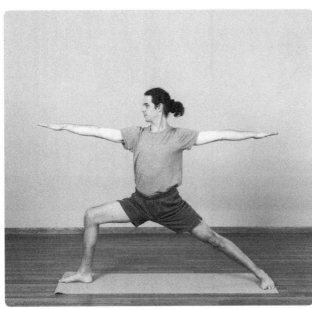
Warrior II

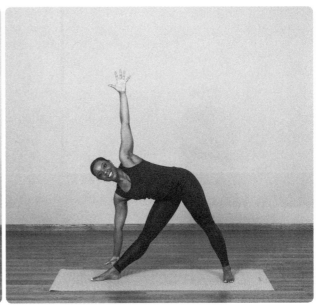
Triangle

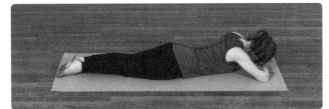
Asvini mudra

## Motivation Off the Mat

To increase first chakra energy, eat foods high in protein and earth-based foods such as root vegetables. Spend time moving the body outdoors. Ride a bike, power walk, or garden.

To decrease the energy in an overactive root chakra, lighten up; increase your exercise regimen, eat less, and smile more. Eat organic, fresh, and locally grown foods, and eliminate processed foods and soda from your diet.

Meditate on the color red. In a seated position, place the thumb to the pinky finger in earth mudra, and rest the backs of the hands on the thighs. Envision the color red glistening at the base of the spine, filling your pelvic floor, legs, and feet with grounding earth energy and strength.

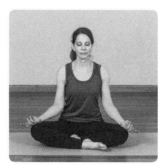

Earth mudra

## Walking Meditation

Take your meditation practice outside. As you walk, concentrate on each foot leaving the earth and re-rooting with each step.

## WISE WORDS

Remember that the word *muladhara* means "support" or "foundation." A solid root chakra foundation provides lifeforce to the six other energy centers; any imbalance in the root will adversely affect all the chakras.

# CHAKRA 2: SVADHISTHANA (SACRUM)

## Intention

To feel the pleasures of the second chakra.

## Lesson

Svadhisthana, the second chakra, is the body's center of motion, located at the lower abdomen, at the lumbar vertebrae in the back. The word *svadhisthana* means "abode of the vital force." Svadhisthana relates to the element of water and vibrates to the color orange.

Pleasure is the motivating principle in chakra 2. Once survival needs are met in the root chakra, we turn toward enjoyment. When this chakra is balanced, we experience happiness, joy, and sensuality. We have a passion for life, and are expressive, trusting, and sexually satisfied.

Imbalance of the second chakra may occur as feelings of guilt, powerlessness, isolation, self-blaming, emotional instability, or manipulative behavior. Physical symptoms of imbalance emerge in the sex organs, large intestines, pelvis, hips, and bladder. Some common physical manifestations of imbalance are impotence, frigidity, infertility, and low-back pain.

When svadhisthana is overactive, it can lead to sexual addictions or obsessive attachments, craving stimulation, and being excessively sensitive. A deficient second chakra manifests as fear of change, poor social skills, stiffness in the body and in life, or guilty feelings.

Today, our practice for opening and balancing the second chakra targets movement in the hips and lower abdomen. Keep the area of the second chakra in your mind's eye, experiencing the joy of motion in the body, awakening to the healthy pleasures of life. Move fluidly, like water, being present to every sensation.

## Asanas for Deepening

○ *Standing pelvic tilts.* Connect with earth energy through the legs, lifting into the second chakra. Tilt the pelvis forward, pushing against the earth. Imagine the energy you're building in the legs flowing like water into your sacral area.

○ *Temple flow.* Free the arms and move from side to side, flowing with pelvic energy and connecting to the water element.

○ *Butterfly with chant.* Exhale as you bend forward in butterfly chanting *vam*, the seed sound of the second chakra, bringing your awareness to the pleasure center. Repeat this movement 3 times.

○ *Pelvic rotations with bhastrika.* From a seated position, move the torso in a clockwise rotation while activating the bhastrika breath. Visualize stirring up the creative forces in the second chakra. Switch directions after 3 rotations.

○ *Reclining hero.* Lean back in hero pose while reflecting on the vibrant orange pulsation within the lower abdomen.

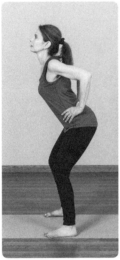

Standing pelvic tilts

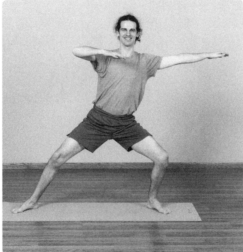

Temple flow

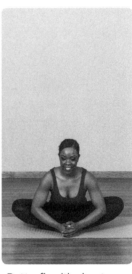

Butterfly with chant

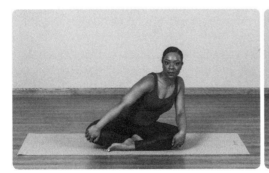

Pelvic rotations

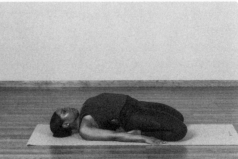

Reclining hero

## Motivation Off the Mat

Drink water.

Move! Walk, dance, run, and stretch. Go with the flow of your creative, expressive body.

Rediscover your sexuality. Fill your sexual journey with passion, romance, and creativity. More than the sexual act, honor the divine spirit of your partner.

Meditate on the pleasure center by visualizing an orange lotus in the second chakra area. Hold that image in your mind for several minutes while breathing deeply.

## WISE WORDS

A balanced second chakra is an expandable resource of energy available for creativity, movement, procreation, and pleasure.

A healthy second chakra connects you to others without becoming codependent or losing your identity.

# CHAKRA 3: MANIPURA (SOLAR PLEXUS)

## Intention

To strengthen the power of will.

## Lesson

Located at the navel center, the third chakra, the body's energy battery, resides at the *manipura* or the *"jewel of the lotus."* Here, prana rising from the first and second chakras, has the potential to become a compelling force within the body. The third chakra is associated with the element of fire and vibrates to the color yellow.

A balanced third chakra ignites inner power, self-confidence, and the ability to take risks. The intensity of the navel center feeds self-esteem, courage, and willpower. While the second chakra may inspire us to make positive changes, like quitting a bad habit or eating healthier, the fiery force from the third chakra motivates us to execute *lasting* change.

When the third chakra is deficient, it leads to fearfulness, burn out or lack of energy, and low self-esteem. When this chakra is overactive, we can be controlling, competitive, and stubborn, putting too much emphasis on power and social status. Ulcers, chronic fatigue, and digestive problems are common ailments associated with the third chakra.

The practice for opening and balancing the manipura chakra embraces poses that fan the flames of the inner fire. The focus is on moving with will and purpose, energizing limbs and torso, and building and storing inner strength.

## Asanas for Deepening

○ *Locust.* Lift the legs, head, and shoulders off the ground while holding the posture for 5 to 10 breaths. Repeat the pose 3 to 5 times. Notice the sensations around the navel.

○ *Seated forward bend with chant.* Exhale into the stretch, chanting the sound *ram*, the seed sound of the third chakra. Hold your awareness at the navel through your exhalation. Repeat the chant 3 times while holding the stretch, igniting the flame of manipura.

○ *Uddiyana bandha (stomach lift and lock).* This bandha guides energy from the first and second chakras and moves it upward to the purifying fires of the third chakra. From a standing position, bend forward and rest your hands above your knees. Exhale completely, pulling the belly back toward the spine. Apply mula bandha (the root lock). Lift the lower abdomen upward, under the rib cavity until the navel center appears concave. Drop the chin toward the chest. Hold the exhalation. When you need to inhale, lift the chin as you release the stomach lift and mula bandha. Repeat the sequence 3 times.

○ *Warrior spirit flow.* This devotional flow warms the body and encourages the strengthening of the emotions, spreading warrior spirit and confidence.

1. Mountain
2. Warrior I
3. Pyramid
4. Warrior II

5. Triangle
6. Side angle with bind
7. Seated twist
8. Yoga bicycles

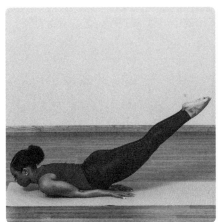

Locust

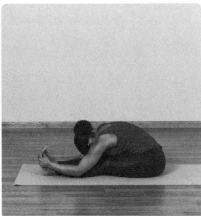

Seated forward bend

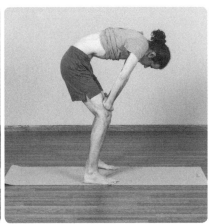

Uddiyana bandha

## WARRIOR SPIRIT FLOW

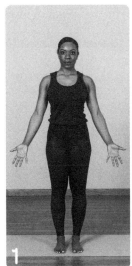

Mountain

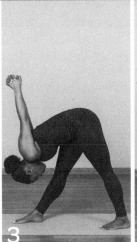

Warrior I

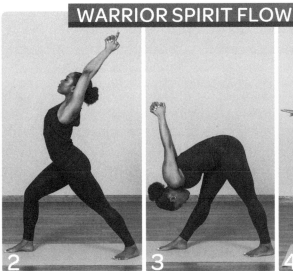

Pyramid

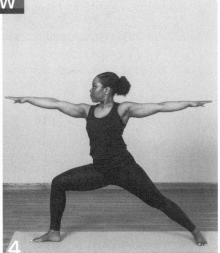

Warrior II

*(continued)*

Chakras    157

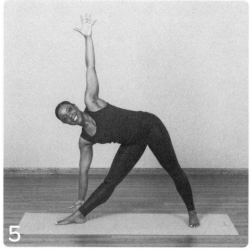

Triangle

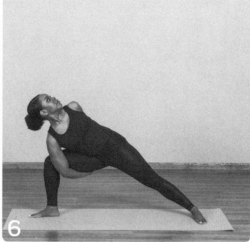

Side angle with bind

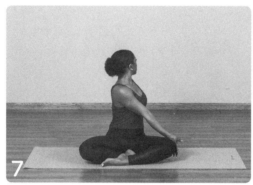

Seated twist

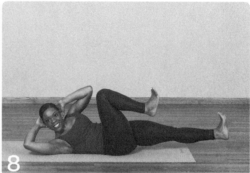

Yoga bicycles

## Motivation Off the Mat

The way to a strong third chakra is to flex the muscles of your inner strength. Take risks; move beyond what feels safe. Weigh the risks in relation to what seems appropriate for the health of your third chakra. This could be anything from asking a server for more ketchup to starting your own business.

Make a list of daily goals, then use the willpower of the third chakra to accomplish each one.

## WISE WORDS

A balanced solar plexus connects you with your internal source of power, the body's energy battery.

The best practice for progress and power comes from discipline and ritual.

Having strong abdominal muscles enhances all the yoga postures and strengthens every system in the body.

# CHAKRA 4: ANAHATA (HEART)

## Intention

To arouse and harmonize the heart center.

## Lesson

The fourth chakra, *anahata*, is the heart center, the center of love. Its physical location is the heart, lungs, thymus gland, upper chest, upper back, shoulders, arms, and hands. The word anahata means "unstuck," "fresh," "clean," or "unhurt." The element of anahata is air, and it vibrates to the color green.

The heart center is the link between the lower three and the upper three chakras, positioned halfway between the earth—our connection to the physical plane, and the sky—our link to the spiritual plane.

Anahata carries the seed of inner peace and harmony. As the heart center expands, the seed opens and grows. When the heart is in balance, we feel caring, compassionate, accepting, and peaceful, and instinctually know how to give and receive love.

When the heart center is lacking energy, we feel shy, lonely, critical, intolerant, resentful, and have difficulty forgiving. Physically, the shoulders are rounded forward, causing the heart to sink away from the world. Symptoms of an overactive fourth chakra include codependency, jealousy, and possessiveness. The physical imbalances of an overactive heart center appear as shallow breathing, asthma, high blood pressure, and heart disease.

Yoga practices for harmonizing the anahata awaken the supporting anatomy around the heart, offering the chest plenty of breathing room. The internal focus is on releasing blocked or flooded emotions. During practice, lead and work from the heart, not from the head.

## Asanas for Deepening

○ *Cobra*. With each inhalation, raise the heart and open to sensation. Maintain the opening as you exhale and release your heart to the earth.

○ *Bow*. The heart desires harmony. The bow develops the physical expansion and surrender required to bring the heart center toward tranquility.

○ *Triangle*. The triangle is considered the posture of joy because it spreads the wings of the shoulders, expands the backdoor of the heart housed between the blades, and releases joy throughout the body.

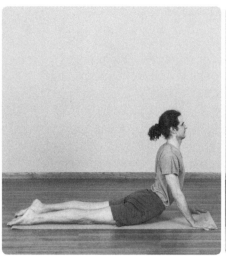

Cobra

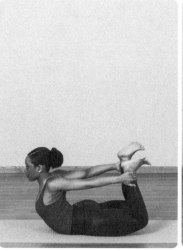

Bow

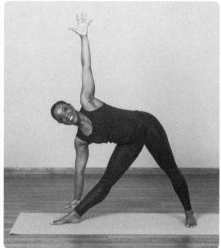

Triangle

○ *Heart-Opening Vinyasa.* Emphasize broadening the shoulders, freeing the chest, lifting the sternum, and expanding the supporting anatomy around the heart. Hold each pose for 5 breaths, meditating on the rhythm of the heartbeat.

1. Easy pose with lotus mudra. *The lotus flower erases sadness and loneliness within the heart.*
2. Easy pose with side stretch
3. Easy pose twist
4. Downward dog twist
5. Fallen triangle
6. Plank
7. Side plank
8. Upward dog
9. Downward dog
10. Warrior I with eagle arms
11. Standing yoga mudra
12. Mountain with anjali mudra

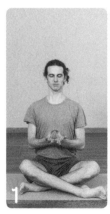

Easy pose with lotus mudra

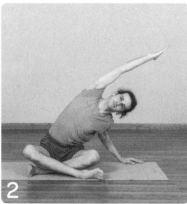

Easy pose with side stretch

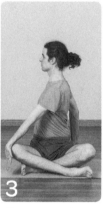

Easy pose twist

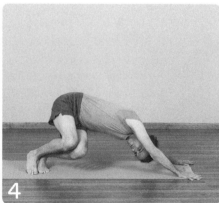

Downward dog twist

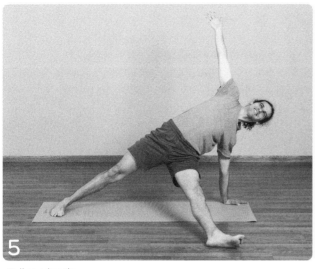

5

Fallen triangle

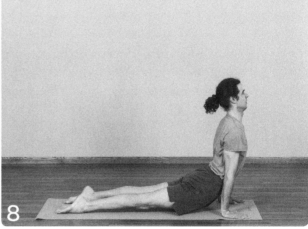

6

Plank

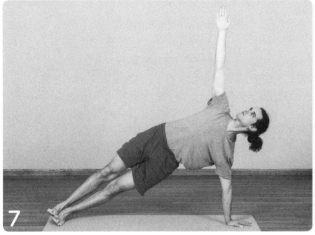

7

Side plank

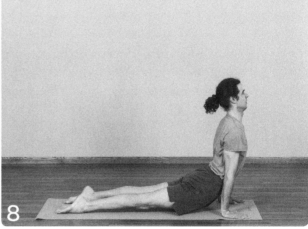

8

Upward dog

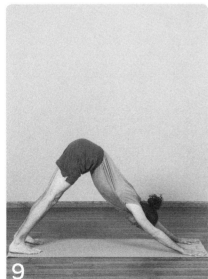

9

Downward dog

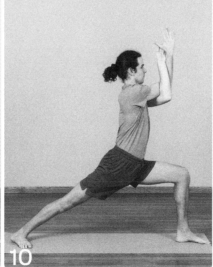

10

Warrior I with eagle arms

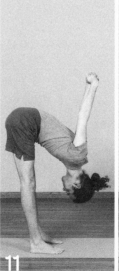

11

Standing yoga mudra

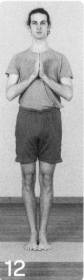

12

Mountain with anjali mudra

## Heart Connection

Anahata governs the sense of touch and rules the hands. Experience the sensation of hand touching hand in anjali mudra. The prayer position completes the energy circuit between the hands and the heart, and harmonizes the two hemispheres of the brain. Focus your awareness on the emerald green chakra. With each exhalation, chant the sound *yam*, awakening the spiritual heart.

## Motivation Off the Mat

**Be grateful:** Honor all that you have to be thankful for. Keep a gratitude journal, and create a nightly ritual of writing down five things that you are grateful for.

**Give of yourself:** Call someone who is lonely, spend time with others who need companionship, or do a favor for a friend without expecting anything in return.

**Forgive:** Forgiveness is essential to a healthy spiritual heart. Forgiveness doesn't mean forgetting. It's simply a method to release the self-sabotaging, destructive thoughts of the past so that you can walk an obstacle-free path.

## WISE WORDS

When fear or depression sets into consciousness, the muscles contract in an effort to defend the body from storing more darkness.

A balanced heart is open to the vibrations of universal love.

*I looked at temples, churches, and mosques. But I found the divine within my heart.*

—Rumi

# CHAKRA 5: VISUDDHA (THROAT)

## Intention

To stimulate the communication center.

## Lesson

*Visuddha*, the fifth chakra, is located at the throat center, and it's the first chakra that focuses on the spiritual plane. The word visuddha means "purification of higher consciousness." It's associated with the element of sound, and it vibrates to the color blue, representing clarity. Vibration, rhythm, voice, and words are connected with this center. Writing, speaking, listening to music, dancing, and singing are all ways of communication and expression within the fifth chakra.

When visuddha is in balance, the voice is clear, listening skills are sharp, and miscommunications are brief. When energy is lacking in the throat center, the voice is soft, and there's often an inability to put feelings into words. Those with an overactive throat center tend to talk too much or too loud, and are inconsiderate or unfocused listeners.

Physical imbalances of the fifth chakra manifest as neck stiffness, teeth grinding, jaw disorders, throat ailments, or as an underactive or overactive thyroid. The asana practice for opening and balancing this chakra includes moving with sound, feeling the vibrations inside the body, and using sound to release blockages.

## Asanas for Deepening

○ *Mountain to standing forward bend.* From mountain *(photo a)* exhale to forward bend, chanting the seed sound of the throat chakra, *ham (photo b)*. Inhale, rise to mountain, tasting the air inside the throat. Repeat the movement and the chant 3 times. The seed sound resonates and activates the center of the throat chakra, clearing away phlegm and emotional blocks.

○ *Side angle with ujjayi.* As you hold side angle, keep the neck long and gaze up, center, or downward. Listen to the *ujjayi* breath moving from the belly to the glottis in the back of the throat.

○ *Neck rolls.* Turn the head from side to side *(photo a)*, bring the ear to the shoulder using the seed sound *ham* on the exhalation *(photo b)*, and move the chin to the chest *(photo c)*.

○ *Plow.* Extend the legs from the sacrum to the heels. Gently compress the throat, stimulating the thyroid gland, while opening the back of the neck.

○ *Bhramari breath.* The droning sound of the bumblebee breath, *bhramari* clears the mind, soothes the nervous system, and vibrates the throat center by simulating the humming of a bumblebee. To practice, exhale with a closed mouth, making a loud humming sound like a bee. Repeat for 5 to 10 exhales sensing the vibration from heart to throat center.

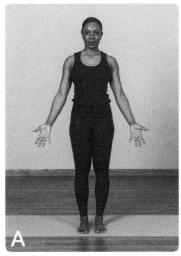

Mountain

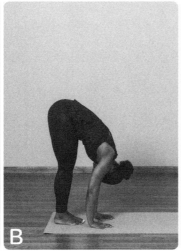

Standing forward bend

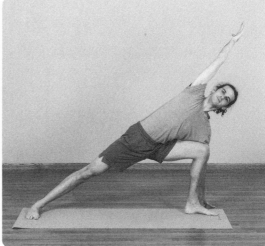

Side angle

**NECK ROLLS**

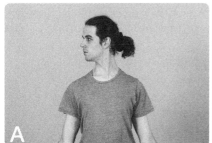

Side to side

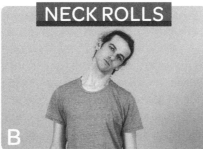

Ear to shoulder with seed sound

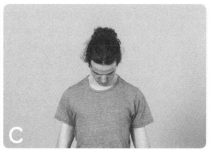

Chin to chest

## Motivation Off the Mat

Listen. For one day, *really* listen to what others are saying. Give them your full attention when they speak, and show interest and enthusiasm in what they're saying. Most importantly, don't interrupt when they talk.

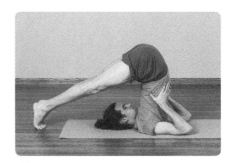
Plow

Avoid complaining and criticizing for one day. This includes criticism of yourself. Notice how much adversity is linked to complaining, while enjoying the freedom from the usual negative energy.

Add a few drops of peppermint essential oil to a glass of water to open the voice, cleanse the throat of mucus, and clear away psychic debris.

Use mantra meditation. Mantra is a tool of the mind that shields you from the traps of nonproductive thought and action. The rhythm of the mantra vibrates and harmonizes subconscious thoughts, and cleanses the root of your thought patterns. If you don't have a mantra, repeat a daily affirmation, goal, prayer, or wish for a loved one.

## WISE WORDS

The release of sound clarifies and organizes the energy in the body.

Sound affects the cellular structure of matter.

The gift of the throat chakra is to be heard, understood, and receive truth.

## Teacher Tip

Wear the color blue (the color of the fifth chakra) while teaching a throat chakra class. Speak clearly, breathe loudly, and lead with your voice.

# CHAKRA 6: AJNA (THIRD EYE)

## Intention

To purify the spiritual eye.

## Lesson

The space between the eyebrows, the spiritual eye, is the home of *ajna*, the sixth chakra. It's here that the journey of consciousness moves into the source of our inner light. Ajna is linked to the element of light, the color indigo, and the seed sound *om*.

The sixth chakra is the home of intuition, dreams, and visions. In children, this chakra is naturally open and active. Children have imaginary playmates and see dragons, witches, and castles. Even colors are more vivid. As we age, the light within ajna dims and we have to work hard to reconnect with our window to the soul.

When the third eye is in balance, we have strong intuition, memory, creativity, and dream recall. A person with an overactive sixth chakra experiences difficulty concentrating and has headaches, hallucinations, or nightmares. If the chakra is deficient, thought energy, memory, and visualization are impaired.

Our asana focus today is on envisioning the energy from the lower chakras moving up into the spiritual eye, cleansing our inner light and window to the soul.

## Asanas for Deepening

- *Eye exercises.* These exercises alleviate eye strain, reduce headaches, and improve concentration.
- *Fish.* The fish stretches and inverts the space between the eyebrows and the forehead.
- *Squat.* Bring the hands to prayer position and place the thumbs at the third eye. Feel the energies of all the chakras from the ground up moving into the spiritual eye.
- *Child's pose with spiritual triangle.* Place the hands on the floor under the forehead. With thumbs and index fingers touching, make a triangle "nest" for the third eye to rest and open.
- *Lotus.* Chant the sound *om*, the seed sound of the third eye. Rest awareness at the eyebrow center, visualizing the energy along the subtle channel between the root and eyebrows.
- *Massage.* Massage the forehead, ears and earlobes, and temples.

## EYE EXERCISES

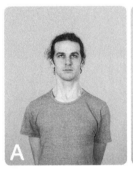

A

Look up

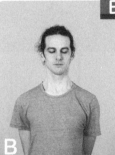

B

Look down

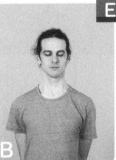

C

Look center

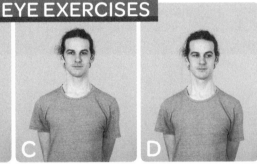

D

Look left

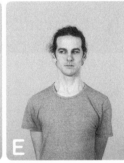

E

Look right

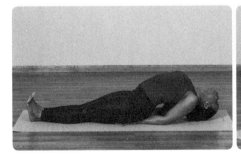

Fish

Squat

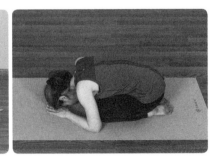

Child's pose with spiritual triangle

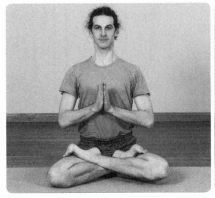

Lotus with chant

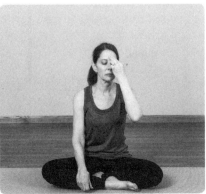

Massage (third eye)

## Motivation Off the Mat

Engage with ajna. Stay present and expand your awareness by visualizing your breath flowing in and out through the third eye.

Light up your life. Light is stimulating to consciousness, awakening emotions, visions, and the link between your inner and outer worlds. Illuminate your home and work space by adding lamps and opening curtains and blinds to let in the natural light.

Keep a dream journal. Record your dreams, even if you can only remember small pieces of them. Dreams reveal the dynamics of the subconscious and train the mind to stay alert.

## WISE WORDS

The word *ajna* means "command," "perception," "knowledge," and "authority."

Clairvoyance is not just for the gifted few. We all have the ability see clearly if we look deeper and trust our instincts.

Awakening ajna opens unexpected realms of transformation, improving your state of consciousness and the ability to perceive your effect on others.

## Teacher Tip

Encourage students to keep their eyes closed during class using *umpada drishti*, the inner gaze toward the eyebrow center. Because the eyes provide 85 percent of sensory input, an eyes-closed practice eliminates all distractions in the practice space.

# CHAKRA 7: SAHASRARA (CROWN)

## Intention

To perceive the crown chakra.

## Lesson

The seventh chakra, *sahasrara,* is the crown of the chakra system located at the top of the head, symbolizing the seat of enlightenment. The word sahasrara means "thousand-petal lotus." The element of the crown chakra is thought, corresponding to the highest functions of the mind. Sahasrara vibrates to the color violet, and its seed sound is *om.*

The crown chakra is the link to divine intelligence, wisdom, and understanding. A person with a balanced crown chakra feels a oneness with a higher universal power, enjoys a spiritual connection to something bigger than the individual self, and is open-minded. A balanced crown chakra allows a sense of peace in the knowledge that life has a deeper meaning than what's on the surface.

The characteristics of an overactive seventh chakra include feeling like a spiritual elitist, having narcissistic tendencies, or feeling detached from one's environment. If the crown center is lacking energy, a person may be a spiritual skeptic, have difficulty thinking, or have a closed mind with a rigid belief system.

Today's asana practice for opening and balancing this chakra is to focus on the awareness gained from witnessing your thoughts, releasing attachments, and connecting to a divine spirit, a higher power, or mother nature.

## Asanas for Deepening

○ Bridge
○ Wheel
○ Handstand
○ Headstand or tripod
○ Nadi shodhana pranayama

○ Lotus chant – While in lotus, chant the seed sound *om* with each exhalation. Rest awareness at the crown center, visualizing energy moving up sushumna between the root and the crown.
○ Massage the crown of the head and the back of the ears while in a seated pose.

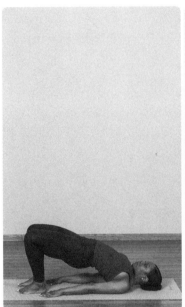
Bridge

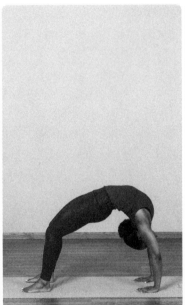
Wheel

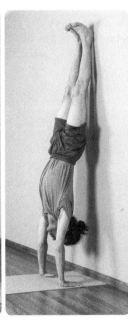
Handstand

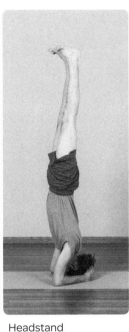
Headstand

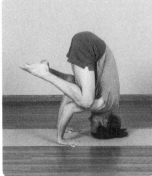
Tripod

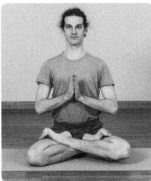
Nadi shodhana

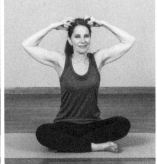
Lotus chant

Massage the crown

## Motivation Off the Mat

*Meditate.* The seventh limb of *raja* yoga is dhyana, meditation. Meditation is the optimal yogic practice for balancing the crown chakra, joining divine energy and expanded consciousness, while empowering the mind to become present, clear, and insightful.

*Sadhana (spiritual practice).* Once a day, connect with your authentic self through meditation, asana, or pranayama. Sadhana is best practiced between 4 a.m. and 7 a.m., when the mind is quiet. Any conscious effort to connect with your authentic self, no matter how long, is magnified in the crown chakra. Visualize your concept of divine spirit, and honor the wonders of nature as you walk to your destination, look out the window, or watch the sunset.

## WISE WORDS

The crown chakra is the meeting point between the finite (the body and the ego) and the infinite (the universe and the soul).

A healthy, balanced development of the lower chakras is a prerequisite for moving spiritual energy up to the crown chakra.

# CHAKRAS AND THE FIVE TIBETANS

## Intention

To maintain the health of the chakras.

## Lesson

For thousands of years, holistic practitioners have known that the body has seven principal energy centers called chakras where the nadis (the body's subtle energy channels) intersect. The chakras are located along the spinal column and are considered transformation centers that regulate the flow of prana. These seven energy centers form the major components of our consciousness and are linked to specific areas of the body and mind.

Prana can be released for physical, emotional, or spiritual functions, or it can be held and ultimately blocked, causing disruptions that interfere with energy flow. As we age, chakra energy slows and we experience this stagnation as pain, discomfort, or emotional suffering. The five Tibetan rites (commonly called the five Tibetans) are a series of 2,500 year-old exercises that when practiced daily, are said to hold the key to lasting youth, health, and vitality by keeping the chakras balanced and in motion.

### Benefits of the Five Tibetans

**Hormonal balance:** When the endocrine glands are healthy, we have more vitality to experience the joys in life. Balanced hormones also help alleviate premenstrual syndrome and menopausal discomforts.

**Enhanced bone mass:** The five Tibetans include a variety of weight-bearing exercises to strengthen the bones.

**Lymph system drainage:** As the five Tibetans compress and stretch the various organs, glands, and muscles, each exercise assists in draining the lymph system, flushing toxins out of the body.

**Sustained energy:** The rites stoke the inner fire in the third chakra and release energy throughout the day. For a restful night's sleep, be sure to practice the rites in the morning rather than the evening.

## The Five Tibetan Rites

It takes about 20 minutes to complete the full 21 repetitions of all the Tibetan rites. Beginners should start with 3 to 5 repetitions a day for the first week, increasing the number by 2 repetitions each week until reaching the 21 repetitions. Today, we'll practice 5 repetitions of each exercise.

*Rite 1: Spinning.* Stand in mountain pose with the arms outstretched, parallel to the floor. Slowly spin in a clockwise motion, keeping a consistent speed. (In the southern hemisphere, spin counterclockwise.) To prevent dizziness, try not to move your head; focus on a point on the wall or floor as you spin.

*Rite 2: Leg lifts.* Lie face up on your mat. Extend the arms along the sides of the body. Inhaling, raise your head and shoulders off the floor, tuck the chin to the chest, and simultaneously lift your legs, aiming the soles of the feet parallel to the sky. If possible, let the legs extend backward over your head *(photo a)*. Exhaling, slowly lower both the head and the legs to the ground.

*Rite 3: Camel.* Stand on your knees with your hands at your sides *(photo a)*. As you exhale, tuck the chin to the chest. Inhale, place the hands to the lower back, move the head and neck backward, arching the spine while pressing the public bone forward and up *(photo b)*.

*Rite 4: Table lift.* Sit on the floor with the legs straight out in front of you and feet about 12 inches (30 centimeters) apart. Place your hands on the floor alongside the hips, exhaling, tuck the chin into the chest. Inhaling, raise the torso, bending the knees into a reverse table, while lowering the head back, extending the neck. Tense every muscle in the body as you press up.

*Rite 5: Upward dog–downward dog.* Lie face down. Place your palms on the floor beneath the shoulders, and turn the toes under. Inhale, lifting into upward dog with the pelvis and the legs hovering over the ground *(photo a)*. Stay on the balls of your feet. Exhaling, bend the knees and lift the hips to downward dog; tuck the chin toward the chest, and stay high on the tiptoes *(photo b)*.

*Savasana.* Relax for 5 minutes.

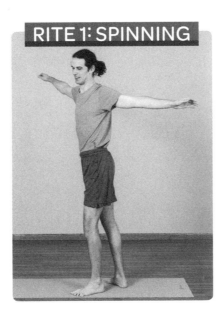

RITE 1: SPINNING

## RITE 2: LEG LIFT

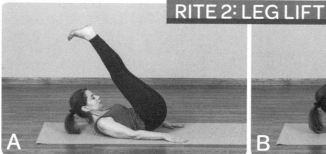

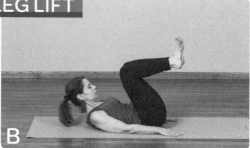

Leg lift (straight legs)

Leg lift variation

## RITE 3: CAMEL

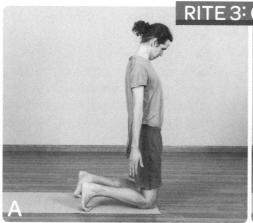

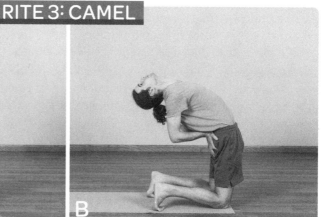

Head down

Head back

## RITE 4: TABLE LIFT

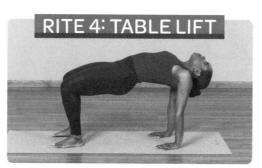

Lifted table

## RITE 5: UPWARD DOG–DOWNWARD DOG

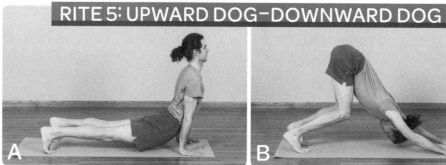

Downward dog on tiptoes

Upward dog with toes curled

## Teacher Tip

Guide students through several sun salutation warm-ups prior to introducing the five Tibetans.

# 11

# Mindfulness

*When you realize how perfect everything is you will tilt your head back and laugh at the sky.*

—Buddha

Have you ever driven somewhere and neglected the journey? You drove, but you didn't see the scenery. You may have missed out on other experiences because you didn't pay attention. When you assign mindfulness to daily activities like driving, brushing your teeth, or eating a bowl of cereal, the journey of life becomes a moving meditation.

The lessons that follow illustrate how to practice mindfulness by paying attention. Once you cultivate attention, you'll be amazed at how much life you've missed. As the saying goes, *Those who are awake live in a constant state of amazement.*

# VINYASA FOR AWAKENING

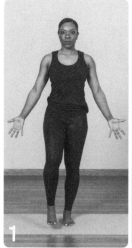

1 Stomp the feet

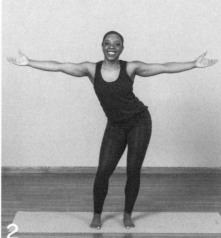

2 Hip circles

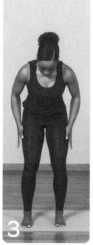

3 Slap the body

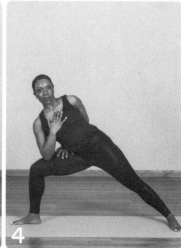

4 Side angle with half bind

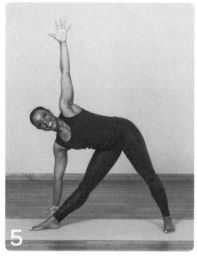

5 Triangle

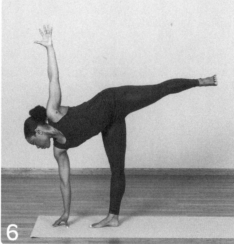

6 Half moon

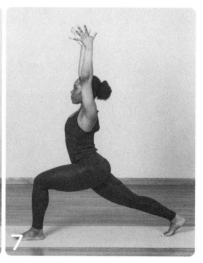

7 Crescent lunge

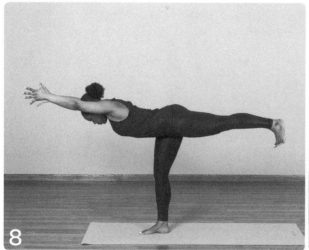

8 Warrior III

9 Squat

10 Mountain

# MINDFULNESS: THE CORE OF PRACTICE

## Intention

To integrate mindfulness into yoga practice.

## Lesson

It's said that to practice yoga, you don't have to be flexible or strong, you just have to be awake. Mindfulness, the awakened state, is at the core of yoga practice. It's what separates practicing asana from a choreographed stretch or movement. Mindfulness means fully experiencing what happens in the here and now. It's the art of becoming deeply aware of the present moment.

The opposite of multitasking, being mindful means doing or thinking about one thing at a time. Whether it's asana practice, meeting with co-workers, or playing golf, when you put your full attention into what you're doing, you are awake in that moment.

When you're mindful, you're not missing what's happening by engaging in the past or future. The purity of your focus is in charge; distractions stay on the periphery of the mind. Focus stays intact, and your immediate experience is fully realized.

The emotional benefits of mindfulness are boundless. Mindfulness helps to turn down the noise in your head and, with that, the feelings of anger or doubt, worries about tomorrow, and ruminating about the past. In yoga asana, mindfulness begins by feeling the pose come to life, sensing the response of the breath, and noticing the body's reaction as well as its boundaries.

Let's lie on the ground. Allow your mind to become absorbed in the sound of the breath; notice the sound of the inhalation and the exhalation. As if you're watching ocean waves, let your mind be drawn into the presence of the experience while the breath continues to move. The breath is always changing; no single breath is the same as the last. Partake in each breath, giving it your full attention.

## Asanas for Deepening

Practice the postures using an internal mantra or a phrase that has meaning to you. If you don't have a mantra, use an affirmation such as *I am strong* or *Patience is my practice*. Inhale and exhale the mantra. For instance, inhaling, think, *I am;* exhaling, think, *strong*.

- *Sun salutation with side plank.* When flowing through postures, stay mindful of the action of muscular energy. Like a full-body stocking, hug the muscle to the bone, and draw your energy toward the midline of the body. Feel the experience in every breath, joint, and thought.

- *Wild thing.* From downward dog split, bend the top knee (photo *a*) and flip the dog, landing the top foot parallel to the standing foot (photo *b*). Let the head delicately drop, and gaze past the fingertips. Enjoy the topsy-turvy adventure!

- *King dancer.* Breathe smoothly, bringing the pose to life. Don't waver from your drishti (the focus point for your gaze). Accept where you are in this moment without striving, comparing, or judging.

- *Reclining leg cradles.* When you're at your edge and can't pull the leg in any tighter, stay where you are. Maintain the action of the pose while breathing into the intensity of the stretch. Close your eyes, and sense the profound openings around the hip, low back, and buttocks.

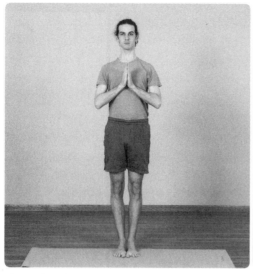

Sun salutation

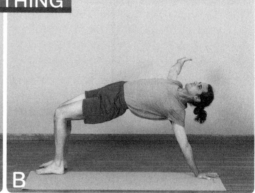

Side plank

## WILD THING

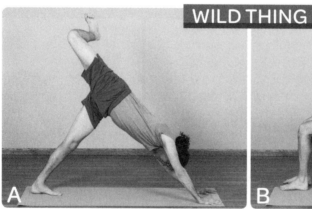

**A** Downward dog split with lifted knee

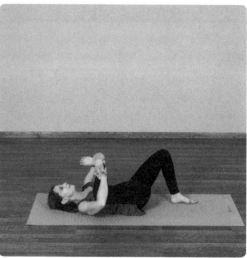

**B** Flipping the dog

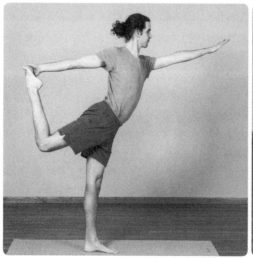

King dancer

Reclining leg cradles

## Motivation Off the Mat

Exercise mindfulness during the routine tasks of your day, such as brushing your teeth, working on your computer, or hugging a loved one.

○ *One-step meditation.* When you're unfocused or too busy to concentrate, try the one-step walking meditation. Walk slowly, taking one step at a time. Use the mantra *One step.* Each time you take a forward step, mentally say and think, *One.* As the opposite foot comes forward, mentally say and think, *step.* Take in everything that's happening at that moment—the feet touching the ground, the knee joints bending, and your weight shifting from left to right. Mindfulness, like all things of merit, can be accomplished one step at a time.

○ *Mindfulness of breath.* Count each set of inhalations and exhalations as 1 until you reach 10. The objective is not to get to 10, instead monitor how quickly the mind becomes impatient as it rambles into the past and the future.

## WISE WORDS

Practice mindfulness to encourage "one day at a time" philosophy.

Yoga is the method that calms the mind so targeted energy can be directed into constructive channels.

Be mindful because this moment will pass. If you're somewhere else, you've missed it.

*The foot feels the foot when it feels the ground.*

—Buddha

# PAYING ATTENTION

## Intention

To learn neutrality of the mind and take a step toward meditation.

## Lesson

Yoga philosophy tells us the world is exactly as it's supposed to be; that everything that's happening in the world right now, personally and globally, is what is meant to occur.

When you look at life this way, with all the elements that are out of your control, on top of all your personal challenges and messy moments, spiritual questions begin to arise. In the yogic tradition, these questions can be answered through clear thinking.

Asana neatly conveys the importance of the now—being in the moment, feeling the present, whether you're sad or anxious or happy or tired. This is the way you naturally become aware of chitta vritti, the fluctuations of the mind. In this lesson, we'll learn to focus first on the gross aspects of the body and then on the more discriminating components of prana and our ability to control it.

Gradually you'll begin to develop the mind's capacity to focus on one thing; this is called dharana, the concentration required to meditate. From here, the mind instinctively flows into dhyana, meditation. Today, our intention is to practice training the mind to pay attention, awakening our inner and outer worlds.

## Asanas for Deepening

Work with the internal mantra *Breathing, grounding, lengthening*. Exhale, breathing and grounding down to the toes. Inhale, breathing up to the crown of the head, lengthening, and sensing the breath move through you.

- *Inverted table*. Observe the hands and feet strongly reaching down, the spine lengthening in both directions, and shoulders opening and moving away from each other.
- *Fish*. Blissfully lift the heart throughout the pose. Fill the lungs with a gratifying breath as the spine soars into the back.
- *Lotus*. Free the weight of the body into the earth, awakening the crown toward the sky. Step away from the thinking process and watch what unfolds.
- *Crescent lunge with raised front heel*. Once you're stable in crescent lunge, lift the front heel, supporting the weight of the front leg on the ball of the foot. Enjoy using a new set of muscles in this pose.

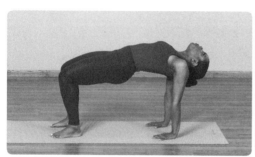

Inverted table

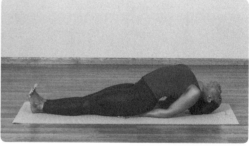

Fish

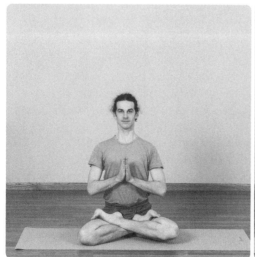

Lotus

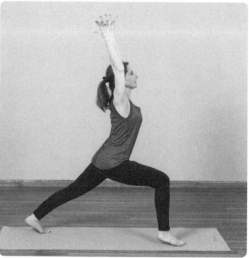

Crescent lunge with raised front heel

## Motivation Off the Mat

Sit with the eyes closed. Focus your attention on your breath, a mantra, or a visual focal point such as a candle or deity. After a few minutes, take stock of your inner world. What's happening? Do you notice a pain in your back? Do you hear your breath? Do you feel your heart beating? Are you thirsty? Listen. Where does the mind go? Witness these thoughts and sensations without changing or judging them. Sit for several minutes. How long are you able to sit in mindfulness before your thoughts cloud the open spaces of consciousness? The idea is to step back from your thoughts and be the observer.

## WISE WORDS

Guard your available prana. People squander loads of mental energy by unknowingly drifting to random thoughts.

Only through continuous and vigilant practice can you develop the objectivity of the mind.

# DHARANA

## Intention

To apply concentration to asana.

## Lesson

Dharana (complete concentration) is the sixth limb of raja yoga. The objective of dharana is to hold focus in one direction, like a mantra or the breath, in order to stop the mind from rambling. When you practice dharana, you're highlighting one particular activity of the mind. The brighter the activity becomes, the clearer the mind.

During asana, the attention to internal body adjustments automatically brings one-pointed awareness to the muscles, joints, and organs, turning the mind's focus to the sensation of the present moment. When you consciously drop the shoulders, the mind becomes present. When the mind wanders, the shoulders rise.

Our class today will focus on the practice of dharana in every asana as we integrate the synergies of lifeforce within the body.

## Asanas for Deepening

○ *Eagle.* Bring the focal point to the thumb. Keep the hips steady, as if the integrity of the pose depends on it.

○ *Candle.* Squat with the hands in steeple position over the head. Release any exertion or tension, especially in the legs and feet. Flow with what happens, and focus the mind on the support of the toes.

○ *Seated angle.* Adjust for subtle areas of strain, using the breath to soften and relax while moving toward deep concentration.

○ *Hero.* Reclining hero *(photo a)* and seated hero *(photo b)* cultivate stillness and inner stability. Inhaling, draw the breath up through the front of the spine. Exhaling, feel the pelvic bones spread toward the earth.

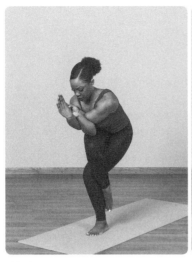

Eagle

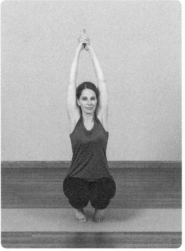

Candle

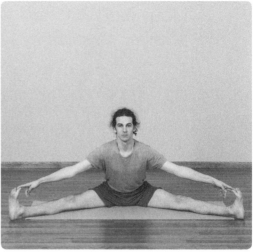

Seated angle

**HERO**

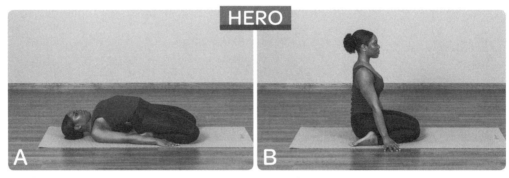

A

Reclining

B

Seated

## Motivation Off the Mat

If you want to live an awakened life, break the patterns of fear that cause you to avoid discomfort or unpleasantness.

To practice dharana, become aware of the breath. Place your attention on your abdomen, and let it rest lightly on the diaphragm muscle. Once you can feel the breath, let it move through you, with your inner eye watching it expand and contract. Stay with each breath; breathing out, breathing in. When the mind wanders off the path, send it back and begin again. Your only objective is to surrender to the movement of the breath. Let it come, let it go. Notice each inhalation, each exhalation, moving on through to the next one, and the one after that.

Practice this exercise daily, while working at your computer, sitting in a waiting room, attending to your family, or virtually anywhere, and you'll encounter the beauty of santosha (contentment).

## WISE WORDS

When the mind is purified by yoga practices, inner healing naturally occurs.

The moment you start to force, you begin to lose awareness of the nervous system and the present moment.

Every physical adjustment in asana tells the mind, "Be here, not somewhere else."

# MINDFULNESS OF GRATITUDE

## Intention

To live in a state of gratitude.

## Lesson

A gratitude practice can be extraordinarily beneficial for people with mild depression or those carrying feelings of anger or doubt about how their lives have unfolded. Some choose a melancholy existence because they don't know any other way. For them, it's easy to go to a negative state of being because it's a familiar place.

Our asana class brings the miracle of the body to the forefront of the practice. Let's not forget that it's important to be grateful for having a body and a brain to boot!

When you make asana a daily ritual, a natural antidepressant kicks in. With mindful breathing, anxiety levels decrease, endorphins are released, and the mood lifts. The more you practice, the deeper you relax. Quieting the mind while generating a strong connection to the heart adds regenerative energy and an attitude of gratitude to your entire system. Gratitude practice is a buffer against recurring stress or anxiety.

Today we begin our practice with the gratitude of heart breath. This is like an adjustment for your feelings; when you focus on positive, loving emotions such as gratitude and appreciation, your heart rhythms shift. In addition, blood pressure normalizes, stress hormones drop, and the immune system gets stronger. During difficult times, the gratitude of heart breath provides comfort, easing depression and anxiety.

First, close the eyes and let the body relax. The gratitude of heart breath asks you to energetically send out appreciation to your loved ones, producing a cascade of biochemical events that nourish the body and mind. Shift from the outside world to the inside world, bringing your attention to the area around your heart center in the mid-chest. Put your right hand on your heart, and envision your breath moving in and out through the heart center. Take slow, intentional, deep breaths.

Now imagine something or someone that you appreciate, such as your children, friends, parents, partner, the divine, or a pet. Send them genuine gratitude and love as you breathe through your heart. See them in your mind's eye. Feel the emotion, not just the thought. [Pause for several minutes.]

After you've finished the gratitude of heart breath, hold on to those qualities of appreciation and love for the remainder of your practice.

## Asanas for Deepening

- *Reclined butterfly.* This pose opens the chest, quiets the mind, and helps relieve anxiety and stress in the hips, groin, and lower back. Rest in the pose for 2 to 3 minutes, propping the knees with blocks or blankets.
- *Rabbit.* Succumb to an attitude of admiration for your life just as it is.
- *Cobra.* Elevate the spine, lengthen the collarbones outward, and pour the chest into the heart center. Notice the prana concentrated in the front and back of the heart. Breathe with compassion and gratitude for this sacred center.
- *Wheel or bridge.* Let the circulation go into full spin, stimulating the nervous system while generating a feeling of well-being, counteracting depression.
- *Tripod variation.* Snuggle one knee behind the opposite knee. Enjoy this moment, marveling at the wonder of your amazing body.
- *Child's pose.* As you take the shape of the child, pause in reverence for the blessings in your life.

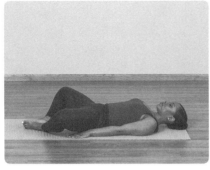
Reclining butterfly

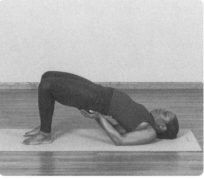
Rabbit

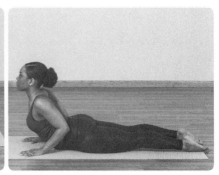
Cobra

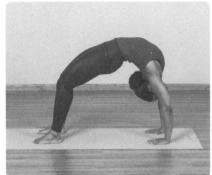
Wheel

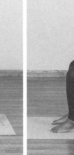
Bridge with hands supporting the low back

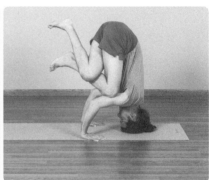
Tripod variation

## Motivation Off the Mat

Every evening at bedtime, take time for reflection. Write down five things you're grateful for on that day. Feel free to include the obvious, such as your health, family, or job, but the entries can be as simple (and just as important) as having running water, clean clothes, or the ability to see the beauty of a rosebud. Within a week, your daily gratitude status will heighten, your role in life will be more realistic, and your anxiety level will decrease. Perspective is powerful medicine.

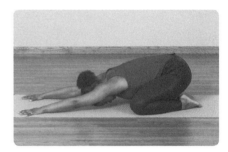
Child's pose

For an entire day, be the messenger of good news. Every time you speak, let it be of something pleasant or uplifting, and make a conscious effort to notice and acknowledge what's good about the day. Next time, try it for 2 days!

## WISE WORDS

Living in appreciation makes every day better.

May you be awake to the gifts you receive and give.

## Teacher Tip

At the end of class, ask your students to say a silent thank you to the other yogis in the room. Then, aloud, say, "Thank you for joining me today to share your practice."

# HOLIDAY GRATITUDE

## Intention

To feel the gratitude of another year of life on Earth with your loved ones.

## Lesson

[This lesson is recommended for use during Thanksgiving through the New Year classes.] At this time of year we're taught to count our blessings and be grateful for what we have. Having gratitude is a choice. When we choose gratitude, we choose to focus on the things that are going well in our lives as opposed to the things that aren't. To practice gratitude in yoga class, we focus on things our body *can* do, not what it can't. With mindfulness of gratitude, we see our entire existence—our bodies, our family, our ability to gather together year after year, as a miracle, rather than simply as the passing of time.

The practice of gratitude is empowering, and it can change the way you perceive life.

Let's come into a comfortable seated position. Close the eyes, bring the hands to prayer, and gently attend to the heart center. Focus on the rise and fall of the chest as you breathe in and out. Think about the people and things in your life that fill you with happiness and joy, and whatever you feel grateful for. As you focus on these things, you may begin to feel warm, calm, and content. Next, send these healing energies to a loved one who needs them today. [Pause for several minutes.]

You are now in a state of gratitude.

## Asanas for Deepening

Be grateful that you're able to come to yoga class to move and appreciate the miracles of the body. With gratitude, you can practice any posture with compassion and wisdom.

- *Child's pose.* This calming, steadying pose brings you into submission to the present, grounding you in ease and appreciation.
- *Resting pigeon.* Indulge the internal organs with a natural massage. Give thanks to your strong diaphragm muscle that helps you breathe. With the forehead on the ground, the senses take a rest, the mind turns to calm, and the back of the heart softens. [To comfort your students, offer them a gentle adjustment on the lower back to ease any tension they may be holding in the hips or thighs.]
- *Horse.* From a kneeling position, bring one heel to the opposite hip and place the arms in eagle position. Both satisfying and humbling, horse pose highlights the bountiful inner structure of the skeletal system.
- *Happy baby.* Come into happy baby and rejoice in the playfulness of the stretch.

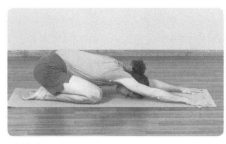

Child's pose

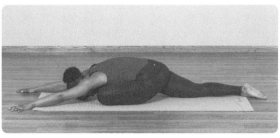

Resting pigeon

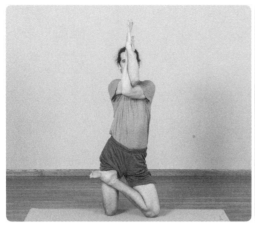

Horse

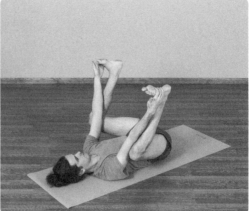

Happy baby

## Motivation Off the Mat

Strengthen your spirit all year long by being mindful of the blessings of your daily life and of your loved ones.

At family gatherings such as holiday dinners, find a poem or prayer that offers a message of love. While many families gather just to eat and return to their homes, your prayer will change the memory of the holiday dinner by planting the seeds of love and gratitude.

If you have children, remind them (and yourself) to be grateful for food, clothing, shelter, and love.

Never take anything or anyone for granted, for life can change in an instant. Things that we have today may not be here tomorrow.

After spending time with a good friend, send them a text or email letting them know how important they are to you.

Don't forget birthdays, including your own. Everyone gets one day a year to celebrate the day they came into this world. Celebrate yours with joy and enthusiasm by throwing yourself a party!

## WISE WORDS

Yoga practices are spiritual catalysts that put us in touch with our dharma (life purpose).

A quiet mind gains access to inner wisdom. Listen to know what feels most useful, fulfilling, and complete in your life.

Celebrate the ordinary.

# MINDFUL EATING

## Intention

To experience the awareness and gratitude of eating.

## Lesson

Have you ever had a full meal but only tasted the first bite because your mind was somewhere else? Mindlessness can disrupt our connection between the mind and the mouth.

Healthy eating requires a thoughtful, loving approach because the foods we eat sustain life. When you eat calmly, with full awareness and gratitude, you're feeding the mind and spirit as well as the body. A healthy body becomes more sensitive to *what* you eat and *how* you eat. This new perspective will help you make better food choices.

From the yogic view, food has properties that influence the physical, emotional, and spiritual life. Stale, processed, or overripe foods have lost their prana, and ingesting them can lead to a dull or lethargic state. Foods with a high concentration of sugar or caffeine overstimulate the nervous and hormonal systems, and counteract the balancing effects of your asana practice.

But foods that originate as close to the earth as possible, like fresh vegetables, whole grains, and fruits, are neither depressing nor stimulating. Like your asana and pranayama practices, they nourish and energize you, bringing balance and harmony to your body, mind, and spirit.

It's also important to pay attention to *how much* you eat. The yogi practices Brahmacharya (moderation) and never comes to a point of complete satiation. Instead of cramming the belly full of food and drink, try to fill yourself to only three-fourths full at each meal, leaving space for healthy digestion.

Enjoy your relationship to food. If you devote yourself to the pleasure and appreciation of the food itself and its source, you'll find what truly nourishes you, and you'll no longer want what doesn't.

## Asanas for Deepening

Focus on asanas that help food assimilate, digest, and eventually move through the system.

- *Reclining easy pose.* Relax and let the pose soothe heartburn and improve digestion by increasing blood supply to the intestines.
- *Belly massage.* The belly massage is excellent for improving digestion and elimination problems, including constipation. Lie on your back, and rub your hands together until they feel hot. Place one hand flat on the navel. Next, using the fingertips and applying firm pressure, rub the belly in small clockwise circles around the navel, gradually widening the circles. Focus on the heat building in the navel center as you massage.
- *Bound seated twist.* The twist massages and tones the internal organs, and maintains space and mobility in the spine.
- *Shoulderstand or inverted action pose.* The change in the body's relationship to gravity from turning upside down helps relieve constipation and indigestion.

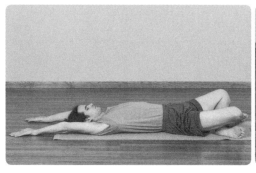
Reclining easy pose

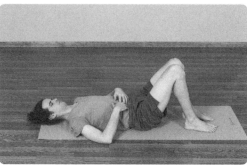
Belly massage

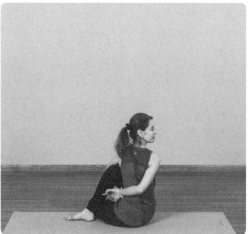
Bound seated twist

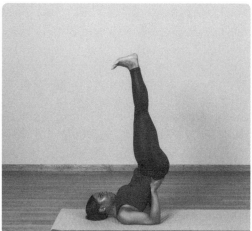
Shoulderstand/inverted action pose

## Motivation Off the Mat

Enjoy a mindful meal by eating a small piece of food, such as a bite of a sandwich, as slowly as possible. Relish the touch and taste of each morsel as you delight in the sensation of the food in your mouth.

Eat by yourself without distractions from your phone, other people, or reading material. Simply sit, just you and your food, being attentive to the nourishment your body is receiving.

If you want to give your friends a meal they'll never forget, invite them over for a silent dinner. Eliminate all distractions such as music, television, and phones. The meal can get even more interesting if you serve crunchy foods, like celery or hard-shell tacos, and slurpy foods, like stews and soups. If your friends are game for a more mindful adventure, next time, try eating in the dark!

Just for fun, place your eating utensil in your non-dominant hand while you eat your meal.

## WISE WORDS

Before eating, take a moment to quietly give thanks, reflecting on the source of your food and its purpose in your life.

Is your food nourishing you? Is it stimulating, filling, or does it make you sleepy? Are you aware when you're full, or do you overeat until you're stuffed? Practicing mindfulness in asana helps you recognize when you overeat, teaching you the sensation of fullness.

# 12

# Lessons of the Heart Center

*Teach this triple truth to all: A generous heart, kind speech, and a life of service and compassion are the things that renew humanity.*

—Buddha

The heart is the temple of the soul, holding the secret to self-knowledge. Unlike the brain, the heart, the center of love, doesn't need words to express itself; it speaks in sensation, feeling, and emotion.

The transformational powers of love ignited by yoga practice extend beyond yourself, and they grace the universe with compassion and kindness.

## Teacher Tip

*Create Connection.* Introduce your students to each other. Remember their names and at the end of every class, thank them for joining you on the yoga journey.

*Teach with a Full Heart.* We never know what someone else's story is, or what difficulty they're bringing to the mat. Practice unconditional compassion, especially for difficult students.

# HEART CENTER VINYASA

1. Thread the needle
2. Cat–cow
3. Downward dog
4. Downward dog split with hip rotation
5. Plank
6. Side plank flip
7. Downward dog

8. Plank
9. Unsupported cobra with hands interlaced at the back
10. Downward dog
11. Camel
12. Child's pose

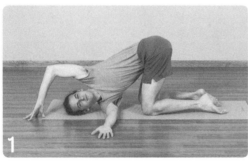

Thread the needle

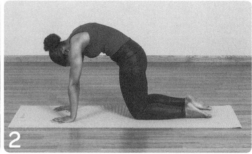

Cat-cow

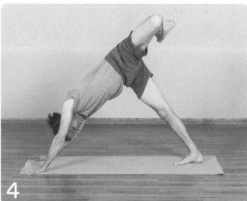

Downward dog

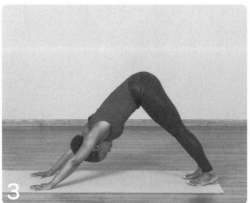

Downward dog split with hip rotation

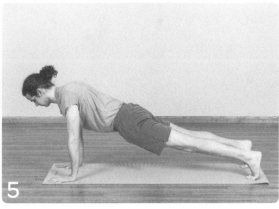

5

Plank

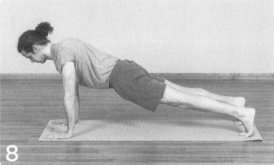

6

Side plank flip

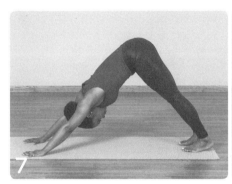

7

Downward dog

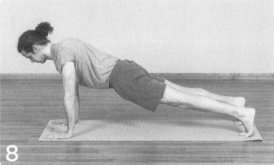

8

Plank

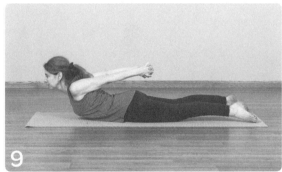

9

Unsupported cobra with hands interlaced

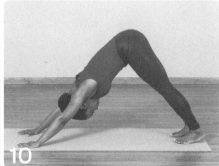

10

Downward dog

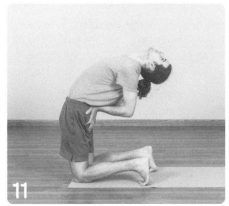

11

Camel

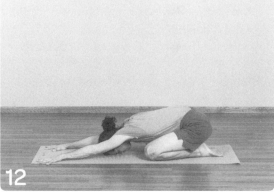

12

Child's pose

# ANJALI MUDRA: NAMASTE

## Intention

To learn the namaste salutation.

## Lesson

Most yoga classes end with the teacher and students bringing their hands together and bowing to one another while saying the word *namaste*, which translates to "The light in me bows to the light in you." Namaste is a greeting in many cultures and the nucleus of our practice, highlighting the internal light within all of creation. The hand position used in the greeting is called *anjali* mudra.

The word anjali stems from the Sanskrit root *anj*, meaning "to honor" or "to celebrate." The word *mudra* means "seal." The prayer hand gesture is used in many asanas, such as tadasana (mountain pose) at the beginning and end of sun salutations, in warrior I, and in balance poses such as tree.

Bringing your hands together at the heart connects the right and left hemispheres of the brain, linking the active and receptive natures, right and left sides, masculine and feminine energies, logic and intuition, and the strengths and weaknesses of our dual nature. Yoga philosophers have stated that the right hand represents the higher Self (the divine), while the left hand represents the lower, worldly nature of self.

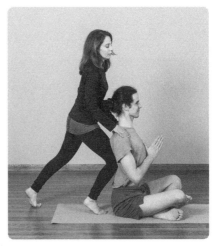

Seated heart lift with teacher adjustment

Let's begin in easy pose. Lengthen the spine out of the pelvis, broaden the shoulder blades, and on the inhalation, spread your chest open. Lift upward through the crown of your head, extending the back of your neck by dropping your chin slightly. Be aware of energy rising up from your tailbone as you follow your breath to the crown. Inhaling, reach farther. Feel the space between the ribs broaden, and listen to your breath until there's nothing left to inhale; then exhale until there is no breath left to exhale. On the next inhalation, cross your legs the opposite way.

Now, with open palms, lift the arms out to the sides, extending your heart center; your heart and hands are connected. Slowly draw your hands together at the center of your chest, observing both sides of your nature converge at the heart center.

## Asanas for Deepening

Anjali mudra can be included within many asanas as a way to come back to center. As you bring your hands together, the mudra is a reminder to ground your intentions within your heart.

- *Sun salutation with twist.* (Refer to chapter 4, Sun Salutation. Substitute high lunge twist for lunge.) Practice anjali mudra in mountain pose at the beginning and end of the salutation, and during the high lunge twist.

- *Warrior I.* Join the hands together over the head.
- *Tree.* Merge with the earth's energy through an upward flow into the heart and above.
- *Side angle.* Connect the shoulder blade (known as the wing of the heart) to the inside of the bent knee, placing the hands in anjali mudra.
- *Fish.* Rejoice in the spiritual interface between the pelvic center and the heart center.

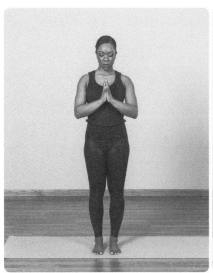

Sun salutation

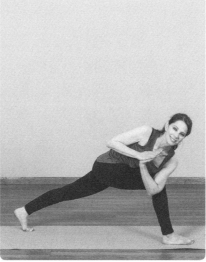

High lunge twist

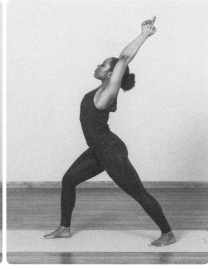

Warrior I

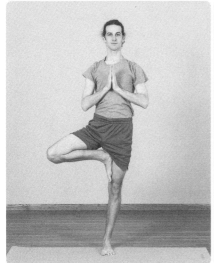

Tree

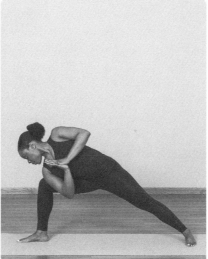

Side angle

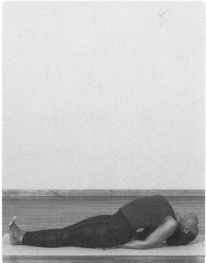

Fish

## Motivation Off the Mat

Anjali mudra is a gesture of composure that eases the symptoms of stress. It's also used as a greeting, communicating heartfelt energy and respect.

## WISE WORDS

In the yoga tradition, the energetic heart is illuminated as a lotus at the center of the chest. Anjali mudra acknowledges the lotus heart, directing it to open to the light. It balances and harmonizes your energies, keeping you centered, clear, and positive.

## Teacher Tip

When you greet your students, say, "Namaste" with hands in anjali mudra. As you bow and show respect for the light and love within, this salutation represents the equality of all your students.

# SEEDS OF LOVE

## Intention

To cultivate the seeds of love.

## Lesson

By practicing asana, we organically tap into the physical attributes of the heart center and surrounding anatomy. As our journey progresses, the subtle energies of the spiritual heart begin to emerge. Just as one drop can send ripples through an entire body of water, the seeds of love can create a sacred surge of emotion felt by the collective consciousness.

Let's put our hands in anjali mudra. Breathe into the heart, and visualize the seeds of your love spreading out into your world—to your family, friends, neighbors, coworkers, teachers, doctors, soldiers, and anyone else who needs it. Now lower your hands to your lap with palms up, and let your fingers curl naturally, resembling the bud of a lotus flower. Using your heart–mind connection, plant a love-seed prayer or affirmation, such as *Peace, Compassion,* or *Good health,* within your anjali mudra flower. Drop your chin, and visualize the manifestation of your prayer. Let's begin our asana practice with a newly awakened sense of humility and respect for the powers of love within us.

## Asanas for Deepening

- ○ *Standing forward bend with big-toe hold.* Surrender to your love of the Earth.
- ○ *Downward dog.* Drop the head below the heart.
- ○ *Tabletop twist.* Reach the heart center to the sky.
- ○ *Half-lotus bound twist.* Squeeze the heart to release the seeds of love.
- ○ *Crown bridge.* Interlace the hands behind the neck and lift the heart from beyond the rib cage while moving the crown of the head toward the floor.
- ○ *Side bow.* Roll from bow to side bow, leading with one side of the heart, then the other.

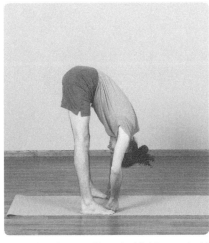

Standing forward bend with big-toe hold

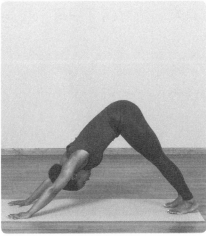

Downward dog

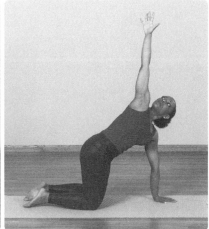

Tabletop twist

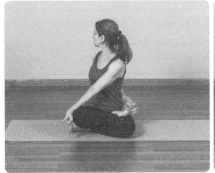

Half-lotus bound twist

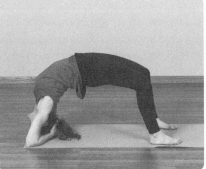

Crown bridge

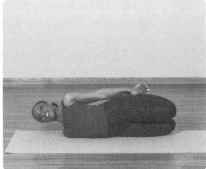

Side bow

## Motivation Off the Mat

Send a note of appreciation to a member of your staff or a coworker for a job well done.

Look into the eyes of each person you talk to. Radiate compassion and love through your energy, voice, and smile. Does the conversation take a different turn?

Plant flower seeds. When they bloom, pick some and give a bouquet to someone you love.

Love your trash. Each time you take out your garbage, give thanks for the goods, services, and blessings you've received from each item before it became trash.

## WISE WORDS

The vibrations of love get smoother and steadier as we become more in touch with the heart.

Lead by example; embody the energy you want to receive.

Living in a state of appreciation turns an ordinary day into a blessing.

# EXPANDING THE HEART

## Intention

To honor the wisdom of the heart center.

## Lesson

We are what we think; and because energy follows each thought, what we think will grow. Optimism grows positive thoughts.; pessimism grows negative thoughts.

You can shift your heart rhythms by directing your thoughts to practical and loving emotions. This shift induces a series of physiological events that assist the whole body. Blood pressure normalizes, stress hormones drop, and the immune system gets a boost. Even anti-aging hormones stabilize, suggesting that negative thinking (such as worry) has an influence on how we age.

To fully experience the yoga journey, asana practice requires awareness of an open heart. Let's begin our heart awareness practice by expanding compassion to everyone in your life with an exercise that opens the delicate passages of the heart chakra.

Close your eyes. Place your right hand over your heart and your left hand below your navel. Spreading your fingers, breathe into your left hand and let the right hand feel the warmth arising from your heart. Visualize your breath moving into and through an emerald-green heart chakra. Now focus on someone you're grateful for, as well as the many good things you have in your life. Send them love, appreciation, and happiness as you breathe through your heart.

Now, sense a white light filled with the vital energy of peace and love entering through the crown of your head, gathering in the heart center. Explore the emotion of love with benevolence and kindness arising as you begin your asana practice. Take a deep breath; on an exhalation, let's chant *Om mani padme hum,* which means "The wisdom of the jewel of the lotus resides in my heart," 3 times.

## Asanas for Deepening

Focus your intentions on expanding the wisdom of the sacred heart, connecting with the loving spirit that resides within you.

○ *King dancer.*  ○ *Wall bridge.*

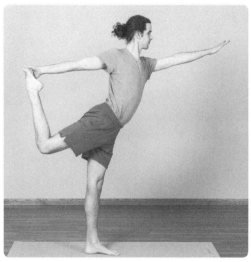 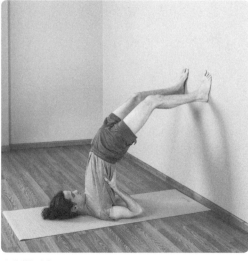

King dancer

Wall bridge

○ *Plank to lunge.*
○ *Plank to wild thing.*

○ *Shoulderstand lotus.*
○ *Gate.*

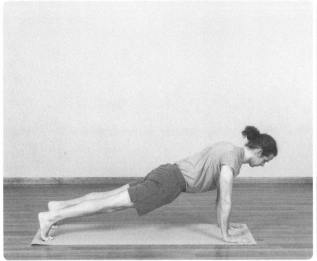

Plank

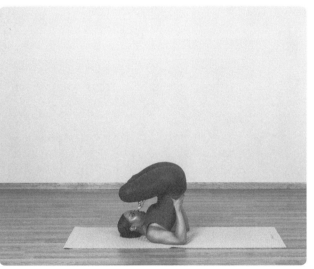 — Lunge

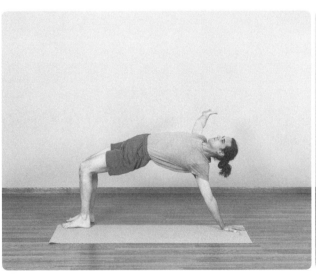

Wild thing

Shoulderstand lotus

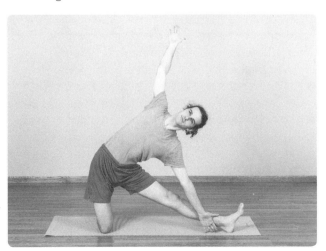

Gate

## Motivation Off the Mat

Today's experiences set the groundwork for future healing. Release negative emotions as you speak, act, and think, and experience the positive, free-flowing love, light, and laughter flourishing within.

Do one loving gesture today that your future self will thank you for later.

## WISE WORDS

Remember the opportunities that are born of love.

When you practice asana, focus on "thinking" through your heart center instead of through the brain's anatomical-alignment instructions. Recognize how that mind-set changes the flow of prana.

# REVERSING NEGATIVE EMOTIONS

## Intention

To reverse negative emotions.

## Lesson

Welcoming the energy of negative emotions, including the old stories that may be at their root, is the opposite of what we usually do: we avoid them. But sitting and staying present with these uncomfortable feelings can lead us to a new place of spaciousness and growth.

When you quiet the mind while sustaining a solid connection with the power of the heart, you can reverse the stress effects of negative emotions. During times of anxiety and crisis, breathe through the heart with the intention of easing your sadness, tension, and fear.

Take a moment now to listen to your thoughts. When you get close and observe your dark emotions without getting caught in your reactions to them, they lose their power over you.

Close your eyes, and bring the feeling of a bad experience into your heart. Hold it there, and identify how you're feeling. For example, you might be thinking, *I'm angry* or *This situation makes me anxious* or *I'm not good enough*. Focus on your breathing as it moves in and out through your nostrils, then turn your thoughts to your heart rate. Do you feel your heart beating faster? Concentrate on your heart center, and visualize it expanding until you have the sensation that you're holding actual space between your heart and the negative feelings. Now, notice what's happening. The emotional activity shifts. Your sadness or anger begins to soften. Stay present to the space, color, and texture of the feeling.

As we sit with our toxic emotions, we learn to shift our perspective on them. Our intention is to explore the energy of these feelings and observe how much power we decide to give them.

And now, through asana, let's work the physical sensations of these dark emotions out of the body.

## Asanas for Deepening

○ *Downward dog at the wall.* Press the heels of the hands into the wall extending the area between the shoulder blades. Breathe and let go of trapped emotions in the backdoor of the heart.

○ *Downward dog in half lotus.* The downward inversion, coupled with the hip opening of the half lotus, acts as an elixir for negative emotions.

○ *Pyramid with cow face arms.* Add the powerful shoulder opener of the cow face to your forward fold.

○ *Standing backbend at the wall.* Standing with your back to the wall, reach the arms overhead and walk the hands down the wall toward the floor behind you.

○ *Reclining hero.* Lean back bringing your head to the ground. If you experience pain in the knees or ankles, do not lean all the way back.

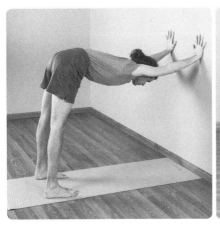
Downward dog at the wall

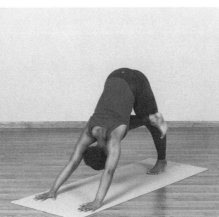
Downward dog in half lotus

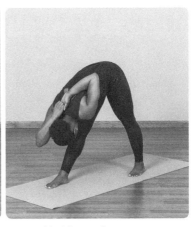
Pyramid with cow face arms

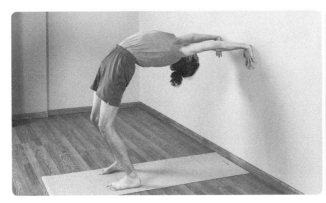
Standing backbend at the wall

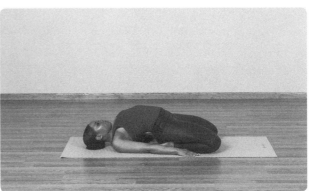
Reclining hero

## Pranayama for Anxiety

The anuloma krama breath (see chapter 6) expands the chest and deepens the inhalation. An ideal practice for replacing the energy that's snatched by sadness and regret, anoloma krama builds confidence and inner strength.

## Motivation Off the Mat

Let self-compassion be your constant companion, especially while you're going through a healing process.

Practice daily self-kindness to reduce nervous system overload.

Don't close your heart in an effort to protect it; meditate on the heart chakra, where fear can get trapped. Imagine that you're holding the key, and unlock the gate of the heart.

## WISE WORDS

Asana puts your body in a position to explore and change your consciousness.

Pay it forward; give in proportion to what you receive.

Choose forgiveness, not because someone else deserves it, but because you deserve peace.

When you harbor bitterness, the only person you hurt is yourself.

*Holding on to anger is like grasping a hot coal with the intent of throwing it at someone else; you get burned.*

—Buddha

## Teacher Tip

Before class begins, hold space for yourself to release surface worries, hostility, guilt, and other unwanted emotions. This pre-class cleansing primes your spirit and enables you to teach from a place of compassion.

# SELF-LOVE

## Intention

Learning to love yourself.

*No one is more deserving of your love than you.*

—Buddha

One of the most substantial outcomes of practicing yoga is learning to love yourself. That's why the self-love lesson is a favorite lesson of mine; it's a class for people who thoughtlessly practice self-sabotage or believe they're not worthy of love.

Focus your class on the awareness of self-judgment, insecurity, and self-deprecation. Begin by asking your students to name three things they love about themselves. The answers (or lack thereof) will quickly determine one's own barometer of self-love.

Self-love yoga classes are frequently charged with emotional curveballs and deep spiritual cleansing. Don't be surprised if you contribute to your students' release of buried emotions; these classes can incite crying, laughing, and lots of sighing.

## Uncovering the Obstacles to Self-Love

The heart chakra is guided by sensation, feeling, and emotion. When we live with fear, depression, or worry, the body contracts in an effort to protect and defend itself. The physical practice for the heart involves stretching its supporting anatomy to give the chest some breathing room. Teach your students to activate their layers of physical heart consciousness by helping them uncover the obstacles to self-love, while releasing blocked or flooded emotions with the following meditation.

# Lesson

## Open-Heart Meditation

Take a comfortable seated position, settling into the weight of your bones and relaxing the jaw, tongue, and throat. Gradually bring your awareness into the cave of your heart. Observe the outside surface of your heart, the side that faces outward toward the world. Think of any events within the last several days that have had an impact on your emotional state.

Next, bring awareness to your inner heart, feeling how these events affect your breathing, heart rate, and energy body. Observe the impression of pain, pleasure, body temperature, and circulation. Note any dark sensations such as humiliation, anger, panic, embarrassment, or guilt. Be patient with yourself while practicing nonjudgmental awareness.

Finally, bring mindfulness to the entire surface of the heart. Feel the space and lightness in your chest. Meditate on a glorious emerald green field inside the heart chakra, where the only thought that exists is love and appreciation for yourself.

## Opening To Self-Love Vinyasa

Guide your students to broaden the shoulders, open the chest, and lift the sternum, reciting the following silent affirmation: *I love myself exactly as I am, right here, right now.*

1. Easy pose with anjali mudra.
2. Easy pose twist.
3. Chest expansion. Kneeling, interlace the hands behind the back, squeezing the elbows and shoulder blades together. Open the collarbones, and lift the heart.
4. Rabbit pose. Bow forward, bringing the forehead to the ground and arms overhead.
5. Downward dog with knee lifted to the side–upward dog. Repeat the movement, alternating the knee, 4 to 6 times.
6. Breathing bridge. Inhaling, reach the arms over the head lifting up to bridge; exhaling, lower the arms to your sides and back to the ground. Repeat the movement 3 to 5 times.
7. Child's pose. Send the breath into the back doors (shoulder wings) of the heart.
8. Easy pose with hug. Give yourself a big, long, loving hug.

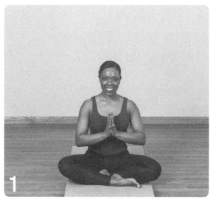

Easy pose with anjali mudra

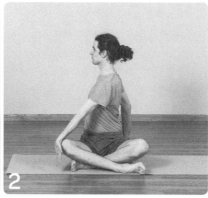

Easy pose twist

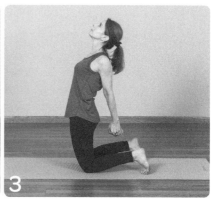

Chest expansion

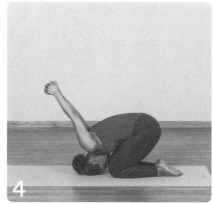

Rabbit

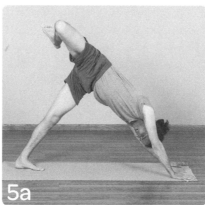

Downward dog with knee lifted

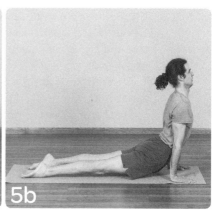

Upward dog

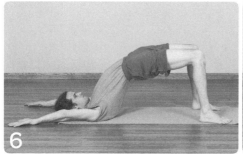

Breathing bridge

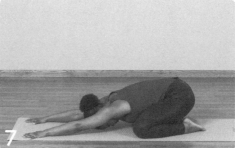

Child's pose

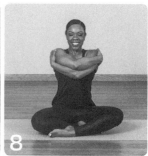

Easy pose with hug

## Teacher Tip

The practice of self-love is an ongoing process. Avoid negative self-talk or making fun of yourself during class.

# CHAPTER 13

# Emotions

*What we think, we become.*

—Buddha

Yoga asana is a position that is both steady and comfortable, a place where you feel completely present. Asana offers a perfect view of the agitated mind, where practice becomes a purifying experience of listening to the inner workings of your thoughts and emotions. Through yoga's colossal awakening response, you evolve, becoming more sensitized, perceptive, and responsive both on and off the mat.

The lessons in this chapter are created to help you recognize the emotions that arise during practice. There's no place for judgment here. Just look, listen, and be aware.

Pay attention.

# EMOTIONAL EFFECTS OF ASANA

## Intention

To bring emotions into harmony.

## Lesson

Have you noticed the effect that yoga practice has on your emotions? It can feel like a welcome sense of spaciousness, as though you've cleaned the room inside of yourself, drawing light and healing to shine through you.

As you consume the practice and let go of frustration, fear, and worry, you start to feel freedom; positive emotions are rekindled through your sense of humor, patience, and a calm mind.

But there's a yin–yang relationship to everything in life, especially within our ever-changing emotions. If we're cleansing and releasing, feeling unwanted emotions is paramount to the process of renewal. When this happens, recognize and name those emotions for what they are—negative sensations rising to the surface. Instead of suppressing them, acknowledge that these feelings arose for a purpose. Stay mindful, observe them, and give yourself time to process these emotions; eventually setting these feelings free.

Different types of poses strongly influence emotional states. For instance, back-bending, which indulges us with an expansive inhalation and opening of the chest, is a stimulating practice that can often elevate a low mood. Exhalation-intensive poses such as forward bends tend to calm an agitated mind. In any balanced practice, sama vritti (balanced breath) is recommended to create equilibrium in both sides of the body and gain emotional harmony.

Today's class is dedicated to restoring equipoise, empowering yourself to release emotionally and take full responsibility for making progress in your life.

## Teacher Tip

Remind your students that negative emotions often come disguised as distraction, impatience, or low energy.

## Asanas for Deepening

- *Shoulderstand and Plow.* In general, inversions help reverse energy blocks such as inflexible thinking, stuck emotions, and sadness.
- *Child's pose.* Be aware of the relaxation vibrations sent to the nervous system.
- *Eagle.* Find your balance to relieve the scattered mind while harmonizing your physical and mental worlds.
- *Seated twist.* One of yoga's greatest asana equalizers, this pose calms the mind and liberates sluggishness from the body.
- *Head to knee.* On exhalation, let the torso sink farther toward the legs relieving emotional energy blocks.
- *Bow.* This inhalation-intensive pose stimulates the thrusting of energy up through the sushumna, breaking through emotional limitations.
- *Woodchopper.* Chop away your frustration and anger. While standing, inhale, lifting the imaginary ax *(photo a)*. With a forceful and audible open-mouthed "Ha!" sound on the exhalation, chop the imaginary wood *(photo b)*.

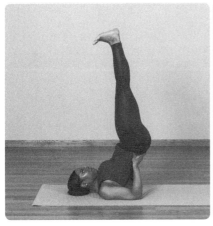

Shoulderstand

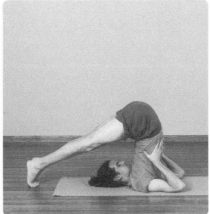

Plow

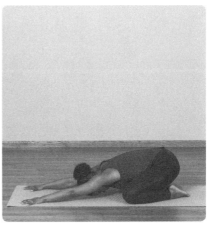

Child's pose

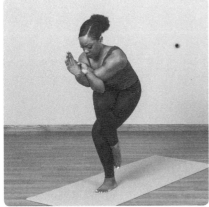

Eagle

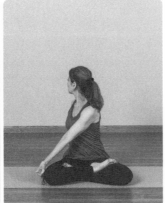

Seated twist

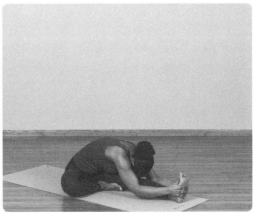

Head to knee

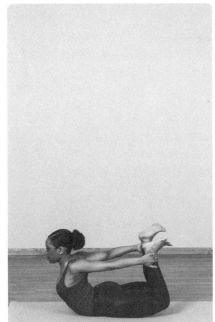

Bow

## WOODCHOPPER

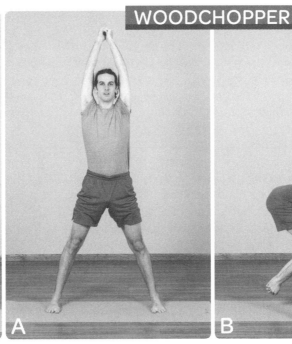

A

Arms overhead

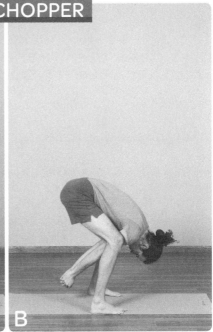

B

Chopping through legs

## Motivation Off the Mat

Notice circumstances that create tension. Just thinking about them may bring on a physiological reaction. Are you an anxious driver or parent? Are you angry at a friend? You don't have to be in the situation to feel the stress it causes.

## WISE WORDS

Following the path of yoga cuts through the roots of suffering.

Hatha yoga teaches control of breath and body. Through awareness you learn concentration, control of thought patterns, and emotional control.

# FRUSTRATION IN THE BODY

## Intention

To identify body frustration.

## Lesson

The physical feeling of frustration often stems from pushing away a situation, resisting change, or being angry with someone, including ourselves.

For instance, discomfort in the shoulders represents the feeling of overwhelm, or the delusion of having to carry the weight of the world. Issues in the back are related to worry, hurtful situations, and grief. Repressed anger can create stiffness in the neck as feelings are forced down the throat instead of coming out as words. Resentment and feeling out of control are often linked to issues in the hips.

For today's practice, let's set the intention to clear away any discomfort that stems from frustration.

Please lie on your back. Breathe deeply into the belly. Feel the response of your respiratory system—the air in the nostrils, throat, and chest; and the belly and chest rising and falling. Notice the rib cage expanding to the front, the sides beneath the armpits, and down into the lower back. Hold your attention on the breath, and observe your emotional state.

## Asanas for Deepening

○ *Reclining twist.* Holding this pose for several breaths clears frustration in the hips and helps relieve sciatic nerve pain, headaches, and low-back stiffness. Inhaling, bend the knees to the chest. Exhaling, twist the knees to the opposite side, revealing an *Ahhhh* breath. Pause for up to 10 breaths. Inhaling, return to your back. Switch sides. Practice the twist 3 times on each side.

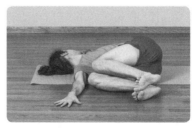

Reclining twist

○ *Arm circles.* Hold a shoulder-width length of strap in front of you. Inhale, moving the arms forward and up toward the sky. Exhale, bringing the arms behind you, using the full range of motion in the shoulder joints.

- *Arm pulls.* Raise the left arm up alongside the left ear. Reach the right arm down toward the ground, stretching through the fingers. Inhale, sending energy upward through the left arm. Exhale, reaching through the right arm and hand. Feel the flow of energy between the left and right arms. Hold for 3 breaths before alternating arms.

- *Collarbone stretch.* Interlace the fingers behind you. Open the chest, bend the elbows, and pull the knuckles to the right side of the waist. Feel the left shoulder blade moving inward toward the spine. Roll the shoulders back while squeezing the elbows together. Switch sides.

- *Leg cradle.* Soothe tension in tight hips as you stretch the thigh, hamstrings, and low back. It also helps provide a more stable and effortless meditation seat.

- *Cat–cow.* Leading the movements with the breath loosens frustration in the back, pelvic floor, abdomen, and neck.

- *Superman.* Fly high as you apply acupressure to points related to general bodily frustration, body aches, digestive problems, and fear. Hold for 3 to 6 breaths.

- *Neck stretches.* Relieve a literal pain in the neck by practicing these variations of neck movements: ear to shoulder *(photo a)*, look over the shoulder *(photo b)*, and chin to chest *(photo c)*.

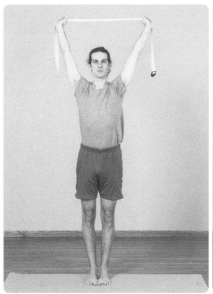

Arm circles

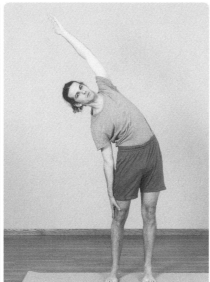

Arm pulls

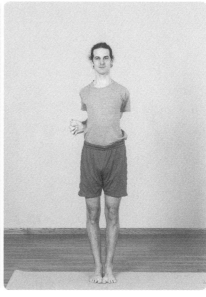

Collarbone stretch

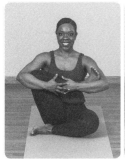

Leg cradle

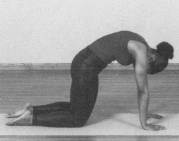

Cat–cow

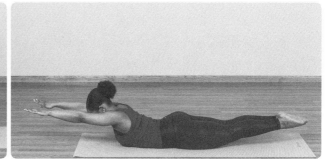

Superman

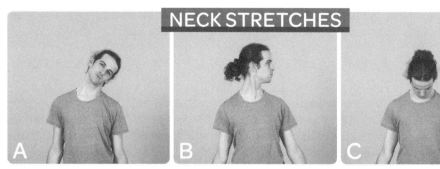

**NECK STRETCHES**

A — Ear to shoulder

B — Look over the shoulder

C — Chin to chest

## Motivation Off the Mat

Body language is the nonverbal and often incognizant communication of emotion and energy used to convey information. Do you hunch your shoulders to protect or shield yourself? Do you put your hands on your hips when you want control over a conversation? Do you avoid making eye contact? Notice what state you're in now, then observe how you communicate to the world through the language of your body.

## WISE WORDS

With daily practice, patience, and determination, energy blocks dissolve, liberating toxins in the body tissues.

The feeling of stress is unique for everyone. Whether or not you feel a situation as stressful depends on your habitual thought patterns and how you process the world around you.

Center your practice by finding the newness in the now.

Stand with confidence and poise.

## Teacher Tip

Warm up your teaching voice and passionate presence by meditating on your contented and loving heart.

# EMPOWERMENT OF CHANGE

## Intention

To learn to welcome change.

## Lesson

Everything in the world is constantly changing—the breath, your state of mind, your family, and the phases of the moon. The lesson of constant change is an abstruse revelation and a harsh reminder that nothing lasts forever. Even our bodies let us down in the end.

Until we accept the changes that occur in our bodies and surrender to the natural course of existence, little progress can be made along the yoga path. The ego resists change and struggles to hold on to the way things are now. The body responds by contracting and holding onto the past, slowing the natural flow of prana, and leaving behind dark barriers in the form of a tight hip or a stiff neck.

In asana, we stand witness to how our bodies, minds, and the world around us are constantly changing. Today, with a watchful eye, we'll awaken to life unfolding moment by moment, as we embrace the realities of change.

## Asanas for Deepening

From the first stretch in the morning to the mindful and heated sun salutation, observe the immediate transformation in the body. Ground your awareness in the subtle changes in breath, circulation, and body heat, as well as strength and flexibility.

- ○ *Inverted poses: headstand (photo a), shoulderstand (photo b), plow (photo c).* Inverted postures reverse the flow of energy and change your perspective on gravity.
- ○ *Revolved triangle.* Begin the pose by twisting from the waist with your arms extending out to the sides *(photo a)*, returning to center several times until you sense the opening in the lower back and waist. Then, take the full posture *(photo b)*.
- ○ *Half-bound lotus twist.* Remain in lotus, discovering new edges within each breath.

**INVERTED POSES**

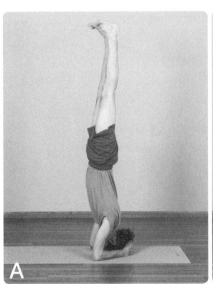
Headstand

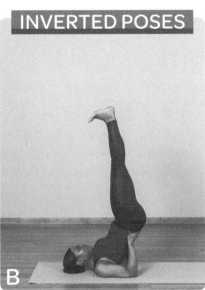
Shoulderstand

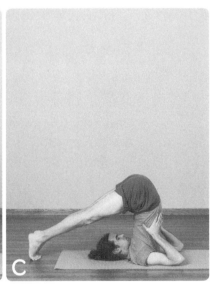
Plow

**REVOLVED TRIANGLE**

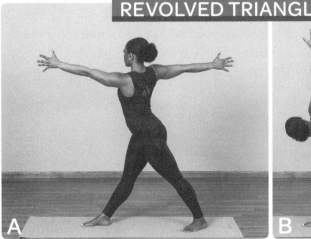
Revolved triangle (prep)

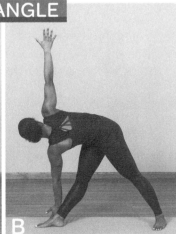
Revolved triangle

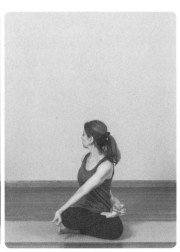
Half-bound lotus twist

## Motivation Off the Mat

Practice being receptive to change, even when it feels uncomfortable.

When plans for a night out suddenly change, take it in stride, knowing that nothing remains without change.

Change can be as simple as getting a new haircut or taking a different route to work.

Look back at all the twists and turns in your life. Observe how these experiences created exciting opportunities, introduced you to new people, and forced you into conquering your biggest fears.

Celebrate the changes of the seasons with a gathering of friends and family on the first day of summer, or throw a vernal equinox tea party on the first day of spring.

During times of change, remain a warrior by adopting a victory power pose, the physical expression of winning, to change your physiology and promote confidence and courage. Hold your arms up in a "V" shape for 2 minutes to lower the stress hormone cortisol and increase testosterone.

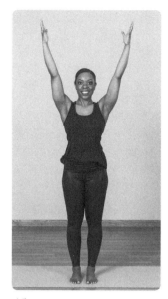
Victory pose

## WISE WORDS

Embracing change with grace generates ease and freedom in your world.

Don't paint yourself into a psychological corner, assuming your life has to go according to your aspirations. The universe may have other plans for you.

# THE ONLY CONSTANT IS CHANGE

## Intention

To embrace the unavoidable changes in life.

## Lesson

Whether you lose a job, fall in love, or get a flat tire, eventually you learn that life can change in an instant. Yoga practice teaches you to remain tranquil and accept life's frequent roller coaster of events, despite knowing that pleasure, pain, good, and bad don't last forever.

The Buddhist parable about a wise farmer illustrates how life can quickly turn around for the better and for the worse.

> *There was once a farmer who had a magnificent prize-winning stallion that he planned to sell for a large profit. One week before the horse was to be sold, a hurricane swept through the farmer's land. It tore down the barn where the horse lived, and the stallion ran off.*
>
> *"What bad luck!" the farmer's wife said.*
>
> *"Good luck, bad luck, who knows? We'll have to see," said the farmer.*

*The next week, the farmer and his wife saw a herd of horses galloping toward the farm with their prize-winning stallion leading a pack of four horses.*

*"What good luck!" said the farmer's wife.*

*"Good luck, bad luck, who knows? We'll have to see," said the farmer.*

*Soon the farmer and his son were training the new horses until one day the son was thrown from one and broke both his legs. The farmer's wife was distraught and sobbing, "My only son! We should have never let those horses in. This is very bad luck," she said.*

*"Good luck, bad luck, who knows? We'll have to see," said the farmer.*

*The next week, soldiers came to the farm. Their king had declared war and the soldiers were drafting every young man in the country. The soldiers saw that the farmer's son had two broken legs and left him at home. The farmer's wife was relieved. "Oh, what good luck we have!" she said.*

*As expected, the farmer said, "Good luck, bad luck, who knows? We'll have to see."*

Detached from life's peaks and valleys, knowing that change is the *only* certainty, the farmer accepted the ever-changing events with an open and objective mind.

Today, let's accept and be thankful for what's true in our bodies, in our minds, and in our lives at this moment. Know that change can be just a call, a text, or a breath away.

## Asanas for Deepening

Take your time, noticing energetic fluctuations on all levels of your being. The posture may appear comfortable (good luck?) then quickly change to discomfort (bad luck?).

○ *Hamstring stretch.* At the start of asana practice, explore the reclining hamstrings using a strap under the ball of the foot on the extended leg or, for the more flexible, the big-toe hold. At the end of class, do it again, noting the difference in the character of your muscles and energy.

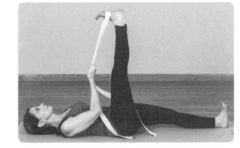

Hamstring stretch

○ *Log.* Invite your hips to melt into the earth. Take in the changing sensation. Can you sense softening?

○ *Boat.* Savor the balance (however temporary), the strength of your core, and your powerful breath.

○ *Winged dragon.* Bring the forearms to mat on the inside of the front leg, wing the front knee outward, resting on the knife-edge of the foot. Note how the energy of the body changes with every breath.

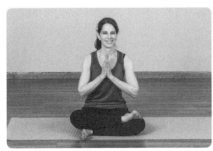

Log

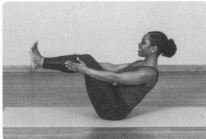

Boat

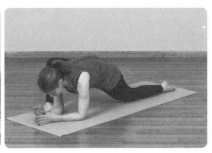

Winged dragon

## Motivation Off the Mat

Keep a journal of daily change, noting what's different about today than yesterday.

Consider the times when bad luck turned out to be good luck in disguise. Perhaps you didn't get the promotion you wanted, but 3 months later you found a better job.

The receptionist at your doctor's office just announced that your doctor is running 15 minutes late. Is it bad luck because you have to wait another 15 minutes? Is it good luck because it gives you time for pranayama to clear your mind and lower your blood pressure?

## WISE WORDS

We can only learn and grow through changing circumstances.

With awareness of the constant fluctuations of life, we cultivate an expansive mind, open to unexpected passages.

Impermanence is life's only guarantee.

Nothing lasts forever. The groceries you bought a few days ago, your childhood pet, even the headache you had this morning, are now gone.

## Teacher Tip

Choose a pose to return to again and again throughout class. Build a progression of that pose, holding the pose longer each time you do it, or gradually increasing the challenge of the pose to the next level. Try chair, chair on the toes, and chair twist.

# FEAR

## Intention

To release fear in order to live your fullest life.

## Lesson

What happens when a yogi is afraid?

Fear suffocates the third chakra, the center of will, courage, and inner strength. When this chakra becomes deficient, we're less willing to take risks, and often hide from life's unlimited possibilities. Living a fearful existence keeps potential at bay.

Yogis take a pragmatic view of the world, understanding that fear and uncertainty are part of the human existence. Whether you lived in a cave thousands of years ago fearing the attack of a bear, are afraid of bad news from your doctor, or have a fear of commitment, the fact is, violence, suffering, and fear of the unknown have always been part of the world.

Asana and pranayama are two of the most potent practices for detaching from the fear, anxiety, and anger that gets trapped in the body's tissues. The path of yoga is the tool for liberation from suffering.

Today's class will reconnect and balance the solar plexus and open the armor that covers the heart center chakra. Instead of letting fear lead you and lock you in a self-imposed prison, fill your heart with the energy of love and gratitude to live your life with freedom.

## Asanas for Deepening

What yoga practices should you engage in if you live in fear of violence, suffering, or even the more mundane events such as job interviews or confrontations with store clerks? Start by untying the armor around the solar plexus and heart center with a series of gentle backbends to relieve depression caused by anxiety.

○ *Cobra.* Practice holding the inhale as you rise to cobra for 2 to 4 seconds.

○ *Locust.* Lift your legs and acknowledge the strength from your solar plexus.

○ *Lunge.* Sink deep into the earth as you courageously raise the arms in confidence.

○ *Standing backbend.* Lean back into the unknown, trusting your body's intuition.

○ *Bridge and camel.* Imagine your heart lifting out of its cage, flourishing in heroic strength and wisdom.

○ *Crow.* If crow is scary for you, first notice your reaction to it. Then, to chip away at the fear, try lifting one foot at a time. The crow develops courage and balances the third chakra.

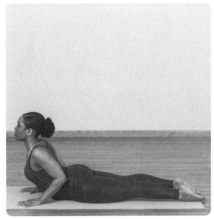

Cobra

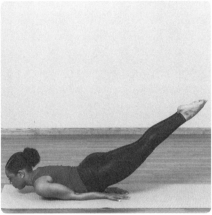

Locust

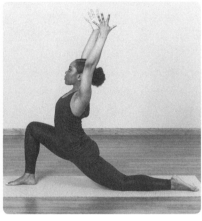

Lunge

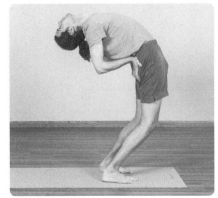

Standing backbend

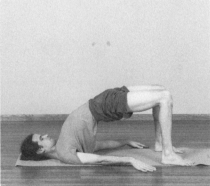

Bridge

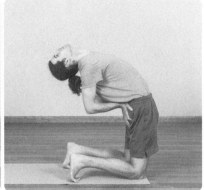

Camel

CROW

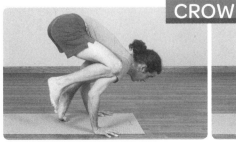

Crow preparation (*lift one leg*)

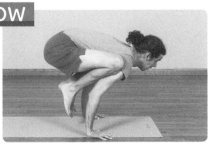

Crow

## Motivation Off the Mat

When an anxiety attack approaches, stop what you're doing, identify the feeling as anxiety, and catch your breath. At the moment of mindfulness, practice two-to-one breathing (exhaling twice as long as you inhale) for 10 breaths. Follow with 20 to 30 left-nostril breaths, closing the right nostril with the right thumb. Repeat the breathing sequence until you feel calm washing over you.

When you're in a state of fear, visualize being in a different place and time. For instance, imagine relaxing on the sands of a safe, warm, tropical beach with a loved one. With each exhalation, feel a wave of cleansing energy rolling through the body, wiping away panic and worry. Add the mantra, *I am stronger than my fear.* Repeat until the fear subsides.

Practice to liberate fear. Check in with your emotions throughout your day. If you feel the butterflies of fear in the solar plexus, welcome the feeling. Take a deep breath, and greet your thoughts of dread and worry with interest and curiosity as if the thoughts were only coming for a short visit. Then, sit with your eyes closed and breathe into your fear, finding its roots, and letting it go, rendering it powerless, until it leaves your body.

## WISE WORDS

> Your mindful practice develops a tenacious ability to concentrate on reality, leading to control of emotions.
>
> You can choose to be afraid of death your whole life, or you can recognize that death is part of life.
>
> When the chakras are in balance, sit in gratitude of the present moment. It's nearly impossible to feel anxiety and fear when you're in a gratitude state.
>
> Choosing love over fear fills the now with appreciation for the present moment.
>
> Fear is **F**alse **E**vidence **A**ppearing **R**eal.

# LETTING GO

## Intention

To abandon emotional baggage.

## Lesson

Carrying emotional baggage is part of the human experience, but for some, their baggage defines who they are. "The River," a Buddhist a parable about the baggage we carry, tells the story about the importance of lightening our loads and leaving our worries behind.

> *Two monks, one old and one young, were about to cross a river when they noticed a woman at the riverbank waiting for someone to help her get across.*
>
> *The young monk said to the old monk, "That woman needs help. Shall we take her across the river with us?" In those days, monks were forbidden to have any contact with women. The old monk angrily replied, "We can't do that. We'd be breaking our*

*sacred vows!" The young monk thought for a moment, then lifted the woman onto his back and carried her across the river.*

*Later that day, after walking a great distance, the old monk bemoaned the young monk's contact with the woman, complaining they had broken their vows. "What are we to do? How will we explain this to our brothers at the monastery?" The young monk stopped, looked at the old monk, and said, "Brother, I left that woman two miles back. Why are you still carrying her?"*

The yama aparigraha (nonpossessiveness) teaches us to stop clinging to bad memories and self-sabotaging behaviors, prompting us to let down our guard and recognize that when something isn't making us happy, it's time to make a change. Clinging to outdated or inflexible ideals imprisons us in a chosen state of suffering.

Think of your yoga mat as a sacred place where you can unearth your buried bags and gift them to the universe. Intentionally let go of emotional drama; forgive and give up guilt, anger, and bad memories so that you can live in this moment. Let life unfold to its full potential.

## Asanas for Deepening

Invite openness and receptivity into the deeper experience of releasing the obstacles that cause the experience of suffering.

- ○ *Tortoise.* Feel the freedom in the stretch, breath, and open state of mind.
- ○ *Butterfly with a block.* Wait for an inner cue, then choose the moment to expel baggage trapped in the groin, hips, and back. Surrender to the outcome.
- ○ *Twist with eagle legs.* Practice the willingness to be present and watch the body unravel.

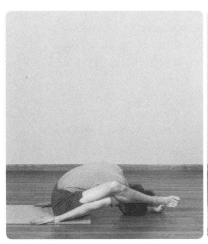

Tortoise

Butterfly with a block

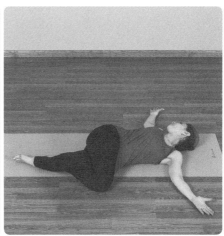

Twist with eagle legs

## Motivation Off the Mat

Create a list of your emotional baggage, and carry it with you in your purse, briefcase, or backpack. Make the list physically heavy by taping it to a small rock reminding you of your self-punishment. After 7 days of literally *carrying your baggage*, let it go. Take the list and say, "I release this emotional baggage from my life. It no longer serves me in any way possible." Then, burn the piece of paper, destroying the baggage and moving forward, free from the heavy issues of the past.

Are you still carrying a grudge over a disagreement with a friend, relative, or business associate? Do you feel the same guilt, betrayal, and anger as you did when it happened? Decide to release that negativity to the universe. You're not necessarily letting this person back into your life. It simply means that you stop giving that dark experience your energy and power, and start living a lighter, burden-free life.

## WISE WORDS

Negative self-identifying behaviors will always hold you back from maximizing your potential.

Letting go allows space to gather new insights, move forward, and attract positive changes and transformation.

Surrender your attachment to memories of failure and mistakes.

When we choose to let go, we fall in love with the present moment, creating a clear path for progress.

# CLINGING TO HAPPINESS

## Intention

To uncover the path of temporary happiness.

## Lesson

A yoga student of mine unexpectedly discovered the root cause of all her afflictions. During a yoga retreat, Marilyn, a bank executive, had an epiphany. She called it a spiritual rocket launched by her retreat teacher. The teacher said, "Yoga is the elimination of clinging. Clinging is want, and to want is to suffer." That was it. In an instant, Marilyn had a flash of insight as to why she was unhappy. She had to stop wanting.

To explain why too much want can be disastrous to our emotional equilibrium, I want to introduce you to the philosophy of *raga*: the attachment that brings temporary satisfaction. The gratification we feel from pleasurable experiences and possessions creates blurred internal vision, emotional ups and downs, and in the long run, is never sustaining.

When we *do* get what we want, we experience unrooted happiness; our feelings of pleasure quickly fade, and we begin a *new* search for pleasure, becoming trapped in an endless cycle of want. If getting what we want makes us happy, even for a short period of time, then when we *don't* get what we want, we suffer.

Raga is the self-induced bad seed that causes an addiction to the buzz of pleasure. You can become addicted to anything—shopping, drugs, sex, gambling, even perfecting yoga poses. These addictions provide a short-lived, illusory comfort. For example, a person may feel confident after the first cocktail, but utterly mindless after the third.

The yogic path to defeating the impediments to happiness is to practice the yama aparigraha (nonpossessiveness) which requires abstinence from greediness, hoarding, and possessing beyond your needs.

The more you look at your own desires, the clearer you see the well in this endless pool of want. The practice of yoga teaches that everything you need is already inside you.

## Asanas for Deepening

Raga shows up on your yoga mat as an attachment to a teacher or an idea of how you want the class to be. When you're open-minded, energetic possibilities flourish.

Attachment to pleasure is a futile grasping at impermanence. People often close the chest to hold the moment, thus shutting down the heart center. An optimal asana remedy is backbends, one of the most concentrated yoga tools to counteract the obstacles to joy. Backbends implore us to strongly focus and open the heart center, balancing the breath and allowing prana to flow into parts of the body that we can't see.

- *Standing forward bend with twisted bind.* This pose encourages the middle way—not too much, not too little.
- *Downward dog.* Explore feeling the vibrations of vitality while stretching through your long torso and spine.
- *Tabletop twist.* This pose provokes a lift through the heart and opens the rib cage and lungs.
- *Lunge with cow face arms.* Practice longer lunge holds with ujjayi breath, mindfully releasing the pelvis toward the ground while expanding your loving heart center.
- *Bridge.* Imagine your heart lifting out of its cage, flourishing with truth and wisdom. Breathe evenly, relieving the static energy caused by the heaviness of discontentment.
- *Supported side plank bow.* Lift and widen the heart center while clearing away deep-seated emotional attachments.

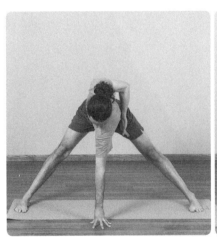

Standing forward bend with twisted bind

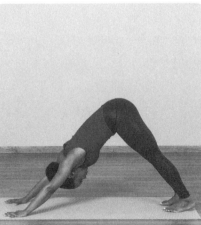

Downward dog

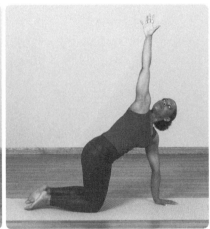

Tabletop twist

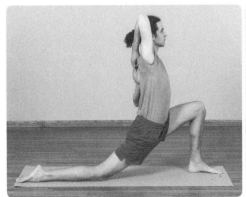

Lunge with cow face arms

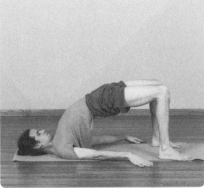

Bridge

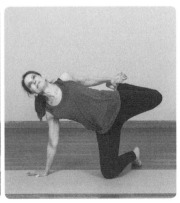

Supported side plank bow

○ *Wheel*. Stay present to the physical effects of the wheel, fine-tuning the sacred flow of prana along the spine.

○ *Lotus twist*. Squeeze the heart, spreading the seeds of love within. Unwind to unleash the fleeting pleasures that consume the mind.

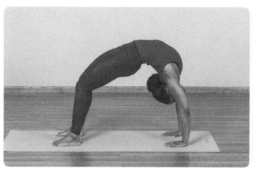

Wheel

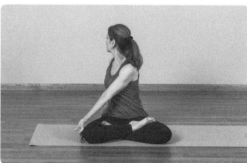

Lotus twist

## Motivation Off the Mat

Reflect on your obstacles. Do you have too much stuff? Do you overspend, overeat, or drink or gamble too much? Do you have a visceral reaction when you don't get what you want? If so, you may be caught in the trap of raga.

When you cling to a person, place, or thing in the hope that it will bring you happiness, it will only bring more want, the root of suffering.

The fiendish call of raga is one of life's biggest distractions, and your spiritual nemesis.

## WISE WORDS

Overcoming raga requires detaching from fleeting pleasure and recognizing that everything in life is impermanent.

Wake up and realize that attaining more possessions and feeding your addictions are running your life. They will never fulfill you, and will only create more want and unhappiness.

What makes us happy is not what we get but who we become.

# PATIENCE

## Intention

To recognize impatience within ourselves.

## Lesson

Of all our negative emotions, impatience is the most prominent. We see it in toddlers, business people, parents, seniors, it even shows up on our yoga mats. Impatience manifests in a variety of directions, and is often interpreted as anger.

> *Stephen was waiting at a popular restaurant to pick up his dinner order. It was a busy evening, and a crowd of customers began to gather in the waiting area. Speaking loudly on her phone, the woman next to him was angrily complaining that her order was taking too long and that the wait was "ridiculous." When the woman's name was called to pick up her order, she yelled at the man behind the counter, "This is a disgrace!" She continued, "You said my order would be ready by 6 o'clock!" The man apologized and said, "I'm so sorry for the wait, Miss, but it is 6 o'clock." "No, it's not," she shouted back, "it's 6:05!"*
>
> *Stephen laughed at the absurdity of this scenario. Yet, how many of us can say we've* never *been this agitated by our own impatience?*

We suffer with impatience because our actions are out of tune with the reality of the now. If our minds are preoccupied with the concerns of yesterday or tomorrow, it's difficult to involve ourselves in the present. Rather than live in the moment, we want things to be faster, better, and smoother. It's as if we're in a cosmic control battle to manage the speed of how things actually happen.

Your yoga practice provides one of the most systematic approaches to improving impatience. As asana brings you back in touch with the physical body, you experience the sensations of impatience and learn how to let yourself open at your own pace. If impatience emerges during today's practice, instead of pushing your restless thoughts away, be mindful that they, like the sensations in your body, are part of the moment.

## Asanas for Deepening

Honor your asana exploration with tolerance and curiosity, the basis of living in the moment.

○ *Seated forward bend.* Don't rush the early stages of the posture waiting to get somewhere that your body is not yet ready for. Find your first place of resistance and adapt before going any farther. Follow the movement of each inhalation and exhalation. When impatience arises (it may rear its ugly head as boredom), bring yourself back to the movement of the breath.

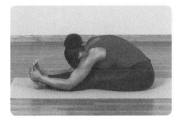

Seated forward bend

○ *Side plank.* Take the posture in as many stages as necessary. First, try it with the bottom knee grounded *(photo a)*. Then extend the legs *(photo b)*. Finally, bring the top leg in a half lotus *(photo c)*.

○ *Child's pose with brahmari breath.* Take a full, broad breath into the muscles along the spine, and hum your long exhalation. The vibration along the back body is like calming medicine.

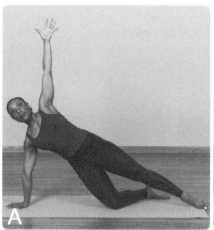

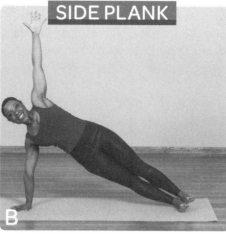

**SIDE PLANK**

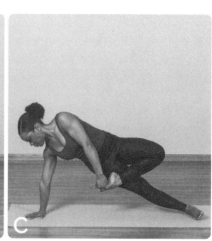

Side plank with knee on ground      Side plank with legs extended      Side plank with half lotus

## Motivation Off the Mat

Watch how others handle a stressful situation. As Stephen observed the impatient customer's reaction, he experienced an awakening of his own impatience. Learning to identify another person's negative emotions will help you recognize them in yourself.

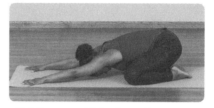

Child's pose with brahmari breath

If you're a parent, check your parenting reactions. Few things can set off a parent's impatience alarm like a misbehaving child. Instead of yelling or acting out on your frustration, set an example for your children by maintaining a calm, centered presence.

Be aware of your tendency to interrupt others when they're talking. Pause and listen to what the other person is saying; don't just wait for them to finish their sentence. You may be missing half the conversation!

### Quick-Calm Breath

When impatience arises, try the 7-4-4-4 quick-calm breath. Exhale to a count of 7, hold the breath on empty for a count of 4; then inhale to a count of 4, and hold for 4. Practice four cycles. Adjust your count if the breath length feels too shallow or long.

## WISE WORDS

Patience is a form of wisdom, helping you accept that everything evolves in its own time.

Impatience is a defensive response to a situation that is out of your control.

# 14

# Workshops

*A man should first direct himself in the way he should go. Only then should he instruct others.*

—Buddha

At some point in your yoga career, you may want to dive deeper into your studies and cover more teaching ground on your most cherished yoga themes. When that happens, it's time to hold a workshop.

Unlike yoga classes, workshops immerse the student in one specific aspect of yoga, revealing the little known details of the topic. Perhaps your passion is for teaching the yamas and niyamas, the chakras, or backbends. Whatever you chose, the students who attend your workshop will be drawn to your subject because they're just like you—curious and longing to know more about maneuvering through the yoga journey.

Before you begin the long, tedious hours of research, take the following guidelines into consideration.

*Plan.* Plan your workshop months in advance. Schedule the date to give yourself plenty of time to work out the details with the studio or facility where the workshop will be held. Use your time wisely to work on your material, promotion, and presentation (including the timing and rehearsal).

*Target.* Know who your audience is, and tailor the entire event from the time of day to the type of workshop to fit their schedule and needs.

*Ask your students.* Your workshop could cover expanded material from what your students already learn in your regular yoga classes. Ask your students if there's something they would like to learn more about.

*Promote.* Have a plan in place to promote your workshop. Whether you choose e-blasts, social media event ads, your website, or calendar items on local news and yoga sites, any kind of promotion that you do requires a link for the reader to get more information and to register. Ask your friends, family, students, and the facility where you're holding the workshop to share the information on their own social media.

*Greet your students.* On workshop day, greet your attendees, introduce yourself, ask them if they're new to yoga, and help them find a space in the room.

*Printed materials.* Give your attendees printed materials with FAQs from the workshop, more reading material on your subject matter, and your contact information.

*Shoot photos.* Hire a photographer or grab a friend to shoot photos of the workshop in action. Repurpose the photos for social media, your website, and other promotional opportunities. Be sure you have everyone's permission to take and use the photos.

*Get names and email addresses.* Collect the names and email addresses of your workshop attendees. After the workshop, send a "Thank you for attending" email to your students, and add additional self-promotion material by mentioning your current schedule of classes and upcoming workshops. And don't forget to ask for a follow on social media!

The workshops included in this chapter are a culmination of months of research on topics that were of interest to me. They were also my best-attended events. Having a workshop already outlined, timed, and scripted will save you hours of preparation.

## WORKSHOP PROMOTION CHECK LIST

✔ Social media outlets

- Facebook posts including ads, event listing, invitations, and post boosts.
- Twitter
- Instagram

✔ Local online calendar event postings

✔ Online yoga site listing

✔ E-blasts: Send 3 to 5 blasts with the majority scheduled 2 weeks prior to the event. If your event is not full by the day before the workshop, schedule an email with a sense of urgency subject line such as "Almost filled—Register now for tomorrow's Joy of Backbends workshop."

✔ Friends and family: It's reassuring to have friends and family surround you with their love, loyalty, and presence. Plus, a full house helps fill the room with good energy.

✔ Flyers: Hand out flyers in your classes, post them on community boards, and have them available for anyone you meet.

# SPRING CLEANING YOGA DETOX

## Intention

To learn and practice holistic cleansing techniques.

**Target:** Yoga students at any level.

**Preparation/props:** Pens, index cards, tissues, printed handouts, peppermint water (for you) to clear your throat, arnica massage oil

**Best time to schedule:** Early spring

**Duration:** 3 hours

**Features:** Self-massage, guided relaxation, pranayama, strong asana practice to move stale energies out of the body.

Prior to the start of the workshop, give each attendee a pen and 10 index cards per person.

## Introduction to the Workshop

Hello, and welcome to our Spring Cleaning Detox workshop. Our detox removes negative energy accumulated over the winter months and prepares the body, mind, and spirit for the positive growth of spring.

Today, in order to put us in a peak state, we're working with cleansing yogic practices to move toxins out of the body through digestion, elimination, breath, as well as the mind.

No matter what kind of yoga you're doing, you're always working with purification. Yoga purifies the system and by extension, your life. *Saucha,* a yogic term that means "purity," "cleanliness," and "clarity," refers to purity of mind, speech, body, and physical surroundings. This concept of clearing out on all levels allows prana to flow freely without obstruction.

> ### WORKSHOP WISDOM
> When we feel good, our confidence rises and we believe we can do anything.

When you're clear, you're able to release and dissolve all kinds of blockages within your consciousness. These may be things that get you stuck in situations where you'd like to make changes, but can't.

For this detox workshop to be effective for you, first get some certainty about what want to get rid of. What are the things that no longer serve you? Your job, toxic people in your life, your weight, your painful thoughts of the past? When you practice with focused intention, you organically create space physically, mentally, and spiritually to manifest something positive into your life.

## Setting the Agenda

We're going to do several types of practices during this workshop.

First, you'll uncover what you'd like to detox physically, emotionally, energetically, and spiritually by writing it down. Knowing your objective and seeing it in your own words is at the root of mindfulness.

Next, we'll practice a variety of pranayama exercises, the breathing practices to physically clear toxic energy patterns.

Then, we'll follow the pranayama with an asana practice to release and negotiate through your tight spaces. Asana helps us feel the physical sensations of moving with intention to open blocked areas, let the dark matter out, and visualize the nadis—the subtle energy channels—expanding and dissolving the mucus, impurities, and distractions that have accumulated over the long winter months.

We have lots of twists on today's asana menu. Twists bring tremendous energy and vitality to the body. Also on tap is a focus on the navel center to awaken the inner body, stoke our emotional and spiritual fire, and help burn off dis-ease.

Finally, we'll do a special meditation on new beginnings to help you visualize your transformation.

Grab one of your index cards, and write down what you'd like to detox. If you're not sure, ask yourself why you came today and what you'd like to achieve. You can make the list as long or short as you'd like. These notes are yours; no one else will see them. They're only here to help guide you. [Pause for students to write their objectives.]

## Opening Movements

Let's start with a short opening movement practice to get your motor running and clear the mind. It's difficult to manifest your greatness when you have a long list of items that are blocking your view.

- ○ Easy pose with one-to-one (equal) breathing followed by two-to-one breathing.
- ○ Easy pose with 11 kapalabhati breaths.
- ○ Gate pose. On the knees, stretch the right arm to the left foot awakening the rib's intercostal muscles; repeat on the opposite side.

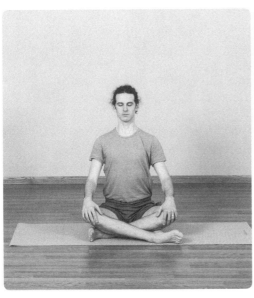

Easy pose                                   Gate pose

### Sun Salutation Warm-Up

1. *Mountain.*
2. *Standing forward bend.*
3. *Low lunge.* Left leg steps back.
4. *Downward dog.*
5. *Cat.*

6. *Downward dog.*
7. *Low lunge.* Left leg steps forward. Repeat the sequence lunging on the opposite side.
8. *Savasana.* Stay for 1 minute.

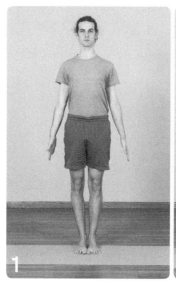

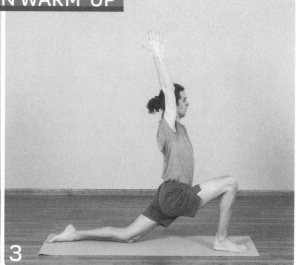

1

Mountain

Standing forward bend

3

Low lunge

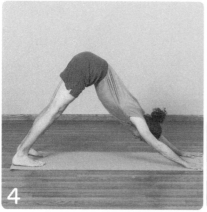

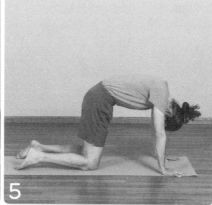

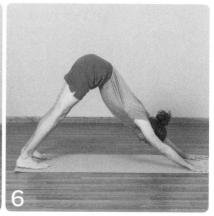

4

Downward dog

Cat

6

Downward dog

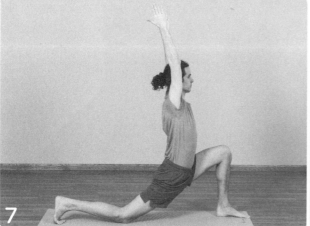

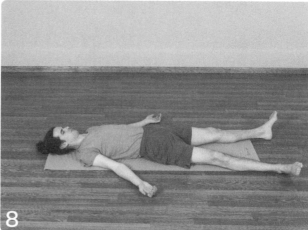

7

Low lunge (opposite leg)

8

Savasana

[Students are seated.] Think about the things you do for spring cleaning. You clean your windows, closets, your desk, and change the baking soda in your refrigerator. You might donate items like clothes and books. The idea of a cleared space in your home, office, or car gives you more room to relax and breathe. The bonus is that you can take this concept of spacious possibility into your life.

Revisit your index cards. Write down what you'd like to detox on a physical, emotional, and spiritual level, and use separate cards for each area. At the top of the first card, write, "Physical detox." At the top of the second card, write, "Emotional detox." And at the top of the third card, write, "Spiritual detox."

On the "Physical detox" card, write down any tight areas such as the shoulders, neck, and back. Make peace with the places in your body that need change. By changing your physiology through asana and mindful movement, you can change your mental state and break through thinking patterns that aren't working for you. An improvement in your physiology leads to balanced emotions, one of the principle ingredients to getting unstuck. [Pause for students to write.]

Let's move on to the second card, "Emotional detox." A toxic emotional state manifests in a variety of unhealthy ways, such as self-doubt, resentment, or the *I'm not good enough* disease. Doubting yourself kills more dreams than failure ever could. What do you want to change today? Do you find it hard to say no, then get angry with yourself? Do you run from confrontation? Along with what you want to detox emotionally, write down what kinds of things you'd like to manifest in your life. [Pause for students to write.]

Now let's take a look at the last card, "Spiritual detox." Spirituality includes a sense of connection to something bigger than yourself, but it may also involve a search for a more meaningful life. For instance, maybe you'd like to be more charitable but you don't make time to help others or pay it forward. Creating small windows in your day to call a friend in need is a way to detox. Look for ways to serve the community, especially volunteer work, that offer no monetary reward. You can even simplify the spiritual objective by smiling at a stranger, making a momentary connection, and sharing your positive energy.

Get clear about anything that weighs you down, closes you off from new ideas, and locks you into negative ways of thinking. Once you focus on what you want to manifest through your detox experience, you can make today's practices a daily ritual. They not only become a part of your life, they become who you are. All you need to do is decide that you're not going to become *retoxed*. Remember that toxic energy—people, food, and things—is always going to be present in your life. How you choose to deal with these situations will make the difference between your detox and retox.

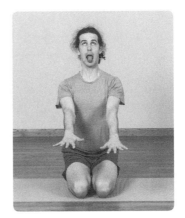

**WORKSHOP WISDOM**

We must be the watcher at the doorway of our minds.

## Breathing, Asana, and Body Awareness

When practiced together, the cousins of meditation—breathing, asana, and relaxation—systematically cleanse us and tame the wild monkey mind.

### PANTING LION BREATH

Besides being fun to practice, this breath removes phlegm from the throat area and stimulates the thyroid to boost energy.

[Students are sitting.] Open the eyes and mouth wide. Stick out your tongue, and begin a panting breath through your mouth, focusing on each exhalation. Draw

Panting Lion

your navel sharply back with each exhalation, and relax it on the inhalation. Continue for 1 to 3 minutes; then close your mouth and your eyes, and inhale deeply into your abdomen. Hold this breath in for as long as you can, resting the focus at your third eye, the point between your eyebrows.

## Asanas for Internal Heating

These poses produce heat from the navel center as they move static energies from the body and breath, initiating transformation on every level.

- *Seated twist in easy pose.*
- *Pelvic tilts in easy pose.*
- *Boat kicks with kapalabhati breaths.* Exhale while extending the legs; repeat the movements 10 times.
- *Seated knee-up twist.*
- *Scrape the barrel with kapalabhati breaths.*
- *Yogi bicycles.* Do 20 repetitions.
- *Leg lifts.* Do single or double lifts.
- *Knees to chest.*
- *Happy baby.*

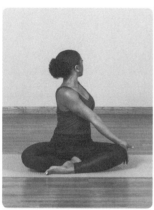
Seated twist in easy pose

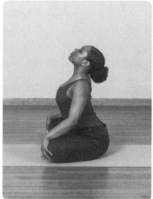
Pelvic tilts in easy pose

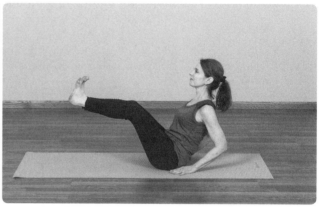
Boat kicks

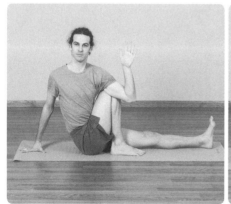
Seated knee-up twist

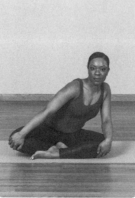
Scrape the barrel

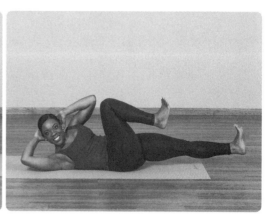
Yogi bicycles

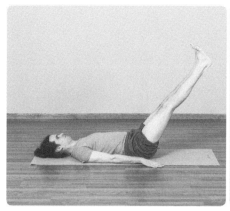
Leg lifts

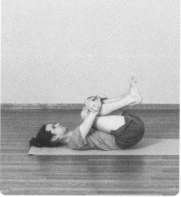
Knees to chest

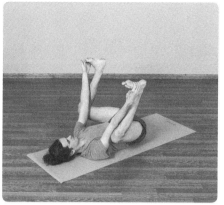
Happy baby

## Asanas with Detoxifying Twists

At the core of the twist is a squeeze-and-soak action. Twists stimulate circulation and have a cleansing and refreshing effect on the torso, abdominal organs, and associated glands.

- ○ *Table twist.* Reach one arm upward, lifting the heart to one side.
- ○ *Table with hip rotation.* Lift one knee to the side body, rotating the hip joint clockwise and counter-clockwise.
- ○ *Cat stretch.* Create heat to burn and sweat out impurities, improve joint mobility, aid digestion and elimination, and increase circulation along the spine. Exhale as you squeeze and lift from the pelvic floor muscles.

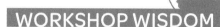

**WORKSHOP WISDOM**

Don't over contract the muscles or compromise the breath by transferring tension into the chest, shoulders, or neck. Detox what you continue to retox— food, stress, work, memories. Get clear, and practice to stay clean.

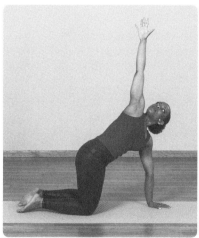
Table twist

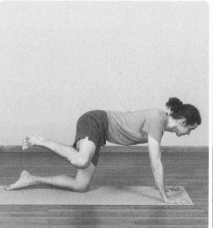
Table with hip rotation

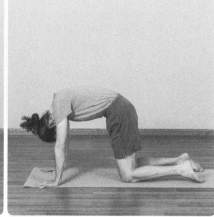
Cat stretch

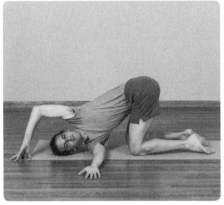
Thread the needle

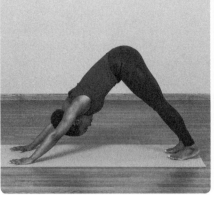
Downward dog

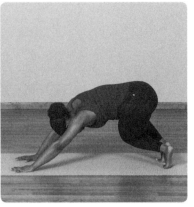
Twisted downward dog

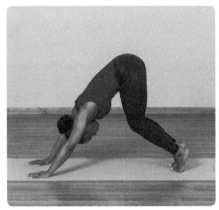
Downward dog with uddiyana bandha

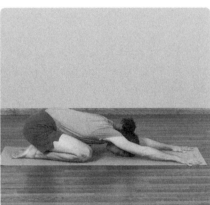
Child's pose

- ○ *Thread the needle.* Reach the "threaded" arm to one side until the opposite shoulder blade touches the ground. Continue to reach with every breath.
- ○ *Downward dog.* Positioning the heart higher than the head reverses the effects of gravity's pull, and helps circulate blood and lymph.
- ○ *Twisted downward dog.* Bend the knees, moving them to the right as the heels move to the left. Reach the sit bones toward the heels to create length in the spine. Repeat the action on the opposite side.
- ○ *Downward dog (or table) with uddiyana bandha.* Squeeze the breath all the way out, pulling the navel center in and back toward the spine. Hold the position until you need to inhale. Repeat 3 times.
- ○ *Child's pose.*

Sit in easy pose and review your cards. Are you working through your objectives? Is there anything you'd like to add or delete from your cards? What will happen if you get rid of these obstacles? Will they come back tomorrow? Can you discover new ways to keep that space open for growth?

**WORKSHOP WISDOM**

Do not take the seeds and throw away the melon.

### Standing Detoxifiers

Standing poses free up sukha, which means "good space," in the pelvis and legs, the densest part of the body. The pelvic area and legs represent the earthy and watery part of the body prone to retaining fat and water.

- *Frog squat.* From standing, bend the knees while exhaling with kapalabhati breaths to squat; inhaling, rise to stand.
- *Sun salutation with high lunge twist.* Synchronizing breathing and movement heats the body and frees circulation.
- *Uddiyana bandha.* The abdominal lift and lock revives your fire essence, and is one of the most important exercises in yoga, practiced for its physical and emotional cleansing values. [See chapter 5 for teaching instructions.] The benefits of this practice are so far reaching that if you have time for only one hatha yoga exercise, practice uddiyana bandha. Hold the breath in as long as possible, then inhale, releasing the bandhas while lifting the head. Repeat 4 times.

## Benefits of Uddiyana Bandha

Massages and tones the internal organs in the abdominal region

Helps relieve constipation, gas, and indigestion

Tones the nerves in the solar plexus region

Massages and strengthens the heart

Reduces abdominal fat and strengthens the abdominal muscles

Energizes the entire system

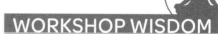

**WORKSHOP WISDOM**

The body is like a self-cleaning oven; you just have to turn it on.

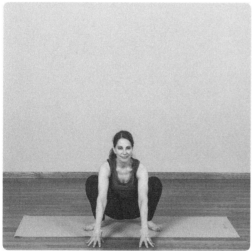

Frog squat

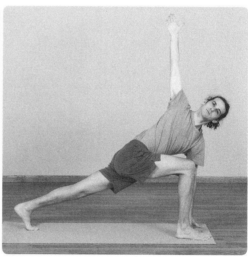

Sun salutation with high lunge twist

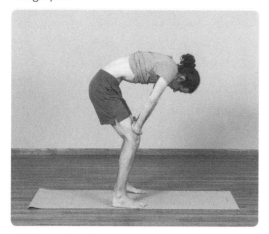

Uddiyana bandha

Sit in easy pose and review your cards. Are you working through your objectives? Don't let your mind get in the way of your outcome.

## SEQUENCE 1: STANDING POSES

1. *Lunge twists.* Do low-lunge and high-lunge variations. Choose a variety of hand and arm positions such as hands in prayer, arms open, or a half bind.

2. *Waterfall warrior with* HA! *breath.* Repeat the breath 6 times.

3. *Elbow plank twist.* While on the forearms, slowly shift the hips side to side, holding the integrity of your long, strong legs, abdomen, and back.

4. *Downward dog split to triangle.* From downward dog split, step the leading foot through the space between the hands, then lift to triangle.

5. *Side angle.* Reach the top arm toward the front of the mat, and twist the heart to the sky.

6. *Revolved triangle.* Squeeze the inner thighs together and upward toward the pelvic floor.

Rest in child's pose or savor a slow vinyasa before repeating the sequence on the opposite side.

## WORKSHOP WISDOM

Do not drive the tiger from the front door while letting the wolf get in the back.

—Hu Zhidang, Han Dynasty

## LUNGE TWISTS

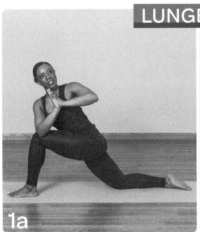

1a

Low lunge twist with hands in prayer

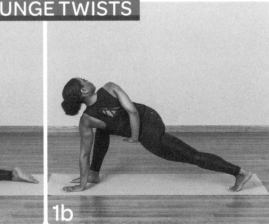

1b

High lunge twist with half bind

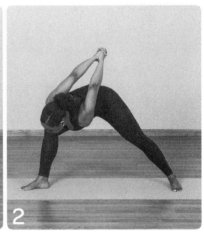

2

Waterfall warrior with *HA!* breath

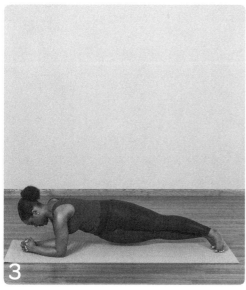

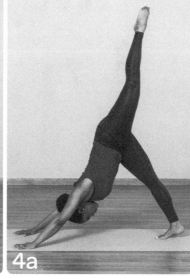

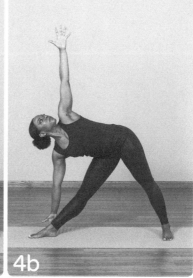

**3**
Elbow plank twist

**4a**
Downward dog split

**4b**
Triangle

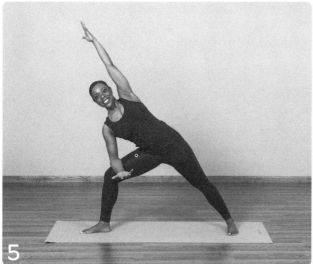

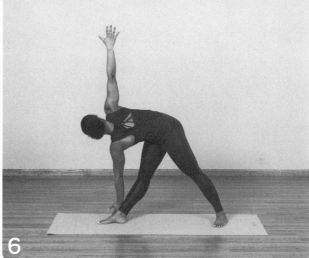

**5**
Side angle

**6**
Revolved triangle

## SEQUENCE 2: STANDING BALANCES

The standing balance poses help control emotions by asking your mind to stay one-pointed on your drishti (visual focal point).

1. *Tree.*
2. *Chair with heels lifted.*
3. *Downward dog.*
4. *Eagle.*
5. *Skier.*
6. *Downward dog.*
7. *Pyramid.*
8. *Side angle with bind.*
9. *Revolved half moon.*
10. *Half moon.*
11. *Hanging forward bend.*

Rest in child's pose or savor a slow vinyasa before repeating the sequence on the opposite side.

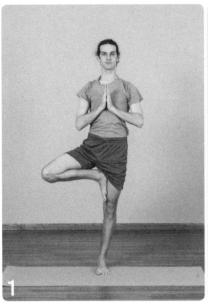

1

Tree

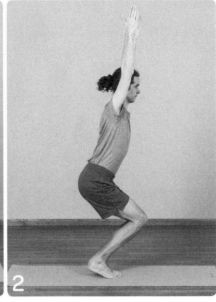

2

Chair with heels lifted

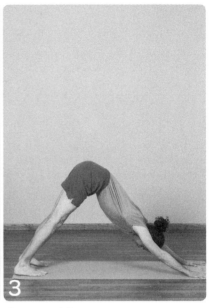

3

Downward dog

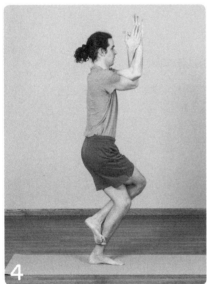

4

Eagle

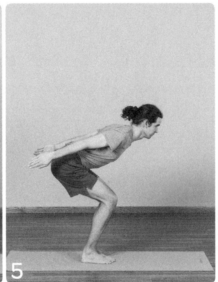

5

Skier

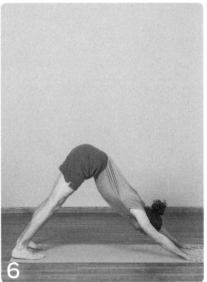

6

Downward dog

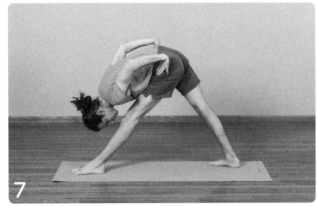

7

Pyramid

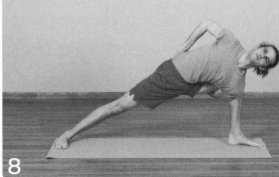

8

Side angle with bind

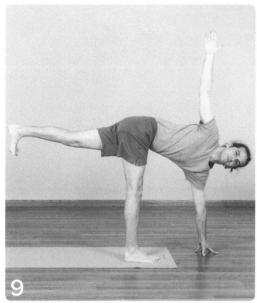

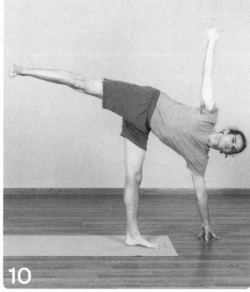

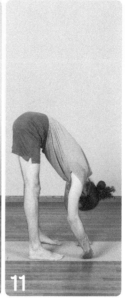

| | | |
|---|---|---|
| Revolved half moon | Half moon | Hanging forward bend |

## Self-Massage

Give each student a few drops of organic massage oil such as arnica or lavender. Instruct students to rub their hands together to warm the oil.

- *Self-massage.* Rub the wrists, arms, shoulders, neck, back, ankles, feet, top of the head, face, and anywhere you have exposed skin.
- *Belly massage.* Sit on your heels. Make fists with the hands, placing them on both sides of the navel center. Move the fists in a circular motion around the pelvic area, then bend forward from the hips, putting the weight of your torso on your fists, nudging the massage deeper into the internal organs.

### Benefits of Self-Massage

Cleanses the lymphatic system: The rubbing and stroking actions dislodge accumulated toxins and impurities from the body and moves them into the digestive system.

Provides a deep feeling of self-love: The skin is one of the primary seats of emotion, feeling, and desire. Touch is 10 times stronger than verbal or emotional contact.

Boosts vitality: Prevents dehydration while providing deep nourishment.

Stimulates the immune system.

Review your objectives. Where are your obstacles now? How can you position your mind to guard you from retoxing?

## SEQUENCE 3: ROLLING HEAT

Let's use the stimulating heating effects of self-massage to push toxins out toward elimination.

1. *Mountain.* Bring the hands to prayer, signifying your objectives coming to life at the heart center.
2. *Chair twist.*
3. *Low lunge twist.*
4. *Warrior II.*
5. *Temple.*
6. *Temple twist.*
7. *Spread-leg forward bend.*
8. *Downward dog.*
9. *Plank.*
10. *Locust.*
11. *Rocking bow.* Rock forward and back (Bow), and side to side (Side bow), massaging the internal organs. [Students will literally roll off their mats.]
12. *Downward dog split.* Lift one leg to prepare for wild thing.
13. *Wild thing.*
14. *Child's pose.*

After resting in child's pose, repeat the sequence on the opposite side.

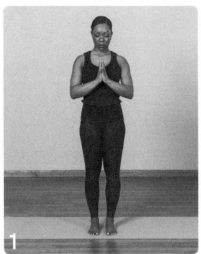

Mountain

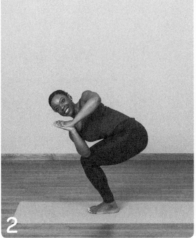

Chair twist

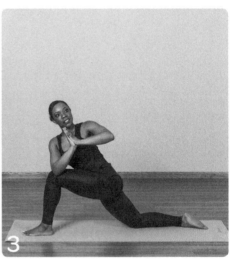

Low lunge twist

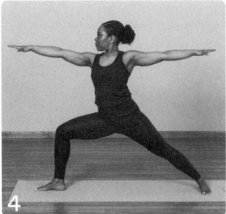

Warrior II

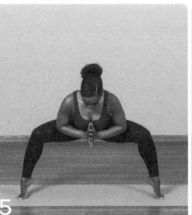

Temple

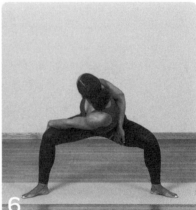

Temple twist

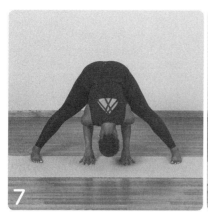

**7** Spread-leg forward bend

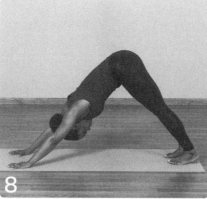

**8** Downward dog

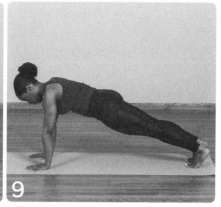

**9** Plank

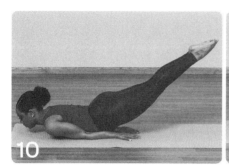

**10** Locust

**ROCKING BOW**

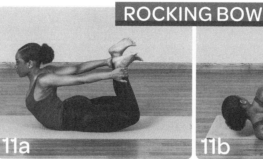

**11a** Bow

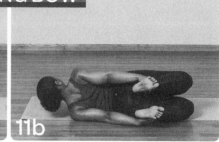

**11b** Side bow

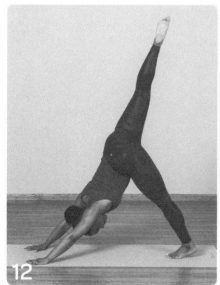

**12** Downward dog split

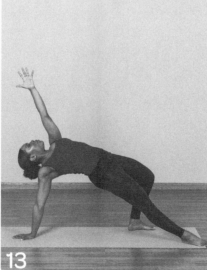

**13** Wild thing

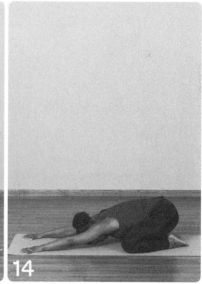

**14** Child's pose

## Seated Detoxifiers

A healthy digestive agni ("fire") is key for good health. Agni provides the physical power of digestion as well as the energy to digest your sensory impressions, thoughts, and feelings. A strong agni boosts courage and prevents you from ingesting and producing more energy blocks.

○ *Churning.*

○ *Seated spread-leg stretch.*

○ *Leg cradles.*

○ *Twist.* Use an equal four-to-four breath. Exhale to a count of 4, and inhale to a count of 4. Hold the twist on each side for 3 complete breaths.

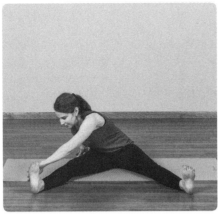

Churning

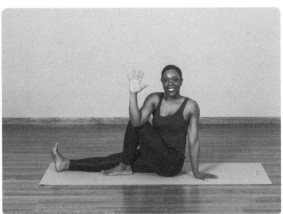

Seated spread-leg stretch

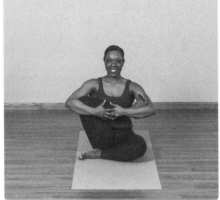

Leg cradles

Twist

## INVERSION: LEGS UP THE WALL

One of the secrets of detoxification is to invert the body. Turning upside down encourages circulation of blood and lymph from the feet and legs to reduce swelling as it bathes the abdomen in fresh blood, and stimulates the digestive organs.

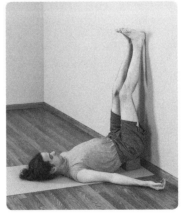

Legs up the wall with a block under the sacrum

### Energies of Pranayama

Let's move on to pranayama, the control of the prana in the consciousness. Pranayama techniques are designed to gain mastery over the breath while recognizing the link between the breath, the mind, and the emotions.

Pranayama practices are tools to help you control the thought waves of the mind. When you inhale, you draw universal energy into the body. When you exhale, you remove toxins from the system, providing more room for prana to exist and expand. There are literally dozens of pranayama exercises; the following are the basic cleansing practices.

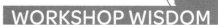

**WORKSHOP WISDOM**

The breath is the barometer for the mind and body.

> These exercises are not recommended for students who have untreated high blood pressure, glaucoma, detached retina, heart conditions, or are pregnant. If students become dizzy, have them stop and return to normal diaphragmatic breathing.

## EQUAL BREATH WITH HOLD

The four-to-four breath consists of inhalations and exhalations of equal duration. After 4 complete breaths, we'll add a 4-count hold on the inhalation. Visualize releasing stagnant energy on the exhalation and creating more open space filled with fresh, nourishing light, clean energy, and oxygen on the inhalation.

1. Inhale to a count of 4. On count one, fill the space from the pelvic floor to the navel center; on count 2, bring the breath to rise from the navel center to the heart center; on count 3, move the breath from the heart center to the throat; and on count 4, move it from the throat to the crown of the head.
2. Exhale to a count of 4, moving the breath in reverse order. On count 1, exhale from the crown of the head to the throat center; on count 2, from the throat to the heart; on count 3, from the heart to the navel center; and on 4, from the navel center to the pelvic floor.
3. Repeat this pattern 3 more times.
4. Let's add the hold on the inhalation. Inhale to a count of 4, then hold the breath in for a count of 4, allowing the oxygen to penetrate to the blood stream, expanding the torso big and round, filling with light energy; follow with the 4-count exhalation.
5. Repeat this pattern 3 more times.

## BHASTRIKA BREATH

Bhastrika (bellows) breath is a rapid, forceful exhalation and inhalation practiced with mouth closed. Over time, you can learn to take the breath rapidly without hyperventilating or feeling dizzy. At the beginning, though, take each breath quickly but completely. Bhastrika tones and detoxifies the organs of digestion, elimination and reproduction, stimulates the adrenals to balance the nervous system and calm anxiety, and helps clear the lungs of phlegm.

1. Begin on an exhalation, pulling the belly in and up.
2. Inhaling, open wide, sending the breath into the pelvic area down into the sit bones.
3. Exhaling, pull the belly in and up. Let go of what's no longer needed.
4. Inhaling wide and strong, imagine a ball of light expanding inside of you.
5. Exhaling, slowly increase the speed of the breath, sharply focusing on pulling in the navel center.
6. On the inhalation, slowly increase the speed of the breath, sipping more air in as you widen the torso.

7. Continue the practice, increasing the speed and fortitude of the breaths for 1 to 2 minutes.

When you've completed the exercise, return to normal diaphragmatic breathing, sitting quietly while noticing the effects of bhastrika.

**NADI SHODHANA**

Practice one round of nadi shodhana (alternate-nostril breathing) before guided relaxation. (For teaching instructions on nadi shodhana, see chapter 2.)

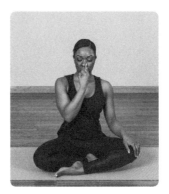

Alternate-nostril breathing

## Moving Forward

[This guided meditation is done while students are in savasana. Allow 1 to 2 minutes for a quiet rest before beginning the meditation script.]

*When you feel ready and cleared of your inner chatter, direct your mind's eye to the crown of your head. Imagine a tiny white light directly above the crown. Visualize it as a small beam of light energy, no bigger than a dime.*

*Imagine that bright white light is pulsating with energy. Focusing on this energy, start to move the light downward through your head, face, neck, shoulders, arms, and chest. The light spreads as it moves through its path. Imagine this light is like an eraser, deleting toxins, tensions, worries, old stories, and waste. All it leaves behind is its pure, glowing white light. Sense your body responding to the natural vibrations of this radiating light.*

*Continue guiding the light through your chest to the abdomen, back muscles, along the spinal column, the pelvic center, groin, thighs, knees, ankles, and the tips of your toes. Allow it to eliminate all the chatter, worries, and emotional garbage. Feel the light pulsing through the veins, muscles, and bones. Now with your exhale, release these toxins out through the soles of your feet. Feel the earth absorb these obstacles as they make their exit.*

*Let all your fears, worries, guilt, regrets, and destructive thoughts surface in your mind, imagining them as a muddy stream flowing out of every pore as you exhale. Feel yourself releasing old hurts, sadness, anger, grief, heaviness, and anxieties. Let go of pain. Feel it dissolving and pouring out of your body. As the old, tangled energy flows out, begin to sense a new lightness. Feel a new power that opens space for gratitude, forgiveness, well-being, and success. This glowing light energy is now in full swing inside you.*

*In your mind's eye, invite the people in your life who are able to respect and honor your growth and change. Dwell in this new space, opening your heart, expressing gratitude for your life, to grow and move forward. Honor yourself for the courage to clean your own house.*

*Breathe in patience, discipline, and action, or any feeling or expression that will help you in this new beginning.*

*Picture what you'd like to receive in your life, and see yourself receiving these gifts. Feel yourself radiating with positive energy as you attract new ideas, resources, situations, and people.*

*Notice how hungry you are for this change. You feel joyful and content with your new reality. You are now living with a new sense of energy, buoyancy, and lightness.*

[Pause several minutes for inner reflection.]

*Begin to come back to your outer world.*

*Open your eyes. Take time to wiggle your toes and fingers, rock the head from side to side, and roll to the right side. At your own pace, rise to a seated position.*

**WORKSHOP WISDOM**

Be transparent in knowing who you are so that you can be as alive as possible!

Today and every day, drink plenty of water to rid the system of waste and flush out the organs of elimination such as the skin, lungs, liver, and kidneys.

Refer to your detox objectives, and make them part of your daily ritual to prohibit the retox effect, especially on the days when you're feeling sluggish. Be curious about your daily well-being. Ask yourself the important questions, such as *Did I get enough sleep?*, *Am I still angry with my partner?*, or *What is the basis for this feeling of worry?* Find out what form this retox is taking so that you can scrub it out as soon as it comes to mind. With these practices, you have the ability to be swept clean.

Have a wonderful day, drink lots of water, and stay quiet and clear of toxic situations and people. Your body and mind did a lot of work, and they need time to acclimate to their new energy.

Thank you for joining me. Remember, no one can go back in time to erase mistakes, but we always have the choice to start where we are now and begin again.

## Teacher Tip

After the workshop, stay to answer questions and check in with your students' results. Use their feedback for the next time you hold the workshop!

# THE JOY OF BACKBENDS

## Intention

To learn the ease and subtleties of gentle to advanced backbends.

**Preparation/props:** Blocks, blankets, bolsters, straps

**Duration:** 2 hours

**Target:** Beginning to advanced yoga students; some yoga experience is recommended.

**Caution:** Not recommended for students with spinal injuries, chronic back pain, or pregnant women.

## Opening

If you're here because you love bending over backwards, you're in the right place. If you're here because you want to *learn* to love bending over backwards, you're also in the right place. Yoga backbends work on the great unknown—the part of the body that you can't actually see, you can only feel—the back. This workshop will stimulate, energize, and awaken your heart, body, and spine. That's why it's called the *Joy* of Backbends. At the end of this practice, you're going to feel good.

Healthy backbends are stimulating and exciting. They deliver quick relief from low energy and mild depression because they provide openness and confidence in the body. It feels like you're unlocking the heavy armor around the heart and lungs, freeing yourself from hidden fears and difficulties. Backbends have the ability to bolster a new sense of expansion and determination.

As I mentioned, backbends can strongly influence your emotional states. For instance, as you move your energy up the spine, backbends thrust your full lifeforce up through a central channel called sushumna, and along the way, it burns through blockages and stuck tissues.

To experience the exhilaration of backbends though, we first need to properly establish the groundwork for a safe, stable, and strong pose. Once we get inside the stability of a sound base with warmed muscles, we're ready to go to new levels of energetic freedom.

Backbends infiltrate many poses, including warrior I, cat, crescent lunge, low lunge, cobra, sphinx, upward dog, camel, bow, locust, bridge, and wheel. When done safely with awareness, backbends help preserve the health of the vertebrae and spinal discs, and they open the body to deep diaphragmatic breathing.

Whether you want to drop back into wheel or find a pain-free upward dog, today's workshop gives you the opportunity to get playful with your practice and try things you might believe you can't do, or don't know *how* to do. We'll work through a progression of poses as we learn and experience the principles of building the backbend.

Yoga is about oneness and the integration of the body, mind, and spirit. So, when areas of the front, back, and sides of the body are closed down, it creates a feeling of disjointedness and limits the flow of energy. Low energy is a common cause of mild depression, fear, and even self-doubt. You're not going to conquer the world or even show up to a social engagement when you can barely get off the couch!

The backbend is a natural rejuvenator. The physical aspects of backbends work counter to negative impressions, because they improve circulation along the spine, which lifts your body as well as your spirits, and relieves symptoms of feeling closed off from the world.

### WORKSHOP WISDOM

A consistent and properly executed yoga practice that includes a variety of backbends can relieve fear and anxiety, increase the body's resilience helping maintain its youth, and eliminate chronic back pain.

### Three Steps to Healthy Backbends

1. *Get ready.* A healthy backbend starts in the mind. Begin by closing the eyes, feeling all the possibilities within the body, and open to receive a new challenge. Set your mind on lengthening the body before any movement begins.

2. *Lead with the breath.* Backbends aren't any different than any other posture; the breath leads the mind and the movement. Much more than an inhalation and exhalation, the breath is the most powerful conscious force in your body.

Most students who strain in a pose are often holding the breath. They're probably holding the breath off the mat as well. Backbends are inhalation-focused poses, so even and steady breathing while concentrating on completing the exhalation inhibits overstimulation of the sympathetic nervous system. This focus makes for a calmer, energetic result.

3. *Respect your energetic space.* Sheer willpower is a force to make progress in life. However, don't let your will *exceed* your available energetic space. You don't organically "breakthrough" into a backbend, so go slow, working at your edge. The backbend is about unfolding and evolving your energy, not forcing it into a position it's not ready for. Keep working the musculature and alignment gently, without presuming to know the final shape your body will take.

Backbending opens up the heart space, which is linked to your sense of well-being and connection with others. Backbends shake you out of your comfort zone. For most people, their daily movements are usually limited to moving forward. People rarely spend time defying gravity by going upside down, backward, or even sideways. It feels natural to bend forward. It's also the instinctive movement when sitting, standing, or picking up something off the floor. Doing backbends offers an exciting way to break up the rigidity of the spine.

## The Practice: Warm Up to Bend Back

○ *Supported reclining pose.* Lie down on the back with one block behind the head and another across the shoulder blades. Practice even breathing for 2 to 3 minutes.

○ *Breathing bridge.* Inhale to press the feet to the floor while peeling the back off the ground; exhale to lower to the ground one vertebra at a time. Repeat the sequence for 6 cycles of breath.

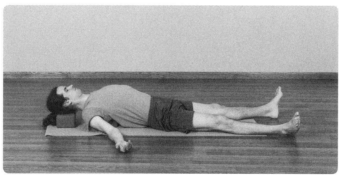

Supported reclining pose

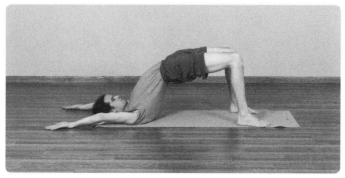

Breathing bridge

## EASY POSE MOVEMENTS

1. *Twist.*
2. *Side bend.*
3. *Arm circles.*
4. *Clam.*

5. *Seated cat.*
6. *Seated cow.*
7. *Rocking chair to standing.*
8. *Mountain.* Ground the feet, and feel the wave in the spine.

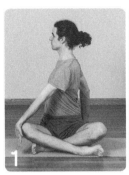

Twist

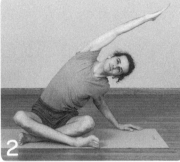

Side bend

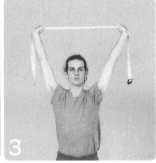

Arm circles

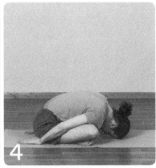

Clam pose

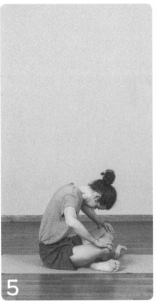

Seated cat

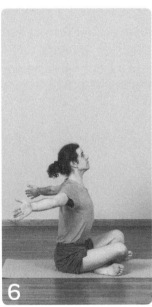

Seated cow

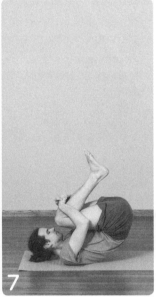

Rocking chair to standing

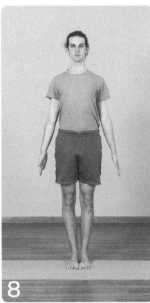

Mountain

## ADDING HEAT TO DEEPEN THE FLOW

The lumbar and cervical spine are the most flexible parts of the spine and do the lion's share of bending, which makes them the most prone to injury.

1. *Downward dog with bent knees.* Bend the knees, bring the heels off the ground, and press the palms into the ground to lengthen through the spine.

2. *Warrior I.*

3. *Warrior II.*

4. *Reverse warrior.*

5. *Side angle.*

6. *High lunge.*

7. *High lunge twist.* Focus on stretching the back quadriceps.

8. *Thread the needle.*

9. *Happy baby.*

Rest in happy baby before repeating the sequence on the opposite side.

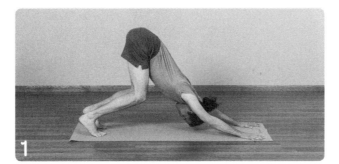

Downward dog with bent knees

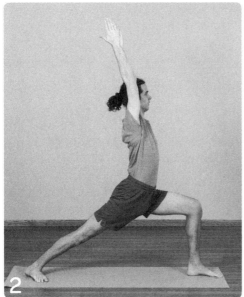

Warrior I

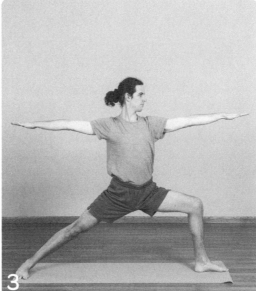

Warrior II

*(continued)*

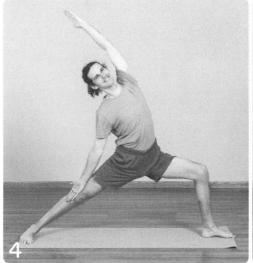

**4**

Reverse warrior

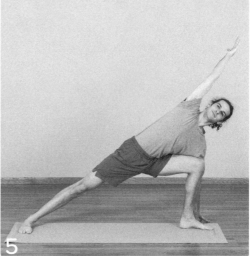

**5**

Side angle

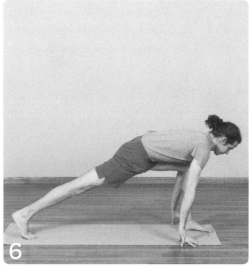

**6**

High lunge

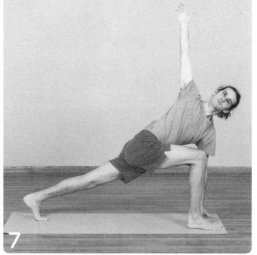

**7**

High lunge twist

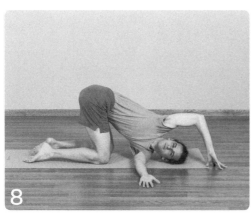

**8**

Thread the needle

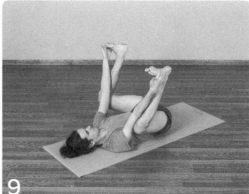

**9**

Happy baby

Don't yank or contort your body while in a pose; instead, keep your body animated with light and breath. Create more breadth by extending, widening, spreading, and unrolling the inner layers of the body. A healthy posture will have the quality of freedom.

1. *Downward dog.*

2. *Plank.* Lift the heart, press the heels back, and lift the kneecaps.

3. *Plank with knees down.* From plank, release the knees to the mat. Bend the elbows and lower the thighs, pelvic area, and belly to the ground.

4. *Sphinx.* Lift onto the forearms, press through the tops of the feet, and brighten the heart center.

5. *Unsupported cobra.* Press the tailbone down while arching the pelvis upward.

6. *Twisted downward dog.*

7. *Wild thing.*

8. *Side plank.* For supported side plank, lower the bottom knee to the ground.

9. *Downward dog.*

10. *Triangle.* Place one hand on the side of the leading leg, on the ground, or on a block, while lifting and lengthening the front and back of the pelvis. Reach up through the front and back of the heart.

11. *Child's pose.* Stretch the arms long, and breathe deeply into the lower back.

Repeat the sequence on the opposite side.

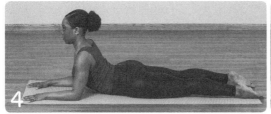

Downward dog

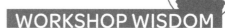

## WORKSHOP WISDOM

Unsupported cobra and locust contribute to a strong and healthy spine by strengthening the back muscles.

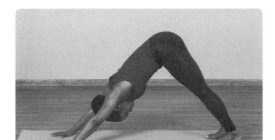

Plank

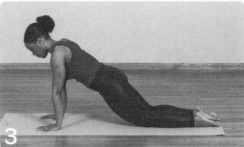

Plank with knees down

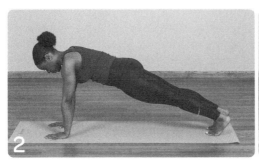

Sphinx

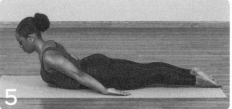

Unsupported cobra

*(continued)*

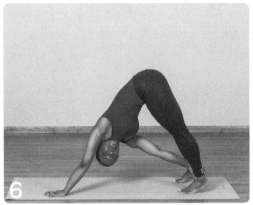

6 Twisted downward dog

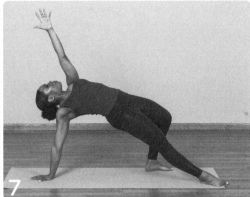

7 Wild thing

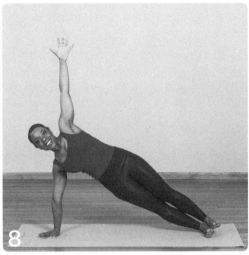

8 Side plank

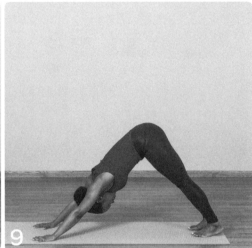

9 Downward dog

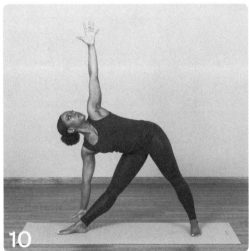

10 Triangle

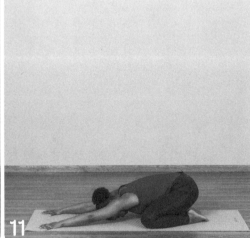

11 Child's pose

## Backbending

When you move into any spinal extension (backbend), feel for an even sensation of curving through the whole back. Each section of the spine has its own unique amount of extension available. For example, the neck and lumbar spine are naturally able to bend more than the mid- and upper back areas. Rest in child's pose between backbends.

○ *Camel.* To avoid compressing and shortening the spine, first lengthen it before pressing the hips and thighs forward. Activate the navel center by lifting from the lower belly, and avoid any sensation of compression in the spine. Place your hands on either side of the low back, or, if flexibility allows, grab the heels. Gently pull back at the base of the skull and open the throat, reaching the heart upward and quadriceps forward. To come out of the pose, lead with the heart center to rise to a vertical position, then sit on the heels to release the back. Rest in child's pose.

○ *Camel at the wall.* Place the front of the body flush to the wall, pressing the thighs forward, while moving into camel. Don't let the thighs lose contact with the wall.

○ *Upward dog.* Place the hands on blocks to add more lift and extension in the body. With the elbows tucked into the ribs, lift the pelvis toward a vertical position, pulling the chest through the arms. Once you feel the sensation of broadness in your chest, draw your shoulder blades back and lift the breastbone up. Use the leg muscles to draw the quadriceps up, squeezing the inner thighs. Rest on the belly for several breaths before taking child's pose.

○ *Bow.* Catch the ankles or feet, and lift the back of the skull, heart center, and thighs. Rise up on inhale; lower and release on exhale. Repeat 3x or take rocking bow. Rest on the belly for several breaths before taking child's pose.

○ *Bow with bolster.* Place the bolster under the front of the pelvis, across the pubic bone. The bolster presses into the abdomen and adds height to lift the thighs high off the ground.

○ *King Arthur's pose/lunge at the wall with blocks.* Facing away from the wall, first take a low lunge with the right foot forward. Next, bend the left knee and place the shin against the wall. [For students with sensitive knees, place a blanket or pillow beneath the knee.]

1. Take a low lunge with fingertips on the ground.
2. Slide your shin to the wall, placing your hands on blocks and breathe as you acclimate to the stretch.
3. Lift the chest and reach the arms and shoulder blades towards the wall.
4. Sit on the heels for several breaths before taking child's pose. Switch sides.

○ *Wheel with blocks.* This pose is the *Wow!* of backbends. Align your mat against a wall and place two blocks on the mat, flush with the wall. Lie on your back with your head pointing toward the wall and bring your hands to the edge of the blocks. Take a breath in; then exhale, rise using your arms and legs to press up into the pose. Draw your tailbone toward the knees, and lift your breastbone to the sky. Stay up for a few breaths, then slowly lower down, gently resting on the crown of the head, then the back of the skull, and finally releasing the back to the mat. Rest for a few breaths, then pull the knees toward the chest. If you're ready, try it again!

○ *Reclining twist.*

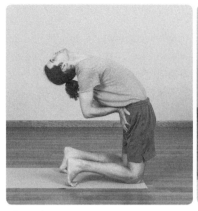

Camel

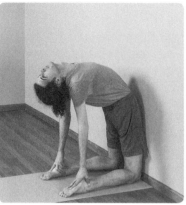

Camel at the wall

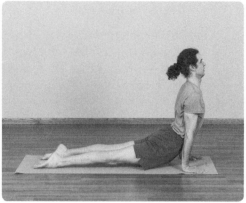

Upward dog

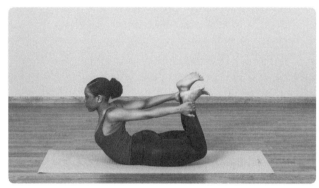

Bow

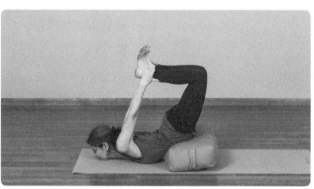

Bow with bolster

## KING ARTHUR'S POSE

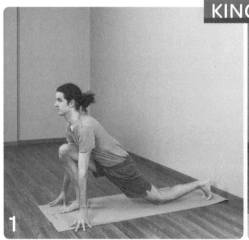

**1** Low lunge prep

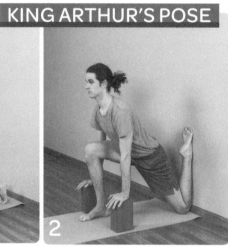

**2** Enhanced quadriceps stretch

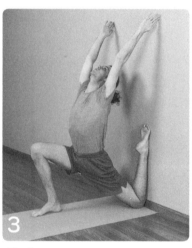

**3** Final pose

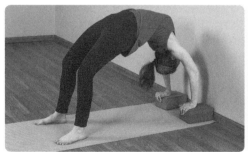

Wheel with blocks

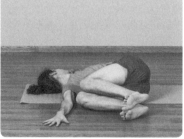

Reclining twist

**DEEP RELAXATION**

Invite relaxation into your body. Close your eyes, and move your attention inward. Feel the belly rising on the inhalation and falling on the exhalation. Let go, relax, get heavier on the mat, and experience deep comfort. Rest your muscles and bones, and allow the wide muscles along the spine to fall toward the ground. Send the breath up and down the spine, from the pelvic floor to the top of the head. Rest in the silence.

[Allow students to rest silently for 5 to 10 minutes as time allows.]

With eyes closed, rub the palms of the hands together to create heat. Place your palms over your eyes, and open the eyes. Roll to one side, and when you're ready, come to seated.

## Closing

Back bending and opening the front of the spine and musculature are exercises we need to engage in every day, otherwise, we'll fall victim to gravity, sinking further into ourselves and into the earth. People actually lose height as the spine becomes older and less flexible. Rather than sink into your soul and grow older, open and lift the heart, and experience everything life has to offer. The yogi's mission is to stay grounded in the earth while lifting up to the heavens.

Thank you so much for joining me today. Remember, if you want to have a healthy body and strong mind, you may have to bend over backwards to achieve them.

# YOGA FOR ABSOLUTE BEGINNERS

**Duration:** 2 hours

**Target:** Neophytes interested in trying a yoga class without a weekly commitment.

**Message:** A complete, nonthreatening, and friendly introduction to people unfamiliar with a yoga class.

## Teacher Tip

Prior to start, introduce yourself and help students set up their yoga mats and props. Ask them about physical difficulties to ensure they have a safe practice.

## Introduction

Hi everyone, and welcome to yoga class. Is everyone here a first timer? There's nothing like your first yoga class because there's nothing like yoga.

There's an ancient proverb, *The best time to plant a tree was twenty years ago; the second best time is now.* Let's plant that tree right now as you start your yoga journey.

Today, we're learning the basics of hatha yoga. When we're done, you'll have enough information that if you decide to join a class, you'll have a clear understanding of its components. Here's what we'll learn today.

## Teacher Tip

Keep it simple, and be approachable. Most people walking into a yoga class have very little experience with body and breath awareness. Speak in English, and skip the Sanskrit.

1. The foundation postures and how to adapt them to your physical needs
2. Simple breathing tools to help you relax and fully experience the movements
3. How to modify postures for your body
4. Guided relaxation techniques

*Yoga* means "to yoke," or to bring together. In the context of our yoga class, yoking means bringing awareness to the body, breath, and mind all at once. For example, in a typical exercise class, we use music for motivation and distraction, and we work out until we sweat and burn. In yoga, we work hard, but we practice learning about our edges, or limits; we follow the breath so that we take complete inhalations and exhalations; and we stay focused on movement. That focus is essential to releasing stress; with yoga practice we don't add stress, we remove it.

Before we start, I'd like to touch on a few essentials to a healthy practice.

- Practice in bare feet so that you can feel all points of contact with the ground for balance.
- Don't eat before coming to class. You won't be very comfortable, especially during twists, and you may even get a stomach ache.
- Turn off your phone.
- There are as many ways to practice yoga as there are people who practice it. No two bodies are alike, so I'll show variations on poses. Let me know about any preexisting injury or special conditions so I can help you.
- Avoid comparing yourself to others. This practice is all about you; there's no team-work or competition in yoga class.
- Never force the posture or the breath. Yoga practice should feel organic and natural to the body. In other words, be productive with the time you have, and don't shove your way through a pose.

You may hear a few words in Sanskrit. *Yoga* is one of them. The word *asana,* for instance, means "pose" or "posture." Another important Sanskrit term is the word *ahimsa.* This is the golden rule and it means "to do no harm." It if hurts, stop doing it or back off the strain.

As a beginner, it can be difficult to distinguish between real pain and discomfort. Discomfort is more like a nagging sensation and may change if, for example, you breathe into it, or your muscles become more flexible as your body heats up. You should not feel pain during yoga practice. Accepting the body as it is in the present moment is integral to the practice. That's how you get to know yourself and your limits. You know your own body better than anyone else. If something feels wrong, it probably is. Err on the side of safety.

Let go of self-judgment and all those little voices in your head that tell you that you're not flexible enough, that you're doing it "wrong," or that someone is better than you. There's no place for negative self-talk here. Be patient; this is new territory.

Most of all, enjoy yourself; have fun. This practice should feel good.

## Yoga and Stress Reduction

Many students come to yoga because it has been praised for its stress-reduction properties. Essentially, stress and tension cause the body to tighten up. Tension blocks energy flow. In yoga, we use the postures and mindful diaphragmatic breathing to open constricted areas of the body and the mind.

These practices help erase tension. As the body relaxes and opens, the mind becomes calmer. When the mind is calm, negative feelings such as anxiety, worry, fear, depression, and anger begin to melt away, releasing stress. This mindful, energized movement will change your physiology and your state of mind. As the mind gets clearer, you start to see the brighter side to things.

Yoga is about simply paying attention. The beginner's mind is approaching something with openness and a lack of preconceptions. It's said that in the beginner's mind there are many possibilities; in the expert's mind there are few. So, what will the possibilities bring you today?

## Breath and Body Awareness

The postures concentrate on the most important parts of a beginning practice—opening the back muscles, elongating the spine, releasing the hip area, feeling the back of the body, and stretching the breathing anatomy where energy gets blocked.

Lie down on your back. If it's more comfortable for you, bend your knees and bring your feet to the floor. Feel the sensation of lying on the ground. Sensation is the language of the body. All you need to do is listen.

Keep your attention on what you're doing. You're lying on the ground, spreading out, feeling the weight of the body, and listening to my voice. When your mind wanders off to matters of the past or of the future—work, family, to-do lists—bring it back to this moment. Just this moment.

Yoga's main ingredient is the breath. In fact, *life's* main ingredient is the breath. The breath leads every pose. You're going to learn how to breathe diaphragmatically to create a complete, deep, cleansing breath. Breathing deeply slows down heart rate, lowers blood pressure, clears the mind, and relaxes muscles. When you're not breathing fully, blood pressure goes up, heart rate increases, muscles become tense, and thinking becomes scattered. Deep breathing is the single most important thing you can do to reduce everyday stress because the breath is the link between the body and mind.

Now, feel the lungs rise and fall with each breath, like a pair of balloons. They fill on the inhalation, and empty on the exhalation. As they fill, they get rounder and longer; they grow in all directions. Feel the breath go into the back and chest, and move sideways down the waist, each breath elongating the spine.

Roughness or shortness of breath is an indicator that you're not getting a full breath and you may be forcing this exercise. Let your breath be your guide. Note the cleansing power of the exhalation and the energy of the inhalation. Slide into breath awareness, naturally.

[Remind your students to continue breathing with awareness throughout the movements.]

## Teacher Tip

After several minutes of breathing practice, guide students into child's pose to offer a safe resting pose and ask about adjustments. For instance, say, "I may give a hands-on adjustment to offer a better alignment in a pose, but please raise your hand to let me know if you would rather not be touched."

◯ *Knee to chest.* Hug one knee into the chest; release; and hug the other knee into the chest.

◯ *Both knees to chest.*

◯ *Reclining twist.*

- *Reclining side stretch.* This shape stretches the intercostal muscles between the ribs.
- *Reclining hamstring stretch with strap.*

- *Reclining leg cradles.*
- Roll to your left side, and come up to a seated position.

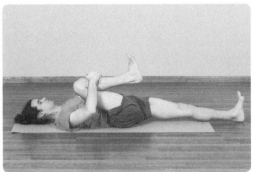
Knee to chest

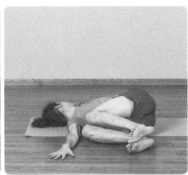
Knees to chest

Reclining twist

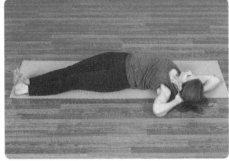
Reclining side stretch

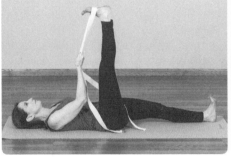
Reclining hamstring stretch with strap

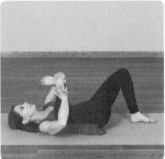
Reclining leg cradles

## Seated Poses

Sit with your head, neck, and trunk in alignment. Roll the shoulders up, back, and down to broaden the collar bones and upper back. Extend the crown of your head upward so that you feel lifted and lighter. Most people have no idea how good their body is supposed to feel until they begin a yoga practice. [Walk around the room and make adjustments on students, gently pulling shoulders back, pressing the back of the heart in and up, and offering props where needed.]

**WORKSHOP WISDOM**

The child's pose is one of gratitude and humility. It's also a pose of wisdom—the wisdom to know when to stop and relax, and when to keep going.

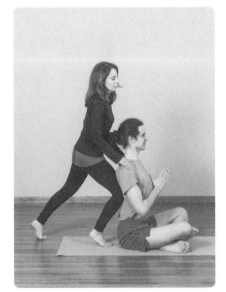
Seated adjustment

- *Neck rolls.*
- *Side stretches.*
- *Clam.*
- *Twist.*
- *Pelvic tilt.*
- *Table balance.*
- *Cat-cow.* Exhale, squeezing the air out through the back; inhale to release the belly and expand the chest, drawing the pubic bone away from the navel.
- *Downward dog with bent knees.* Bend the knees and rise up on the toes, lift the sit bones, and stretch the back body.
- *Child's pose.*
- *Mountain.*
- *Palm tree.*

- *Tree.* Concentrate on a focus point on the floor a few feet in front of you. Grow, extend, and stay put. Notice when your mind meanders.
- *Forward bend.*
- *Low lunge.* Place your fingertips on the floor or on a block. Note where the stretch begins and ends.
- *Rest.* Rest on your back to feel the effects of the new movements.

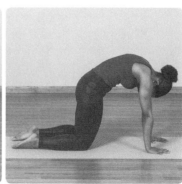

## WORKSHOP WISDOM

Every time you catch yourself saying something negative to yourself, it has a tiny but measurable negative effect on your body. Think about what you think as well as what you say.

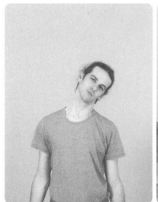

Neck rolls

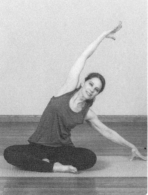

Side stretches

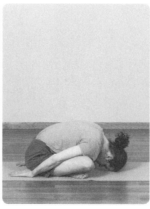

Clam

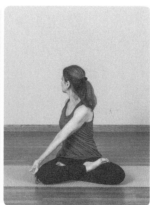

Twist

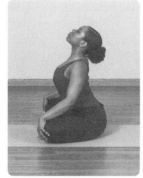

Pelvic tilt

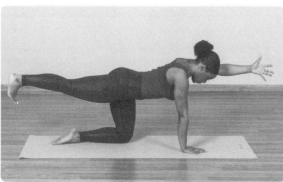

Table balance

Cat-cow

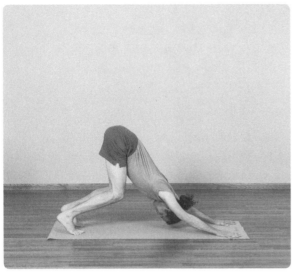

Downward dog with bent knees

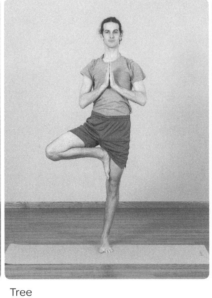

Child's pose

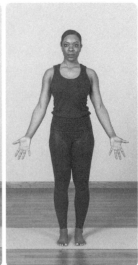

Mountain

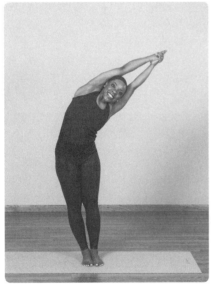

Palm tree

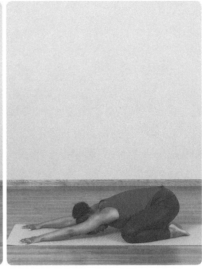

Tree

Forward bend

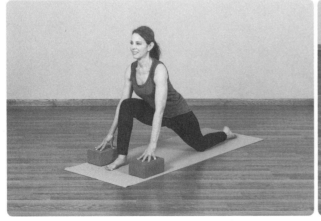

Low lunge

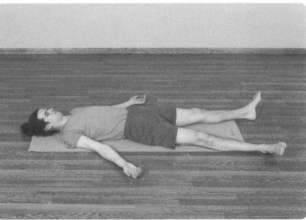

Rest

## Standing Poses

1. *Warrior I.* The spiritual warrior is someone who aims to live life with compassion and strength.
2. *Crescent lunge.*
3. *Warrior II.* Honor and accept life in the present moment without wavering to the past or future.
4. *Side angle.*

5. *Triangle.* Bring the body into energetic observance. Watch the energy flow from the feet, up the legs and spine, through the arms.
6. *Reverse warrior.*
7. *Downward dog.* Choose bent or straight legs.
8. *Child's pose.* Rest for several breaths.

[Repeat the sequence on the opposite side.]

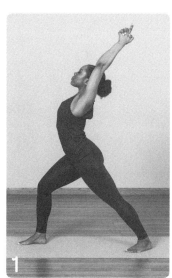

Warrior I

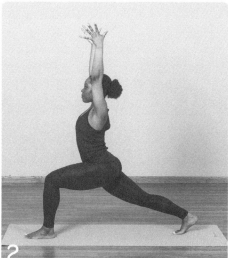

Crescent lunge

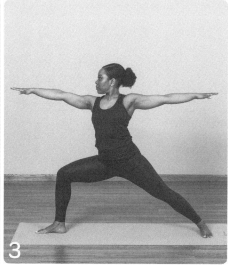

Warrior II

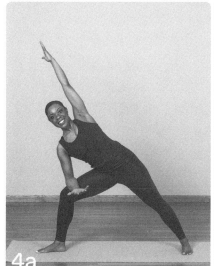

Side angle with arm resting on thigh

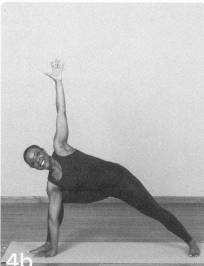

Side angle with hand to inside of foot

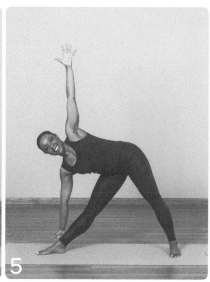

Triangle

*(continued)*

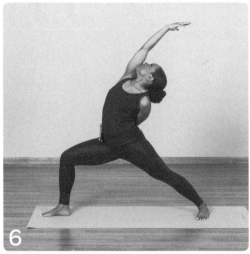

6 Reverse warrior

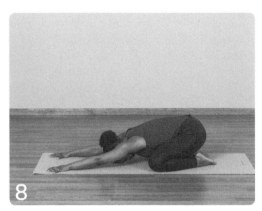

7 Downward dog

8 Child's pose

## COBRA FLOW

1. *Plank.*
2. *Plank with knees on the ground.*
3. *Unsupported cobra.*
4. *Plank with knees on the ground.*
5. *Plank.*
6. *Downward dog.*
7. *Child's pose.*

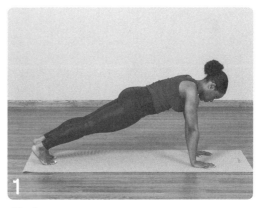

Plank

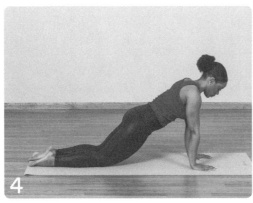

Plank with knees on the ground

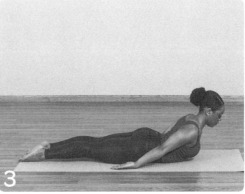

Unsupported cobra

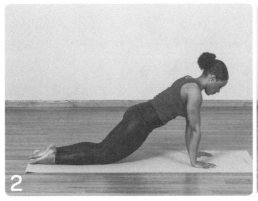

Plank with knees on the ground

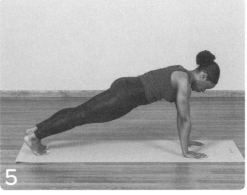

Plank

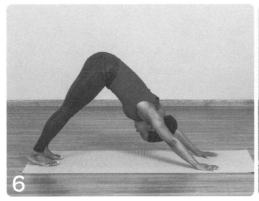

Downward dog

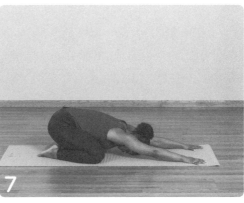

Child's pose

## SUN SALUTATION

[Refer to the instructions and benefits in chapter 4.]

1. *Mountain.*
2. *Forward bend.*
3. *Low lunge.*
4. *Downward dog.*
5. *Plank.*
6. *Plank with knees on the ground.*
7. *Unsupported cobra.*
8. *Plank with knees on the ground.*
9. *Downward dog.*
10. *Low lunge.* The opposite leg is forward.
11. *Forward bend.*
12. *Mountain.*

Repeat on opposite side. (After completing, lie on your back for several breaths to feel the effects of the sun salutation.)

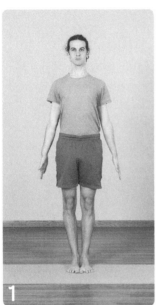

Mountain

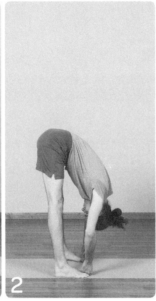

Forward bend

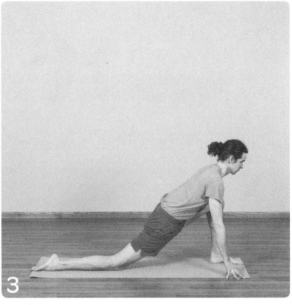

Low lunge

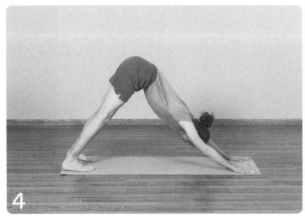

Downward dog

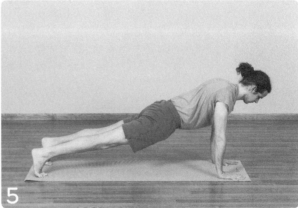

Plank

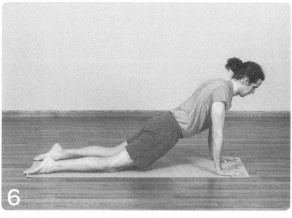

6

Plank with knees on the ground

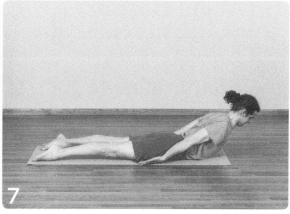

7

Unsupported cobra

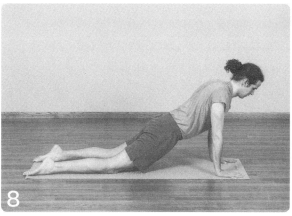

8

Plank with knees on the ground

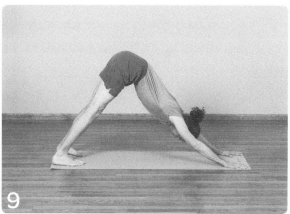

9

Downward dog

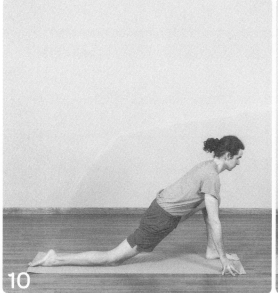

10

Low lunge

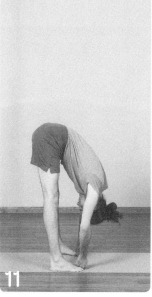

11

Forward bend

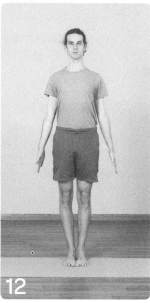

12

Mountain

## Working to the Edge

○ *Dragon.* Dragon permits stagnant energies to move through the hips and back. Ask your body to release what it no longer needs.

○ *Yogi bicycles.*

○ *Single-leg lifts.*

○ *Bridge.*

○ *Reclining butterfly.*

○ *Happy baby.*

○ *Legs up the wall.*

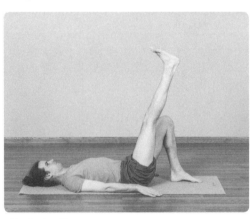

Dragon

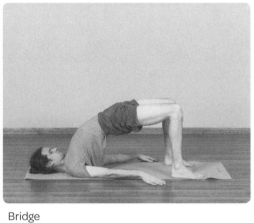

Yogi bicycles

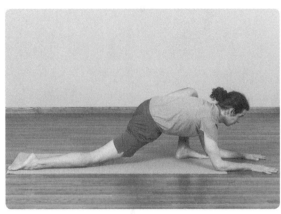

Single-leg lifts

Bridge

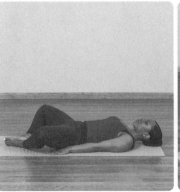

Reclining butterfly

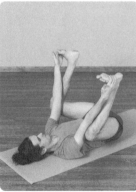

Happy baby

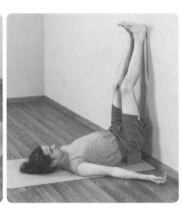

Legs up the wall

### Breathing Practice: Alternate-Nostril Breathing

(For the benefits and teaching instructions on alternate-nostril breathing, refer to chapter 2.)

**RELAXATION**

Stress is cumulative, but so is relaxation. Just like anything else, you have to practice it to be good at it.

Our last pose of the day is called savasana. The word *savasana* means "corpse pose," and it's the closing relaxation pose practiced in most classes. Lie on your back with the palms open and relaxed, arms about 8 to 10 inches from the sides of your body, and place your head on the flat part of the skull. Close your eyes.

Make yourself as comfortable as possible, and remain in this position unless you begin to experience intense discomfort. Constant adjusting or fidgeting will prevent you from experiencing the effects of deep relaxation. If you have any discomfort in your low-back area, place a rolled towel beneath your knees or keep your knees bent with the feet wide and grounded on the mat.

[Refer to the "Be a Corpse" script in chapter 17.]

You cannot always control what happens in the external world, but through mindfulness and a healthy yoga practice, you can always control what happens on the inside.

At the end of a yoga class, we bring our hands together in prayer position, bow to each other, and say the word *Namaste*. It means "the light in me honors the light in you." Thank you so much for joining me today. Namaste.

## Teacher Tip

Allow at least 5 minutes at the end of the workshop for questions.

# INTRODUCTION TO MEDITATION

## Intention

To learn the basics of a mindful meditation practice.

**Tools:** Tissues, pens, paper, raisins, small plastic shot glasses, napkins, handouts, blocks, cushions, and chairs for students who are not comfortable seated on the floor.

**Target:** Open to all.

**Duration:** 2 hours

Before the workshop begins, give each student a pen and a small pad of paper. Place about 5 to 10 raisins in each plastic shot glass, preparing enough shot glasses so that each student has their own. Before beginning the raisin meditation, serve the shot glasses from a tray.

## Opening

*Once upon a time there was student who went before a great sage seeking enlightenment. He asked the sage how to find it, but the sage just sat there. He asked the question again, and again the sage just sat there. The student tried different words and appealed with great emotion. The sage just sat there. Finally, frustrated, the student said, "Why don't you answer me?" The sage looked up, smiled and said, "I have been answering you, but you weren't listening. The answer you seek can only be found within."*

That's what we learn from meditation. Meditation asks us to be still, patient, and listen. Yoga philosophy says that the answers we seek are already inside us. Your enlightenment, joy, and contentment are going to be much different than mine, or anyone else's in the room. Meditation shows you how to access it.

Today, we'll learn meditation from a mindfulness point of view. First, we'll practice asana and breathing exercises to stretch tight areas so we can sit in meditation without body distractions. Then, we'll have several short meditation practices.

You all have paper and pens to journal your meditations. This is a way to track the developments in your practice. I often keep paper and a pen next to me when I sit so that if a "to-do" or new thought comes up that I want to remember, I can write it down and put it aside rather than let it interrupt my flow.

Speaking of which, that's what the mind does really well; it interrupts. All the time. It's called *monkey mind*. It may even be happening right now. Thoughts are like little monkeys swinging from limb to limb, in constant motion. It's like a 3-year-old who wants your attention *NOW*. And that's when you say to the 3-year-old, "Be still. I'll be there when I'm done."

## Meditation 1: Mindfulness

Let's use our first meditation as a baseline for the others yet to come.

This first meditation introduces you to your mind and the little monkey who really wants to distract you. All you have to do is close your eyes and observe your thoughts for about a minute or two. Then, we'll journal about the experience.

*With your eyes closed, notice what you're thinking about. This is the first attempt to listen to your thoughts, judgments, feelings, and physical sensations, including future and past thoughts. Notice where distraction comes from, and watch those thoughts without judgment, and without trying to shut them down.*

*Focus your attention on the breath and on how the body moves with each inhalation and exhalation. Notice the movement of your body as you breathe. Observe your chest, shoulders, rib cage, and belly. Don't try to control your breath; simply focus your attention on the here and now. If your mind wanders, simply return your focus back to your breath.*

*You may be thinking,* My back hurts, *or* I'm hungry, *or you may be wondering if you're doing this right.*

*Just notice all the things that come up both physically and emotionally.*

[Long pause.]

*Notice impatience or frustration.*

[Pause for 1 minute.]

*Begin to come back to the outside world, and to this room.*

**JOURNAL ENTRY #1**

Open your eyes. Take your time to write down all the things that went on in your mind. Draw a picture or write a few key words. Maybe you noticed your heart rate or that you were cold. There's no wrong way to do this.

[After students have completed their journaling:]

So in just about 2 minutes you may have had 4, 5, 20, or 30 completely different thoughts, which is not unusual. It's also not unusual that you can't just shut down those thoughts. In fact, it's said that the mind has between 60,000 and 80,000 thoughts a day, and 90 percent of them are thoughts you've already had.

[To the Class:] Does anyone want to share anything from this first experience?

[Answer questions as needed.]

As you can see, if you want to have a productive meditation practice, you need to learn to tame the wild little monkey mind. Historically, yogis taught seated meditation at the end of the physical practice. That's what asana, the postures, were created for—to prepare you first to sit and listen to your body, then to work deeper into the mind.

The physical yoga practices open your energies, your breath, and your body so that you can surrender your distractions. And it makes sitting so much easier. It's like greasing the wheels of the mind. When you start with the body, the movements becomes the meditation. When you add meditation to your life, it makes everything else you do, *including* your yoga postures, calmer, clearer, healthier, and happier, and it awakens the changes and the joy that lie inside of you. This one aspect of meditation is crucial to the whole of mindful living. Just as we bathe every day to clean our outside body, we meditate to clean the inside. It's like *mental* floss.

If your mind is not at peace, it's difficult to be happy, even if you're living in the very best conditions. You may have good health, a loving family, and money to pay the bills, but it doesn't matter if you don't have clarity. Your mind, if you let it, can be a virtual prison. Your mind is 100 percent dependent on you to be happy.

> **WORKSHOP WISDOM**
>
> As the mind goes, so goes your world.

The most natural way to sit in meditation is to prepare for it, just as you'd prepare to do any task. Before you plant a garden, you get your garden tools and prepare the soil. A physical, meditation-in-motion practice prepares the outer body for the inner experience. In yoga class, postures help you "clean house." You notice at the end of a class, after relaxation, that you don't want to leave your mat. The body and mind are ready to sit and be still.

## Meditation in Motion

Let's explore this concept of the moving meditation. Stand up, and we'll enjoy a gentle practice to release the hips and the back, and open the breathing anatomy.

> **WORKSHOP WISDOM**
>
> Stay in touch with what you're doing now. Don't let distraction rob you of the present moment. If you're driving the car, drive the car. If you're talking to a friend, practice the pause, and listen before you speak.

1. *Mountain with arms up.*
2. *Half forward bend with bent knees.*
3. *Standing twist with arms extended.*
4. *Standing forward bend twist.*
5. *Palm tree.*
6. *Arm circles.*
7. *Swimming.*
8. *High lunge.*
9. *Low lunge to half splits.*
10. *Cat.*
11. *Child's pose.*
12. *Table with hip circles.*
13. *Downward dog.*
14. *Seated pelvic tilts with long exhalation.*
15. *Seated leg cradles.*
16. *Mermaid twist.*
17. *Face and scalp massage.*

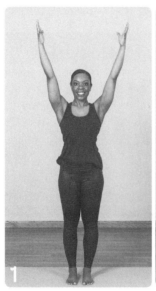

Mountain with arms up

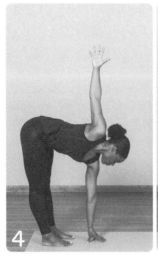

Half forward bend with bent knees

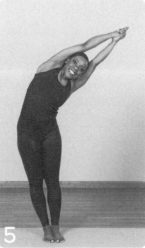

Standing twist with arms extended

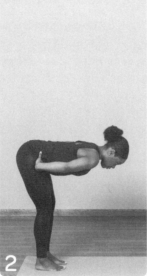

Standing forward-bend twist

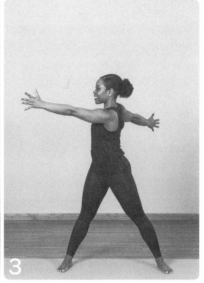

Palm tree

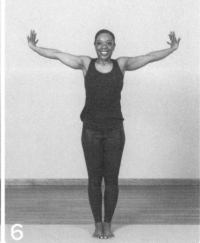

Arm circles

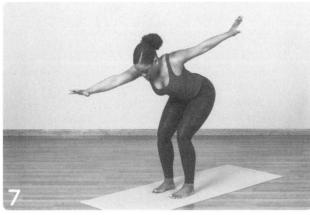

7

Swimming

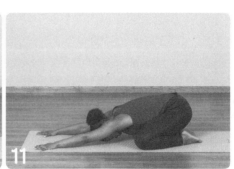

8

High lunge

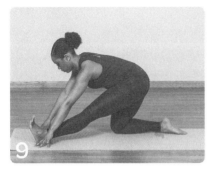

9

Low lunge to half splits

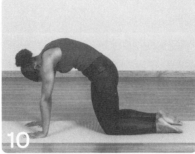

10

Cat

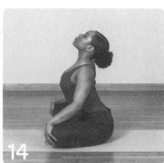

11

Child's pose

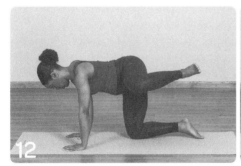

12

Table with hip circles

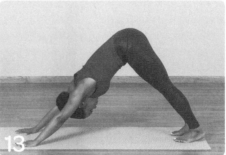

13

Downward dog

14

Seated pelvic tilts

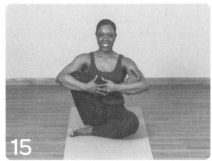

15

Seated leg cradles

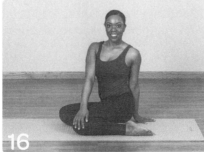

16

Mermaid twist

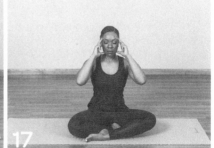

17

Face and scalp massage

## Meditation 2: The Raisin

Distribute the shot glasses of raisins to the class. Offer each student a napkin. Tell your class not to eat the raisins yet.

The raisin meditation is a simple mindfulness practice that was first developed by Jon Kabat-Zinn. It teaches you how to attend to the present moment while you learn to savor the pleasures of food, rather than eating mindlessly. Think about how you eat your meals. Many of us talk, drive, or work through our meals, never really tasting our food because we're too busy doing something else.

This raisin exercise teaches you to taste, sense, and savor your food.

> **WORKSHOP WISDOM**
>
> Mindfulness can help you gain a greater sense of control over your thoughts, feelings, and behavior in the present moment.

1. Pick up a raisin and hold it in your hand.

2. Take a good look at the raisin. Examine every part of it. Notice the softness, color, and folds. Was this *really* once a grape?

3. Using your fingertips, touch and gently squeeze the raisin, reviewing its texture.

4. Now, smell the raisin. Notice if the smell makes you feel hungry or makes your mouth water. Does the smell have any meaning to you?

5. Put the raisin on your tongue. Don't chew it yet, just feel it on your tongue and between your cheeks, and rub it up against your teeth. Explore the impression of this single raisin.

6. Begin to slowly eat the raisin. Notice where you're chewing and how the raisin comes apart in your mouth. Taste and feel its sweetness and texture.

7. When you're finished chewing, consciously swallow the raisin. Feel it in the back of your mouth, going down your throat.

8. Instead of putting another raisin in your mouth right away, notice if you can feel the raisin moving downward into your stomach.

### JOURNAL ENTRY #2

Take a few minutes to journal your experience.

When the mind wanders, bring it back to a focus point. The typical response is to react to all thoughts, which keeps the monkey mind very busy. However, stopping that pattern of busyness with meditation on a focal point, such as a raisin or the breath, is quite simple. You begin by attending to the breath, and, when a thought arises, notice it, be open to it without engaging in it or giving it energy, and allow the thought to pass. It *will* pass!

Meditation brings freedom from the mind's turmoil because it teaches you to attend to thoughts without reacting.

> **WORKSHOP WISDOM**
>
> If one engages in destructive acts or lives in a negative mind state, it's a slow and arduous process to work on one's clarity and health, much less attain inner peace.

## Pranayama Practices

Let's stand up once again, and we'll stretch around the body's breathing anatomy before practicing pranayama exercises.

1. *Standing slaps.* With open hands, gently slap the body from head to toe. Feel the tingling effect on the first layer of skin.
2. *Standing circles with knees bent.*
3. *Side angle.*
4. *Skier.*
5. *Clam.*
6. *Seated twist.*

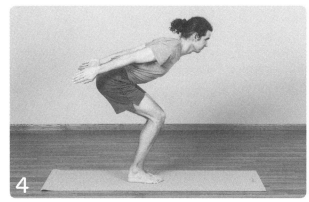

Standing slaps · Standing circles · Side angle

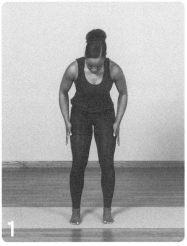
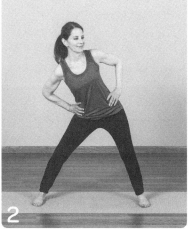
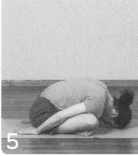
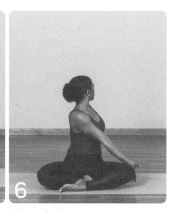

Skier · Clam · Seated twist

Pranayama is control of prana, the body's lifeforce, and it's designed to gain mastery over the breath. In meditation, pranayama is a crucial practice because it's a tool that helps you control the thought waves of the mind. When you control the breath and prana, you control what's *in* the mind. The inhalation is the process of drawing universal energy into the body.

### WORKSHOP WISDOM

Students with chronic diseases, such as untreated high blood pressure, heart patients, and pregnant women, should not practice these exercises. If you feel dizzy or nauseous, please stop and return to normal diaphragmatic breathing.

Exhalation is the removal of toxins from the system, providing room for prana to exist and expand.

There are dozens of pranayama exercises. We'll be working with some basic practices today.

- *Sama vritti.* Sama vritti breathing is when the inhalation is the same length as the exhalation. To practice, inhale to a count of five, and exhale to a count of five. Feel free to change the count to make it slower or faster.

- *Anuloma krama.* This segmented inhalation breath provides your system with more oxygen. To practice, divide the inhalation into 3 equal parts by first inhaling the first third of the breath up from the pelvic floor to the navel. Pause. Inhale the second third of breath from the navel to the heart center. Pause. Finally, inhale the last third of breath from the heart center to the crown. Pause.

    Exhale slowly and fully down to the pelvic floor. Repeat this breath 5 more times. When you've completed the exercise, sit with the eyes closed for several minutes.

- *Nadi shodhana.* Alternate-nostril breathing brings balance to both sides of the brain, body, and emotions. (For teaching and practice instructions, see chapter 2. Take one round beginning with the active or passive nostril.)

- *Kapalabhati.* Kapalabhati is an invigorating and purifying pranayama that cleans the nasal passages and lungs, stimulates the brain, and energizes the body. Following a normal inhalation, force the exhalation deeply and quickly by bringing the navel in and up toward the bottom of the lungs. Take 11 breaths, starting on the exhalation.

    Sit for 1 to 2 minutes, noticing a desirable shift in consciousness.

## Meditation 3: Mindful Body Scan

Now it's time for a meditation on the body. There are many ways to focus the mind including counting from 1 to 10, watching the breath, using a guided visualization or mantra meditation, and even walking meditation. You can add to the practices we're learning today or change them as you'd like.

This next practice combines meditation with relaxation. You can have true breakthroughs in mindfulness when you focus on something familiar, such as the body.

*Please lie on your back. Follow what I'm saying, and notice when the mind wanders.*

*Pay attention to the top of your head and, without looking for anything in particular, feel the sensations there. Then, letting your attention move downward, feel the back of your head, on either side of your head, your ears, your forehead, and inside your eyes, nose and nostrils; feel into the cheeks, mouth, and jaw. Feel your tongue touch the back of your teeth.*

*Connect directly with sensations by feeling the body from the inside.*

*With a relaxed and open awareness, begin a gradual scan of the rest of your body. Place your attention on your neck and throat, noticing the sensations that arise. Then, let your attention move to your shoulders and down your arms, feeling the vitality all the way down to your hands. Notice tingling, pulsing, pressure, warmth, or cold.*

*Watch the mind when it wanders. Notice where it goes, then bring it back to the now.*

*Move on to explore the sensations in your chest, your awareness of your upper back and shoulder blades, then down into your middle and lower back. Feel what's happening in the abdomen, hips, and buttocks. Move slowly downward through the legs and knees, feeling the muscles and bones, then the feet and toes. Notice the areas of contact, pressure, and temperature where the body touches the floor.*

*Be aware of the body as a field of changing sensations. Can you sense the subtle energy field that gives life to every cell and every organ in your body?*

*After you've spent some time with your body consciousness, open your eyes and turn your attention to this room. Then, watch what sensations arise in your body by coming back to your external world.*

*At your own pace, roll to your right side, and come to a seated position.*

**JOURNAL ENTRY #3**

Take a moment to write down any thoughts you experienced and how or when your mind wandered. Get a sense for how your mind works. Maybe you saw your heart beating or felt the muscles in your eyes. Where are you growing more mindful? Were you feeling bored or impatient? It's important to notice when those emotions arise and put them aside. Otherwise you won't grow more mindful, you'll grow more bored and impatient!

**WORKSHOP WISDOM**

Whatever you feed will grow. What you practice grows stronger.

## Meditation 4: Blue Sky Meditation

### Meditation Warm-Up

- ○ *Downward dog at the wall.*
- ○ *Upward dog at the wall.*
- ○ *Downward dog split.*
- ○ *Spread-legged forward bend twist.*

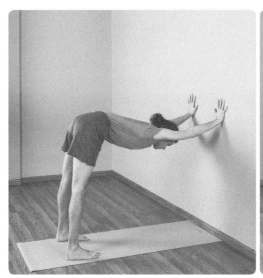

Downward dog, pushing the wall

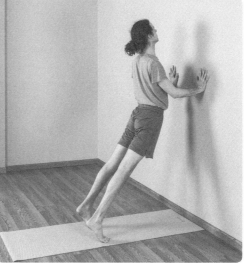

Upward dog, pushing the wall

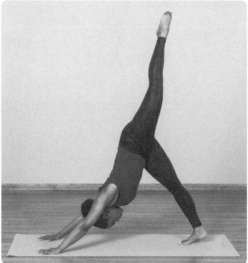

Downward dog split

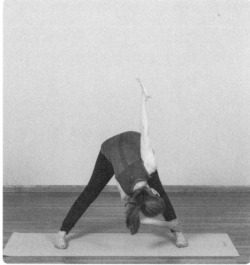

Spread-legged forward bend twist

The mind is often compared to a cup of dirty river water. When it's shaken, the water is cloudy; but when it's still, the sand settles to the bottom of the cup and the water is clear. The practice of meditation is like letting the cup of water—your mind—settle.

We react to experiences in much the same way that we react to our thoughts. If someone says something mean to us, we become angry, defensive, or depressed, and we feel that emotion in the body. If we lose something, we become upset. We become nervous when we're asked to give a speech. We can just *think* about that speech and we feel the butterflies in our stomach.

Our mood usually depends on what's in front of us and, as a result, our life is like a roller coaster of emotion. We react before we've experienced what we're reacting to. We tend to short-circuit these experiences, and we limit ourselves to one or two conditioned responses instead of responding to a situation openly and creatively.

When we use the principles of meditation and apply them to our life's events, we can objectively observe what's taking place. We see our reactions without reacting *to* them. Let yourself be open to experiencing your reactions, and let them move through you.

*Close your eyes and breathe gently through the nose, filling the lungs, then exhale through the mouth, expelling all the breath in your body. Take a few deep breaths, then continue more gently—in through the nose, out through mouth. Focus on the breath, letting go of thoughts with the exhalation.*

*Imagine a beautiful blue sky. When a thought appears, see it as a white cloud; with your exhalation, gently blow the cloud away, leaving a beautiful blue sky in your mind's eye.*

*Continue to focus on the blue sky, blowing away any new thoughts or clouds that appear. Take a look, but don't get involved. You may think,* This is a thought I've had before *or* I'm quite worried about so-and-so. *Don't allow yourself to get caught in the thought. It's a trap. Let it go.*

*Relax and let it be, enjoying the calm and peace.*

*When you feel strong and ready, invite one of the clouds into the blue sky. Look at this one thought all alone, and allow yourself to deal with it in isolation. If you want, continue dealing with each of your thoughts or questions one by one. At any time, you can choose to blow away thoughts you don't want to focus on and enjoy the calm, blue sky once again, or you can choose to look at a different thought.*

*When other thoughts appear, neither reject nor accept them. Don't try to stop thoughts; allow them to arise, but don't pursue them. The goal is not to have any thoughts; the goal is for thoughts to arise yet be rendered powerless.*

*Focus on keeping your attention in the peaceful stillness of your clear blue sky. Whenever you notice yourself residing in the cloud of a thought or a feeling, move your attention back to being the sky. Observe the cloud, and watch it drift away. Bring your mind back to the experience of stillness, of peace.*

*Clouds will come and go; be mindful not to get stuck inside one. Whenever you notice yourself getting stuck, let the cloud float away, then turn your mind to the still and peaceful brightness of your being.*

*Return to the feeling of being seated, the sound of my voice, and the physical sensation of being present in the room. Slowly open your eyes.*

With practice, you'll find that every thought you have will enable you to proceed from blue sky mind. You'll stop running off with your delusions and distractions when they arise. You'll see them as clouds, coming and going all day long. You'll become the watcher of your mind matter. When negative thoughts and emotions arise, they'll only have the power you give them.

**WORKSHOP WISDOM**

The more time you spend with the blue sky, the less time you'll spend in the clouds.

**JOURNAL ENTRY #4**

What did you see in the clouds? Where you able to observe your thoughts, or did you get caught in them? Did you have the same thoughts over and over? Did you have the same thoughts you had during the first meditation? Notice the difference between the first meditation and the last one.

## Closing

I want to leave you with a parable about meditation and nonattachment. Whether things are good or bad, it's inevitable that they'll change. The waves of the mind can be choppy at times, but a consistent practice will help you stay in control of your thoughts.

*A student went to his meditation teacher and said, "My meditation is horrible! I feel so distracted."*

*"It will pass," the teacher said matter-of-factly.*

*A week later, the student came back to his teacher and said, "My meditation is wonderful! I feel so aware, so peaceful, so alive! It's just wonderful!"*

*The teacher replied matter-of-factly, "It will pass."*

Understand there's no wrong way to meditate. If your mind wanders or you have trouble quieting your thoughts, it's easy to think that you're not doing it right and give up. But don't. You can't get meditation wrong.

Remember that you can't avoid problems, but you can change their meaning and your reactions to them.

[Allow time for questions and shared experiences. Make yourself available for one-on-one questions.]

# TRANSFORMATIONAL BREATH

**Duration:** 1.5 hours

**Audience:** Experienced yogis

**Props:** Blocks, bolsters, blankets, tissue

## Opening

Today, we're focusing on pranayama, yogic breathing exercises, to spearhead your yoga practice. The word *pranayama* means "control of lifeforce;" *prana* means "lifeforce" or "energy," and *yama* means "control."

To understand the holistic practices of yoga, recognize the importance of prana in your life. The breath is the most significant way to bring prana into your consciousness. We also receive prana from food, sleep, and love. If your emotions are disturbed or if your sleeping and other habits are unhealthy, prana will be scattered and your valuable lifeforce will be lost or wasted. To be strong and healthy, you have to learn how to maintain your prana.

Prana follows thought. That means if you're thinking negatively, your energy will add to that negativity and help it grow. Be mindful of your lifeforce when you're under stress; you can lose prana. If you're worrying about five different things at once, you may have prana bursting out of you in five different directions. Or, if you're angry with someone, you may be giving that person or just the *thought* of that person, your available energy, your precious lifeforce. Don't feed your problems.

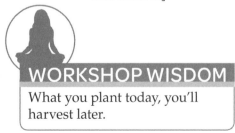

**WORKSHOP WISDOM**

Watch for tension in the body and mind, which restricts the flow of lifeforce.

Breathing practices are the most powerful tools available to achieve mental balance, control stress, create a healthy immune system, and lead a more joyous life. As a stand-alone practice, the results of pranayama are transformational.

The practices in this workshop were designed to help unclog the nadis, the body's subtle energy channels. These channels are like little rivers inside of you where your energy flows. It's said that humans have over 72,000 of these rivers. To keep your energy running smoothly, your practices should clean out any physical and emotional obstacles that keep you from moving forward.

Inhalation, or inspiration, is the process of taking in and filling up with the universe's energy. Exhalation, or expiration, is the removal of toxins, both physical and mental, from the system. Too many toxins and negative thoughts are like weeds in a garden; they take up space where prana should grow.

### Pranayama Practice 1

○ Let's come to stand.

○ *Breath of joy.* [See chapter 4 for practice instructions.]

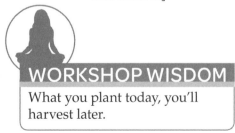

**WORKSHOP WISDOM**

What you plant today, you'll harvest later.

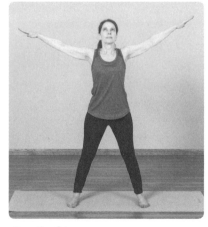

Breath of Joy

### STAGNANT ENERGY RELEASE (SEATED)

The powerful exhalations in this exercise build heat, burn off impurities, and stoke the breath.

1. Take a deep breath into the lower belly.
2. Exhale, pulling the navel in toward the spine to empty out completely.
3. Inhale into the lower belly, filling the pelvic floor, hips, and back with air.
4. Continue for 1 to 2 minutes. Concentrate on the exhalation, emptying completely, as you visualize sweeping away stagnant energy.

### ANULOMA KRAMA

Anuloma krama uses a segmented three-part inhalation to deliver more oxygen into your system. As you inhale, visualize the torso as a tall glass. Each breath fills the glass with more water until it's filled to the top. Exhaling, pour all the water out.

1. Inhale the first third of the breath from the pelvic floor to the navel center. Pause.
2. Inhale the second third of breath from the navel to the heart center. Pause.
3. Inhale the last third of breath from the heart center to crown. Pause.
4. Hold the breath in for a count of 4, savoring the air in the lungs.
5. Exhale slowly and fully down to the pelvic floor.
6. Repeat the sequence 5 times.

## Asana

Asana practice prepares the body for more advanced breathing exercises by reducing body tension, opening the areas that support the breathing anatomy, and bringing awareness to the flow of breath.

One way to motivate your movement is to examine the areas of your life where you want to be most productive. Then consider clearing these areas, which could be physical, professional, financial, spiritual, or emotional, using your mindful ujjayi breath.

### Supine Poses

○ *Knees to chest.* Use ujjayi breath, pulling the knees to the chest on the exhalation and releasing on the inhalation. Repeat 6 times.
○ *Reclining twist.*
○ *Breathing bridge.* Use a three-part inhalation to rise up, hold the breath in for a count of 4, then lower down slowly with the exhalation. Repeat 6 times.
○ *Seated pelvic tilts.*
○ *Side stretch.*
○ *Neck stretches.*

> **WORKSHOP WISDOM**
> Observe how different postures change your breathing patterns and what energetic feelings arise with these changes.

> **WORKSHOP WISDOM**
> If you're filled with toxins, tensions, and closed-down body parts, you won't have room for prana to flow, or the ability to move forward and make progress in your life.

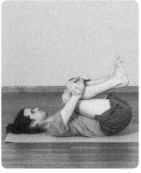
Knees to chest

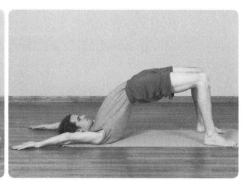
Reclining twist

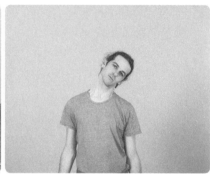
Breathing bridge

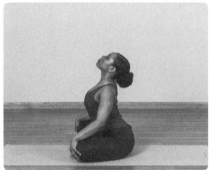
Seated pelvic tilts

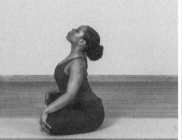
Side stretch

Neck stretch

## LION'S BREATH

The lion's breath eliminates toxins accumulated in the heart and throat center, and frees the mind from pent-up frustration. Sit on the heels, inhale and rise up off the heels, stick out the tongue, look up at the third eye, and on the exhalation, roar like a lion.

Beat the chest and belly. Exhale the lion's breath on every third breath.

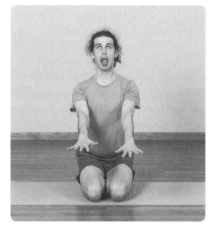
Lion's breath

## ASANA WITH KAPALABHATI

(See chapter 6 for instructions on teaching kapalabhati.) Kapalabhati is a pranayama technique that massages the abdominal organs, improves respiration, and purifies the frontal region of the brain. Thanks to its forceful method of waking up the mind, it's known as the shining skull breath.

1. *Scrape the barrel.* Use kapalabhati breath to circle the breath through the torso.
2. *Cat-cow-dog series.* Exhale kapalabhati as you round the spine; inhale lifting the sit bones, relaxing the belly *(photo a)*. From cat, exhale kapalabhati, holding the breath out of the lungs and belly, soaring the navel toward the spine, and lifting into downward dog *(photo b)*. On the inhalation, lower the knees to the ground, raising the sit bones and heart *(photo c)*. Repeat the sequence 3 times.

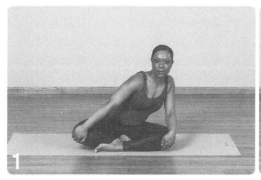

Scrape the barrel

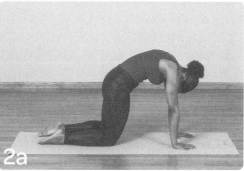

Cat

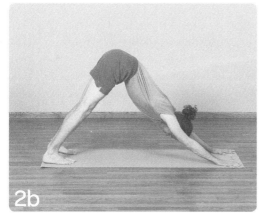

Downward dog

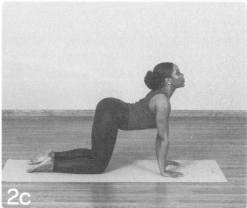

Cow

## Standing Poses

- ○ *Sun salutations.* (See chapter 4 for practice instructions.) Use a smooth, rhythmic ujjayi breath to maintain concentration and ensure that prana spreads heat equally through your body. While facing east, practice 4 to 6 rounds of sun salutations, purifying the body's rivers of energy and empowering the muscles and bones.

- ○ *Crescent lunge twist. (arms spread side to side)*

- ○ *Dragon.*

- ○ *Moon dips with kapalabhati breaths.* Practice 6 times on each side.

- ○ *Stand to squat with kapalabhati breaths.* Practice 6 times.

- ○ *Triangle.*

- ○ *Side angle.*

- ○ *Side angle with reach.*

- ○ *Pyramid.* Use a three-part breath to lift and release. Repeat the breath sequence 6 times.

- ○ *Revolved triangle.*

- ○ *Half moon.*

- ○ *Chair twist.*

**WORKSHOP WISDOM**

Clearing away objects and habits that no longer serve you create openings for greater abundance to enter your life.

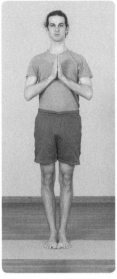
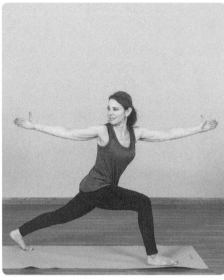
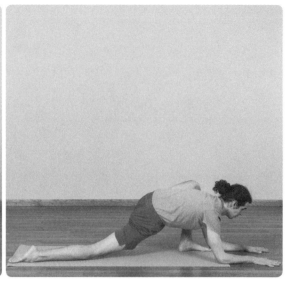

Sun salutation    Crescent lunge twist    Dragon

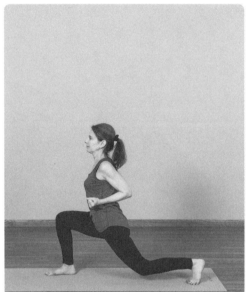
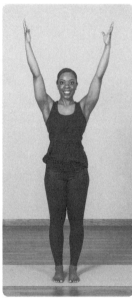
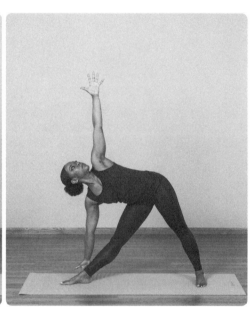

Moon dips with kapalabhati    Stand to squat with kapalabhati    Triangle

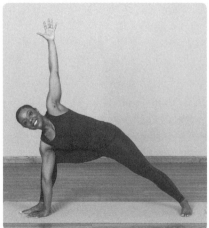
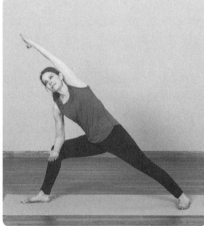
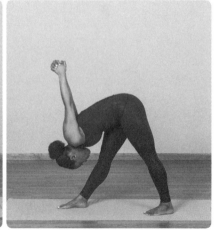

Side angle    Side angle with reach    Pyramid

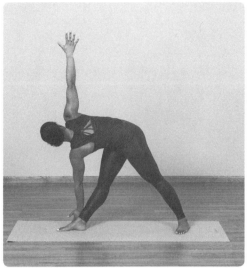

Revolved triangle

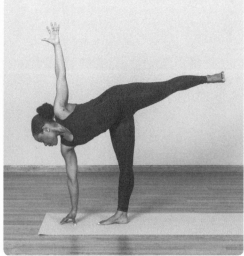

Half moon

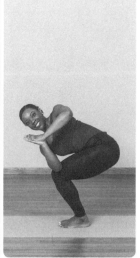

Chair twist

## UDDIYANA BANDHA

Uddiyana bandha, the stomach lift and lock is unrivaled when it comes to massaging the internal organs and stimulating agni (fire). It also relieves constipation, gas, and indigestion, and tones the nerves in the solar plexus as it reduces fat around the abdomen and strengthens the muscles. (See chapter 10 for practice and teaching instructions.)

The stomach lift practices consist of three separate exercises: uddiyana bandha, uddiyana bandha with fanning, and uddiyana bandha with nauli kriya (washing).

○ *Uddiyana bandha.* Practice holding the breath out 3 times. Stand in mountain pose and feel the stimulating heat of agni, the internal fire.

○ *Uddiyana bandha with fanning.* Practice holding the breath out while "fanning" the belly, pulling it in and out. Repeat 3 times. When finished, stand in mountain pose and resume normal breathing.

○ *Uddiyana bandha with nauli kriya.* Practice holding the breath out for 2 breaths, working or "washing" the belly clockwise and counterclockwise.

○ *Boat or half-boat kicks with HA! breath.* Use an audible *HA!* breath on exhale, kicking through the heels.

○ *Seated twist.* Twist on the exhalation until there's no breath left to let go of. Squeeze and hold the twist. As you inhale, release.

○ *Chandrabhedan.* Left-nostril breathing is a benefit for those suffering from insomnia or anxiety. Close the right nostril with your right thumb. Breathe through the left nostril only. Take 10 to 30 breaths. Stop when you begin to feel relaxed.

> ### WORKSHOP WISDOM
> The word *tapas* is derived from the Sanskrit word *tap,* which means "to burn." The traditional interpretation of tapas is "fiery discipline," the focused, constant, intense commitment necessary to burn off the barriers that keep us from being in the true state of yoga—united with the universe.

> ### WORKSHOP WISDOM
> If the body is tied in a knot, so too are the mind and emotions.

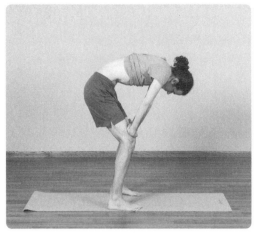
Uddiyana bandha

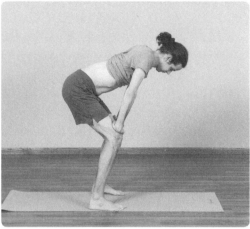
Uddiyana bandha with fanning

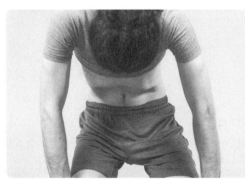
Uddiyana bandha with nauli kriya

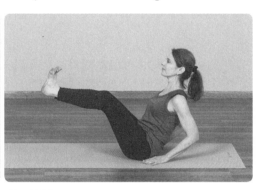
Boat kicks

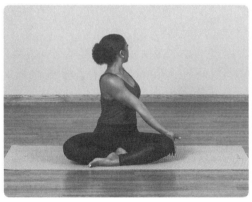
Seated twist

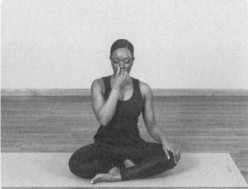
Chandrabhedan

## RELAXATION

*Lie on your back, releasing the body to the earth, softening areas that carry stress, such as the face, eyes, jaw, shoulders, wrists, mid- and lower back, belly, hips, knees, and ankles.*

*Imagine that you can breathe in the qualities that you need for the next chapter of your life. Breathe in courage to be true to yourself. Breathe in patience, discipline, or anything that you feel would help you on your journey. See yourself as strong, determined, and positive. See yourself as lifeforce itself. In your mind's eye, picture what you would like to manifest in your life and imagine yourself receiving these gifts. Feel yourself radiating with magnetic energy as you attract new people, ideas, and situations.*

*Feel your ambition and your transformation.*

*Slowly begin to deepen your breaths. Gently move your fingers and toes. Keeping your eyes closed, take three final deep breaths. When you're ready, open your eyes.*

*At your own pace, rise to a seated position.*

## Closing Pranayama

○ *Suryabhedan.* Right-nostril breathing stimulates the solar nadi and awakens external energy. Close the left nostril with the right ring finger. Breathe through the right nostril for 10 to 30 breaths.

○ *Bhastrika.* Practice bellows breath. (See chapter 5 for practice instructions.) Practice 3 rounds of 22 breaths in a seated position with arms extended overhead. Pause between rounds and take 3 diaphragmatic breaths.

○ *Bhramari breath.* Hum the breath of the bumblebee on your exhalations, breathing for 2 to 3 minutes. Feel the vibrations rising upward through the heart center.

**WORKSHOP WISDOM**

Like the breath, life is a balance of holding on and letting go.

## Teacher Tip

Encourage your students to find their own pace in Bhramari. The bumblebee breath will immerse the class in sound and vibration.

## Closing

Sit in the effervescence of your pranic forces. Yoga practices bring you to new levels of unobstructed confidence and inner strength. When you're clear, you can see that you're just one decision away from a totally different life. Keep going. Remember why you started the practice.

Change is hard. It's easy to stay where you are. So many of us deny ourselves the life we could have had because we're afraid. Yoga practices stoke our courage and belief in ourselves. The real challenge is the commitment to work every day, to do the daily ritual, and realize what we want from this life.

This is just the beginning. If you really want it, don't put your transformation on the back burner. It's right in front of you. Let nothing hold you back from creating the life you've always wanted.

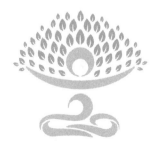

# Yoga for Special Populations

*Health is the greatest gift, contentment the greatest wealth, faithfulness the best relationship.*

—Buddha

Yoga has a plethora of practical tools to assist any person, in any challenge, at any age. As many senior students have proven time and time again, it's never too late to start a yoga practice.

Teaching yoga for special populations targets specific groups to offer appropriate guidance and modifications for a safe practice. The lessons in this chapter can help a variety of people gain access to the healing powers of yoga. Every stage of life is significant.

## Intention

To teach kids how to feel good and have fun with yoga.

## Lesson

Sharing yoga with children is a gift. The positive mindset that yoga encourages leaves kids feeling aligned, focused, and happy. Instead of presenting a weekly script for the class, keep your lesson plans open and flexible. Here are a few tips to make sure your young students stay engaged and have fun.

- *Do a whole-class activity.* Begin class with a focus-based activity. For instance, during the lesson, move around the room and ask about everyone's favorite animal. Later, practice the pose of each animal. If a favorite animal doesn't already have a pose, ask the kids to make one up!

- *Shake it out.* Kids are active and don't sit still for long periods of time. To get rid of the wiggles, have everyone stand up and shake out their hands, arms, and legs.

- *Enjoy the sun.* Practice a sun salutation pretending that you're outside at a park honoring the warmth of the sun.

- *Make breathing fun (and silly).* When practicing bhramari breath, have kids buzz around the room and pretend to be bees. Later, while seated, try the breath again and ask the class to attend to the vibration and sound of the other "bees" in the room.

- *Use a gong or Tibetan singing bowl.* Open and close class with a light touch on a gong or a Tibetan singing bowl. Ask the kids to listen carefully, noticing when the sound ends.

- *Don't give adjustments.* Keep your asana instructions simple and joyful, ensuring that the kids are safe and having fun. Don't concern yourself with how a pose *should* look.

- *Give positive feedback.* A simple goal such as being able to touch one's toes can create a feeling of achievement. Acknowledge even the smallest accomplishments.

- *Let your students teach you.* Play. Create. Wiggle. Tap your toes. Jump up and down. Express your energy and show your joy.

- *Teach kids how to manage stress.* Many adult yoga students report that they wish they'd been taught stress management when they were children. Now, through the privilege of teaching yoga, you can be the one to do it. Stretching and controlled breathing work wonders for stress and anxiety, helping to give kids a sense of calmness and reassurance. Teach your students how to reduce stress and get back in control when they feel anxious by remembering the acronym SBR—Stretching, Breathing, and Relaxation.

- *Make up songs.* For example, use the SBR acronym so kids will remember what to do next time they feel stressed. Make up your own funny tune with these lyrics:

  > *S is for stretching,*
  > *B is breathing,*
  > *R is relaxation.*
  > *We remember our SBR to send our stress on vacation.*

○ *Teach mindfulness.* By using the whole body and remembering to think about the breath in each pose, yoga is the perfect introduction to mindfulness.

○ *Create an on-the-spot lesson plan by asking the group leading questions such as:*

- What do you do when you're feeling sad or angry?

- Do you feel anxious about school work?

- Do you have a hard time falling sleep at night?

- Do you have a favorite saying that helps you when you're scared or nervous?

- What does it feel like in your body when you're scared? What does it feel like in your body when you're happy?

○ *Tell yoga stories.* Dozens of fascinating age-appropriate yoga stories are available for kids. Share a parable, then open the discussion for the children to explain *their* view of the story. Try the following examples:

### A Cup of Tea (or The Busy Mind)

A Zen master had a visitor who came to ask about mindfulness. The Zen master served the visitor a cup of tea. He poured tea into her cup until it was full, and then kept on pouring. Aghast, the visitor watched the Zen master pour the tea until she finally said, "It's overflowing! You can't put any more tea in that cup." "Like this cup," the Zen master said, "you are full of your own opinions and speculations. How can I show you Zen unless you first empty your cup?"

### Right and Wrong

A yoga master held a 2-week meditation retreat. During the retreat, a student was caught stealing. He was reported to the yoga master with the request that the thief be sent home. The yoga master ignored the request.

Later, the student was again caught stealing, and again, the yoga master ignored it. This made the other students angry. They told the yoga master that they wanted the thief to be sent home; otherwise, they said, *they* would leave.

Unwavering, the yoga master said, "You are wise students. You know what is right and what is not right. You may go somewhere else to study if you wish, but this poor student does not even know right from wrong. Who will teach him if I do not? I am going to keep him here even if all the rest of you leave." The thief cried and cried when he heard this truth, and all desire to steal had vanished.

## Asanas for Deepening

Share the benefits of asana from your own yoga practice without losing the connection to your inner child.

- ○ *Neck rolls.*
- ○ *Bow.*
- ○ *Cat–cow.*
- ○ *Inverted table.*
- ○ *Woodchopper.*
- ○ *Lion.*
- ○ *Flapping butterfly and rolling butterfly.* During butterfly, share the parable about the Taoist master who dreamed that he was a butterfly. In the dream, he had no awareness of being a person; he was only a butterfly. When he awoke, he was a person once again. But as he lay there, he thought to himself, *Was I a man who dreamt about being a butterfly, or am I now a butterfly who dreams about being a man?*
- ○ *Spider on the ceiling.*
- ○ *Crow.*
- ○ *Warrior I.*
- ○ *Bridge.*
- ○ *Wheel.*

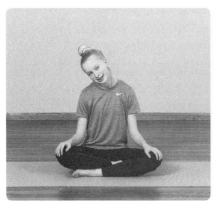

Neck rolls

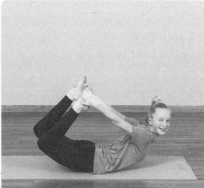

Bow

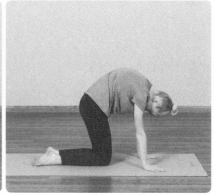

Cat–cow

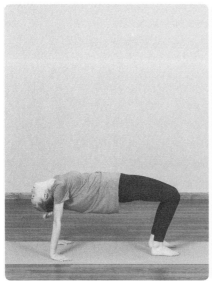

Inverted table

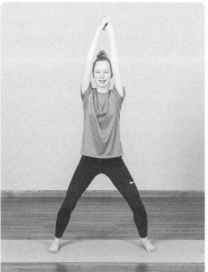

Woodchopper

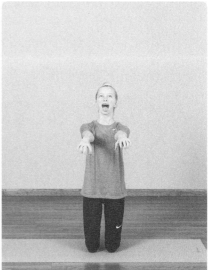

Lion

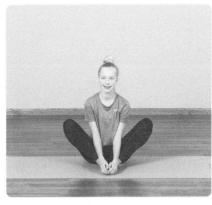
Flapping butterfly

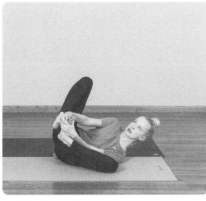
Rolling butterfly

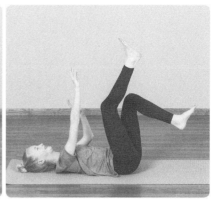
Spider on the ceiling

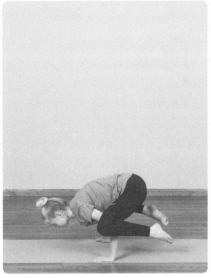
Crow

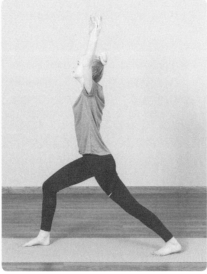
Warrior I

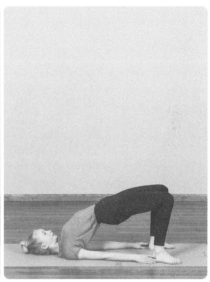
Bridge

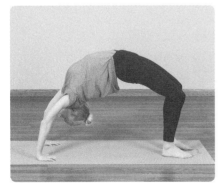
Wheel

## Teacher Tip

Connect with your inner child. Be spontaneous, entertaining, surprising, and childlike. This isn't adult yoga!

# YOGA FOR PREGNANCY

## Intention

To become a mindful mother, be aware of the growing force within the body.

## Lesson

Congratulations to all of you moms, and welcome to prenatal yoga. There is nothing more exciting than growing another human being inside of you. During pregnancy, the body is very busy and alive with new developments, creating the need for physical modifications.

This class focuses on yoga poses and variations of common poses specifically for the pregnant body. You'll also learn proper breathing and relaxation techniques for an easier and more comfortable labor.

If you've had an advanced yoga practice before becoming pregnant, all the rules about pushing and challenging yourself don't apply here. You have another person practicing with you now, and we want to keep the baby happy and safe. Your body is not alone in this.

All things considered, yoga is one of the best mind–body experiences for both you and your baby. Here are some of its benefits:

- Improved sleep
- Reduced stress
- Increased strength, flexibility, balance, and endurance
- Decreased lower-back pain
- Decreased nausea

Another amazing benefit of yoga is that it'll help you prepare for labor. Prenatal yoga addresses the physical challenges inherent to pregnancy, such as a shifted center of gravity and lower-back pain. Yoga poses help alleviate aches and build strength in your legs, back, and abdominal muscles to prepare you for giving birth.

Let's start with a brief meditation for you and your baby.

*In a seated pose, place your hands on your belly, gently cradling the baby. Observe the sensations you feel beneath your hands. Do you feel heat? Movement? Breathe slowly, in and out, sending your baby your love and lifeforce. If your mind wanders, breathe deeply into your belly, as if you were gently stroking your baby's head. If a thought arises, let it float away, like a cloud in the sky.*

## Asana for Deepening

Adhere to the golden rule of prenatal yoga, *Make space for the baby!*

At the second trimester, avoid poses that place weight on the belly such as cobra or bow, and any postures that require moving in or out of a pose quickly, such as vinyasas.

Also avoid inverted poses because circulation and lung capacity are reduced as the baby grows. Use props as needed.

Work slowly, and transition mindfully.

○ *Neck rolls.*

○ *Extended side angle pose.* Place the forearm on the bent leg to open the hips. Extend the upper arm over the head.

○ *Modified triangle pose.* Move the feet about a foot (about 30 cm) closer together than the usual triangle. The triangle will help you regain a sense of balance, strengthen the legs, and stretch the side body and shoulders.

○ *Seated side stretch.* Try to find as much space in the torso as possible. Open the side waist and pelvis, and stretch through the hips.

○ *Cat–cow.* Gently rock between cat and cow to warm the spine and stretch the torso. Cat–cow also helps shift the weight of the baby away from the spine.

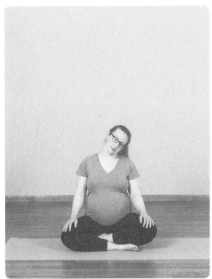

Neck rolls

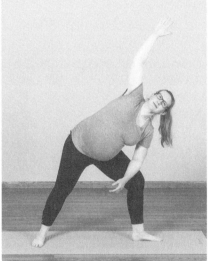

Extended side angle

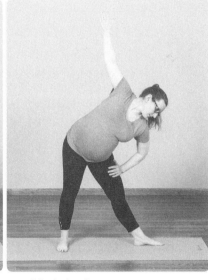

Modified triangle

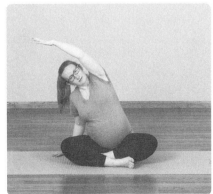

Seated side stretch

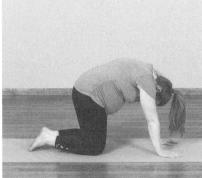

Cat

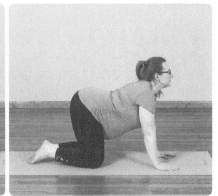

Cow

○ *Push the wall.* Pushing the wall offers many of the same benefits of a downward dog without putting weight on the shoulders, arms, and wrists.

○ *Standing hip circles.* Place one hand on the wall for balance. Lift one foot off the ground, bend the knee, and move the hip in a clockwise and counter-clockwise direction.

○ *Seated twist.* Avoid twisting from the waist. Instead, lead the twist from the shoulders.

○ *Side leg lifts.* These movements work the oblique muscles without causing strain to the deep abdominal muscles.

○ *Candle breath.* Practicing the candle breath helps release anxiety and tension in the body.

   1. Start in a comfortable, seated position.

   2. Draw a deep breath in through the nose.

   3. Exhale through pursed lips, as though blowing out a candle.

   4. Repeat this pattern for 1 to 2 minutes.

○ *Standing squats.* Squats expand the pelvic floor and hips, increasing flexibility throughout pregnancy to allow an easier delivery. Use a wall for support if needed.

○ *Side-lying savasana.* At about 20 weeks into a pregnancy, lying on the back increases the risk of oxygen being cut off to the baby. It's best to rest in savasana on the side instead of the back. Use a bolster, blanket, or block between the legs.

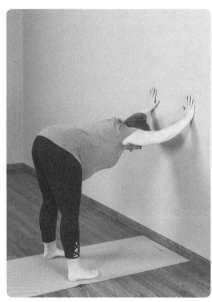

Push the wall

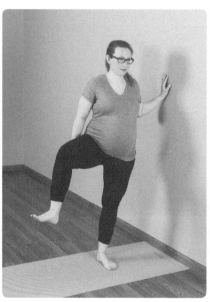

Standing hip circles

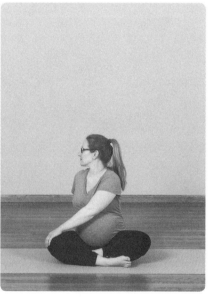

Seated twist

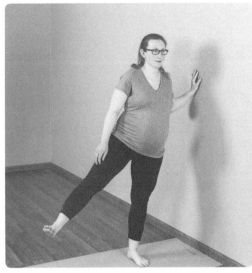

Side leg lifts

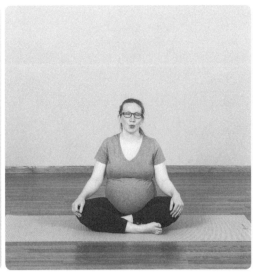

Candle breath

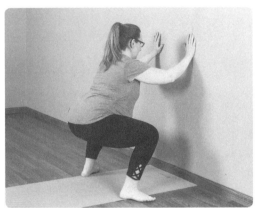

Standing squats

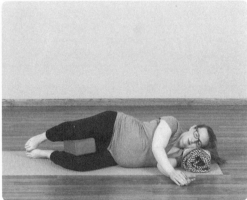

Side savasana with prop between legs

## Motivation Off the Mat

Use positive affirmations such as *Inhale for the baby (or use the baby's name)* or *Exhale a strong mama breath*. Affirmations help you relax, center, and rejuvenate through a difficult pregnancy or labor.

### Talk and Sing to Your Baby

That's right, talk to your baby. At about 23 weeks your baby can hear your voice, your heartbeat, even your growling belly. Hearing your voice while the baby is still in the womb helps her feel attached to you quickly once she's born. She may even remember the songs you sang to her!

## WISE WORDS

Your stress and anxiety affect all of you, especially your baby. For the baby's sake, learn to relax, and practice yoga every day.

Consult your doctor before starting prenatal yoga.

This truth is from my own mother: "Once you bring you bring your baby home, your life will never be the same."

## Teacher Tip

Yoga asana enables the mom-to-be to feel every movement of the life she's growing. But for the experienced yogi, everything they thought they knew about themselves, from breath length, to balance, to flexibility, are in constant flux. One minute they feel a rush of energy, the next they feel tired and nauseated. Teach your students to honor and learn from these continuous changes, and to include their baby's presence in all of their yoga practices.

# YOGA FOR SENIORS

## Intention

To help older adults open their minds, hearts, and bodies to the yogic experience.

*I embraced opening to all of life's possibilities when I began teaching yoga in a retirement community. The residents, aged between 80 and 99, have shown me how to rise above adversity, sharing their inconceivable tales of courage. From enduring the death of a spouse, child, or both, to making the life-altering move from their family homes to communal living, while living with their own illnesses, they remain present, strong, and hopeful. Experience has taught them the power and process of survival.*

*The lesson that follows assumes students have the ability to use a mat and get up and down from the floor. For seated poses, refer to the Chair Yoga lesson later in this chapter.*

## Lesson

This class is designed for your mind and your body. No matter what we do in this class, please first respect your body and its limitations. The stretching, strengthening, and balancing exercises we do in yoga are a way to reap the benefits of conscious breathing, meditation, and relaxation.

Yoga is unlike any other exercise class. As we age, we can't treat the body as we did 20 years ago. Honor your limitations, your balance issues, your joints, and any medical issues you have. One of the most important things to learn in yoga is how to understand what your body needs. If you have arthritis, limited mobility, or any other physical limitation, there's a modification for almost every yoga pose to accommodate you.

Each of you is fortified with the wisdom that comes through a lifetime of experience, and you still have much to learn about yourself. Yoga helps to ease suffering, let go of unresolved issues, and allow healing and acceptance to begin. Many people live their lives half-asleep; it's never too late to open your eyes and pay attention to the things that really matter.

Let's begin today on our backs in a reclining pose. (Add props if needed.)

## Asanas for Deepening

- *Tense and release.*
- *Knees to chest.*
- *Hamstring stretch with strap.*
- *Cat–cow.*
- *Low lunge.*
- *Standing pelvic tilts.*
- *Swimming.*
- *Triangle.* Use a chair or wall for support.
- *Warrior II.* Use a chair or wall for support.
- *Warrior I.* Place the hands on the hips or reach the arms overhead.
- *Tree.* This pose helps to improve balance, preventing falls.
- *Seated leg cradle.* Use a blanket or block if needed.
- *Seated twist.*
- *Sphinx.*
- *Child's pose.* Place a bolster under the torso.
- *Bridge.*
- *Savasana.*

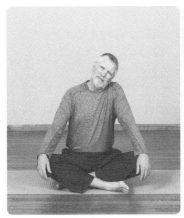

Tense and release

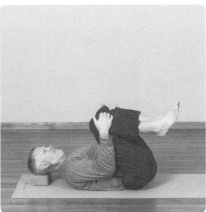

Knees to chest

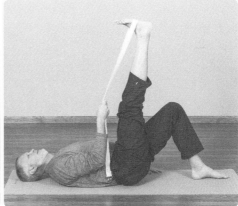

Hamstring stretch with strap

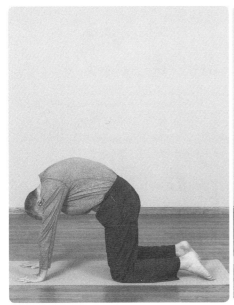

Cat-cow

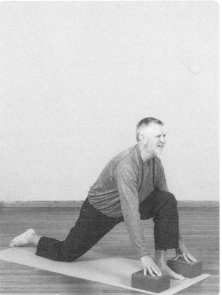

Low lunge

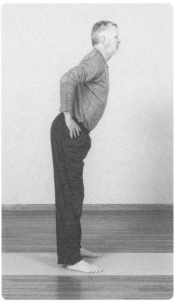

Standing pelvic tilts

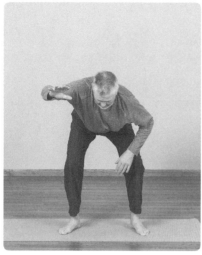

Swimming

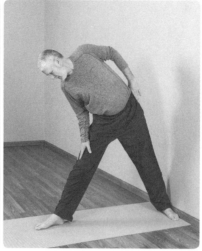

Triangle

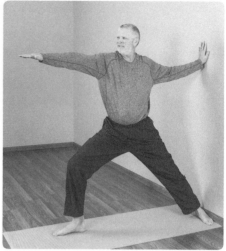

Warrior II with wall for support

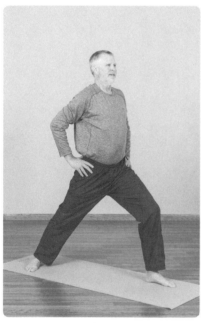

Warrior I with hands on hips

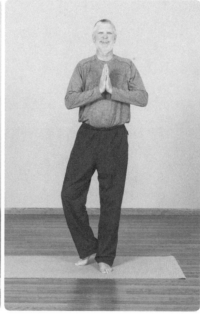

Tree

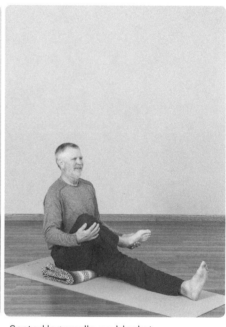

Seated leg cradle, on blanket

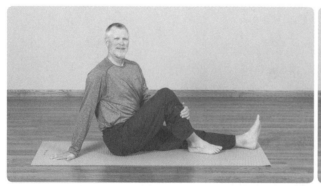

Seated twist

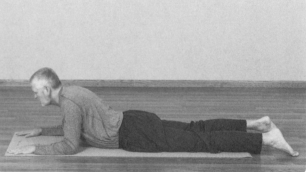

Sphinx

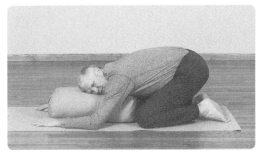
Child's pose with bolster under torso

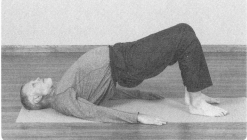
Bridge

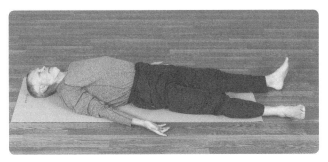
Savasana

## Teacher Tip

Can you teach an old dog new tricks? *Yes*, if you're willing to open your mind to the possibilities of life, and *no* if you're inflexible in your thinking and too set in your ways.

## Motivation Off the Mat

Nothing is impossible. Ninety-year-old Renee, standing strong at 4 feet, 9 inches (about 145 cm), told me her life's philosophy revolves around the bumblebee. Aerodynamically, the bumblebee isn't supposed to be able to fly; its wings are too big for its body. However, the bumblebee doesn't know that and manages to fly anyway. Renee said she has lived her life like the bumblebee. You don't know that you can't do something if you've never tried.

## Teacher Tip

Chanting can be a great way to vent frustrations. Some seniors refer to it as "yoga yelling" and request chanting as an emotional outlet.

## WISE WORDS

Judgmental thinkers limit their options. Gladys, an 87-year-old student with no knowledge of Buddhism, says, "We are only limited by our own minds."

As we age, we must keep moving forward in order to stay the same.

No matter how old you are, the pelvis likes attention. Gentle seated backbends, hula-like hip movements, and a mindful squeeze at the pelvic floor, give senior students a better understanding and awareness of their digestion, elimination, and sexuality.

### Tips for Teaching in a Retirement Community

○ *Talk loudly; soft yoga voices are not effective here.* Many senior yogis have trouble hearing.

○ *Be gentle when offering adjustments.* A hand on the shoulder in a twisting pose or a gentle nudge in a seated forward bend can be enough for the student to feel the edge of the pose.

○ *Try subtle movements.* Movements that may be too slow in other classes are loved, honored, and well-respected in this setting. Add eye exercises, joint rotations, foot stomping, temple and scalp massage, and finger stretches to your lessons.

○ *Smile, open your heart, and share your joy.* Show your students the healing power of yoga.

○ *If possible, stay after class.* Some students have waited all week to share something with you.

○ *Respect and appreciate the strength and perseverance of your students.* Many have had struggles you can't imagine—yet. Learn from them.

# YOGA FOR ATHLETES

## Intention

To experience the benefits of yoga for performance athletes.

## Lesson

Yoga postures are extremely beneficial for athletes because they go beyond simple one-direction stretching by working the muscles and joints through all ranges of motion, activating the little-used muscles that support the primary movers.

Beyond the big stretches, yoga enhances performance and prevents injury. A healthy yoga practice includes flexibility training, core work, strengthening, and balance postures. Yoga helps you recover more quickly after workouts, opens up the tight areas that impede performance, and improves your range of motion.

Yoga is good for you physically, but it also develops your concentration and mental focus. The main emphasis in yoga is on breathing, and the awareness of how your body responds to it. When you're holding a yoga posture, focus on feeling the body's alignment. Sense your physical response, especially with poses that target the hips, the back, and the side body, because these areas are often very tight.

Close the eyes. Notice which muscles you're using to sit. Then, without changing your posture, notice whether you're able to relax those muscles. Drop your shoulders away from your ears. Release your hips and knees. Where do you notice restriction in the breath or in how you're sitting? Be aware of how your body feels right now. Notice what it feels like to breathe intentionally from the belly. Connect with your breathing, and sense how you can calm yourself by bringing awareness to the breath.

## Asanas for Deepening

Yoga practice is much more than the physical postures; but for beginning yogi athletes however, it truly *is* a physical practice. Athletes need a challenging workout sprinkled with energetic stretches and strengtheners. Since strong athletes tend to be less flexible than the average person, avoid teaching advanced flexibility poses such as lotus or full cobra.

- ○ *Squat.*
- ○ *Extended leg squat.*
- ○ *Downward dog twist.*
- ○ *High lunge twist.*
- ○ *Reclining hamstring stretches.*
- ○ *Eagle.*
- ○ *Yogi crunches.*

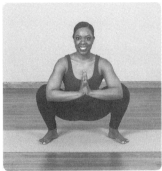

Squat

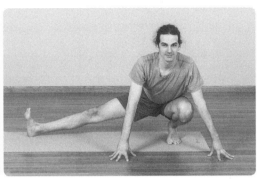

Extended leg squat

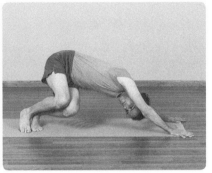

Downward dog twist

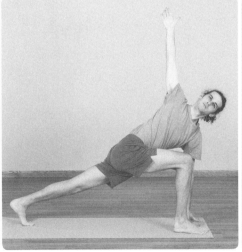

High lunge twist

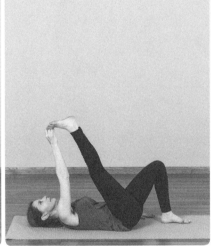

Reclining hamstring stretches

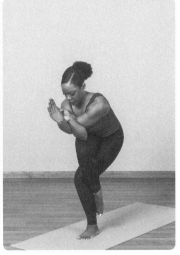

Eagle

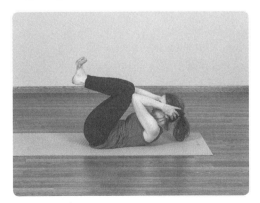

Yogi crunches

## Motivation Off the Mat

Monitor your body by staying in touch with it. Yoga asks you to pay attention to your physical self and stretch to your edge, noticing what hurts and what feels like relief. When you're not on the yoga mat, pay attention, noting which conditions or people make your neck tight or your shoulders hunch. Which situations loosen you up? Strive to cultivate anxiety-free relationships and life events. Feel the tension arrive, then make a conscious decision to let it go.

While practicing, think about how your yoga practice will enhance and elevate your sport. Visualize yourself as faster, more dedicated, conscious of movement, and more flexible.

Get curious about what thoughts generate your confidence, where you feel it, and how your whole body reacts to that feeling. Connect with that strength.

For any athlete who thinks, *I'm too stiff to do yoga,* the opposite is true. The tighter you are, the more you'll benefit from a yoga practice.

# CHAIR YOGA

## Intention

To create a motivating yoga workout for students with physical limitations.

## Lesson

It may seem implausible, but adapting yoga poses to a chair is a lot like a typical yoga class—the possibilities of movement are endless. With the exception of inverted poses, any posture can be modified while seated or standing with support. The emphasis is on body awareness and grounding, such as how you sit and stand, whether you favor one side over another, or how you're treating your injuries.

Now, become very conscious about how you're seated. Move your spine to the back of the chair, and place your feet on the ground. [If a student's feet don't touch the ground, bring the ground to them by placing a block beneath each foot.] Press the soles of the feet into the ground, feeling a slight awakening of the spine. You're suddenly sitting taller. As you press into the feet again, lift this muscle energy into the calves and thighs. Then, plant your sit bones to rise from the seat of the chair. Feel the torso straightening. Lift the belly and the lower back, allowing that lift into your heart center. Draw the shoulders up, back, and down. Raise the head, crown lifted toward the sky, and chin parallel to the ground. Feel the energy from the floor to the top of your head.

Take some deep cleansing breaths by putting your hands on your abdomen and sending a big inhalation into the lower belly, expanding the navel outward. On the exhalation, release the breath, feeling the belly return to normal. Do it again. Inhaling, expand with oxygen, light and energy; exhaling, release toxins, tensions, and worries. The yoga breathing practices will help calm and energize you, and you can practice them at any time.

## Asanas for Deepening

○ *Wrist and ankle rolls.* Subtle movements that may seem too slow in other classes are celebrated in this setting.

○ *Arm and shoulder stretches.* Shoulder rolls, eagle arms, cow face arms (with straps), and face framing (opposite hand to opposite elbow with arms overhead).

○ *Pelvic tilts.* Perform seated cat–cow movements.

○ *Leg exercises*. Include toe curls, ankle rolls, knee lifts, leg lifts with legs crossed and uncrossed to strengthen the hip flexors, and seated leg cradles.

○ *Forward bend*. Spread the feet wide, gently inch forward on the chair away from the back, and rest the forearms on the thighs as you bend at the hips to lengthen the spine. If flexibility allows, slide the hands down the legs to reach the ankles or floor.

○ *Twist*. Turn toward the twisting side, resting a hand on the back of the chair. Lengthen the spine, and gently twist on the exhalation.

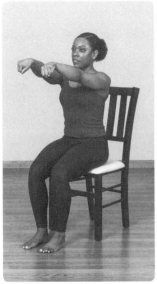

Wrist rolls

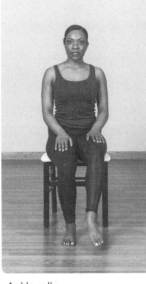

Ankle rolls

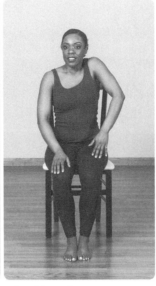

Shoulder rolls

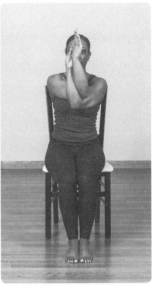

Eagle arms

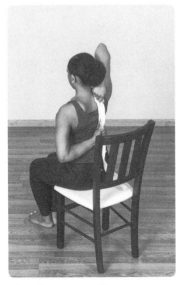

Cow face arms with strap

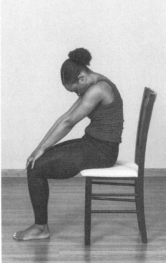

Face framing

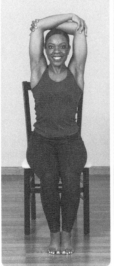

Seated cat

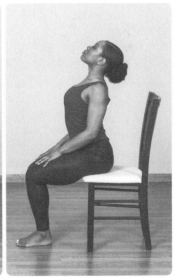

Seated cow

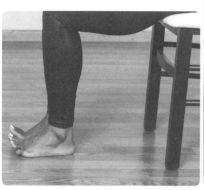

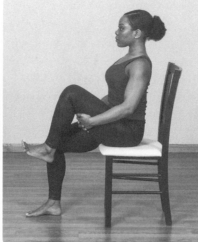

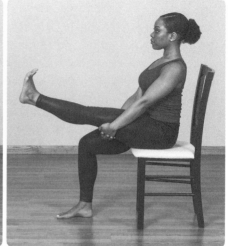

Toe curls

Knee lifts

Leg lifts

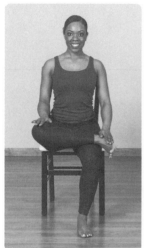

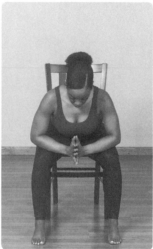

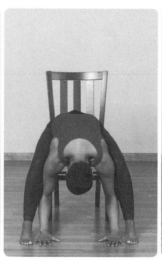

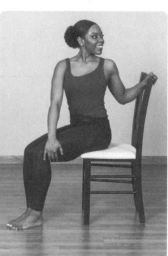

Seated leg cradles

Seated forward bend with arms on thighs

Full seated forward bend with hands to the ground

Twist

## Standing Poses

Use a sturdy chair for support. Where possible, place the chair against the wall.

○ *Mountain.* Stand behind the chair, holding the back of the chair for support. Emphasize the importance of weight being distributed evenly between the left, right, front, and back, of the body. For a variation, rise up on the toes.

○ *Standing forward bend.* Standing with one hip facing the back of the chair, place one hand on the chair and the other hand on the hip. Bend forward at the hips, micro-bending the knees, stopping when you meet resistance.

○ *Warrior II.* Stand behind the chair, and place one hand on the top of the chair for support. Alternate the arm lift.

○ *Triangle.* Stand behind the chair, and place one hand on the chair for support. Once in triangle position, rest the leading hand between the waist and the knee for maximum stability.

○ *Tree.* Stand to the side of the chair, holding the back of the chair with one hand. Root the standing leg, and turn the opposite leg out, keeping the foot on the ground. If balance allows, rest the foot on the ankle or calf.

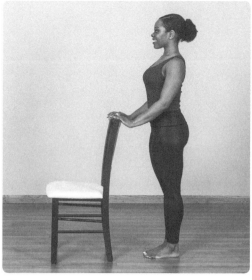

Mountain

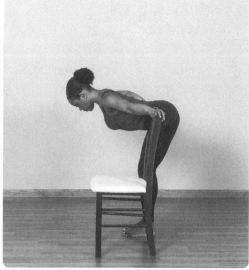

Standing forward bend

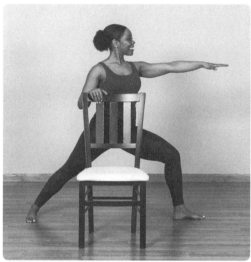

Warrior II

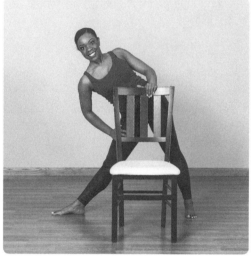

Triangle

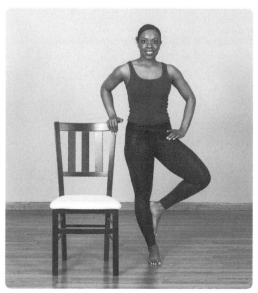

Tree

### Breathing Practices

Lion's breath

*HA!* breath: Fill up with breath lifting the arms above the head; on the exhalation, lean forward, bending at the hips, move the arms toward the back of the room with palms up, and yell "HA!"

Chant *Om* 3 times at the end of practice, extending the *mmm* sound.

## Motivation Off the Mat

The gentle stretching in yoga relieves joint pain and aching muscles. Yoga's focus on deep breathing improves respiration, lowers anxiety, and clears the mind.

## WISE WORDS

Seek progress, not perfection.

Setting an intention at the beginning of yoga practice is an invitation to reframe your thoughts, let go of resistance, and work toward your highest potential.

## Teacher Tip

Divide the class time into segments that include (1) centering, (2) seated movements, (3) modified standing poses using a sturdy chair for support, and (4) relaxation and meditation.

Avoid supine poses. Most chair yogis will have difficulty getting up and down from the floor.

Do not ignore important body signals such as dizziness, vertigo, and faintness, even if there is no danger of a fall. Keep a watchful eye on your students.

Several people may be in wheelchairs or use walkers and won't participate in standing postures. Show chair variations of the supported standing poses.

# 16

# Practices for Home and Office

*Meditate. Live purely. Be quiet. Do your work with mastery.*
*Like the moon, come out from behind the clouds! Shine.*

—Buddha

It's said that the more you practice yoga, the more you'll want to practice yoga.

A daily home practice creates a ritual and encourages the mindfulness of discipline. Plus, it offers you plenty of leeway; the space doesn't have to look or feel like a yoga studio. And because you're alone in your own home, you can make your own rules. The lessons in this chapter are addressed to both teacher and student. Teach these sequences to your class for their home practice, or offer your students suggestions for practicing anywhere they put their intention.

## Designing a Practice that Supports Your Needs

A home practice lets you cater to your needs alone. Do you want to soothe a busy mind, work out the kinks in your shoulders, or relieve today's digestion issues? You decide. On your own turf, you can move at your own pace, wear what you want, and create a practice that best supports your day. You can practice on a yoga mat, your carpet, or a bare floor. If you don't have blocks, use books. If you don't have a strap, use a belt or towel. Keep your mind-set dedicated but informal. It's just you and your practice. Embrace your imperfections; no one's looking but you.

To build the habit of practice, start with a 10-minute daily routine. Soon, your daily sadhana will be as automatic as brushing your teeth.

Despite the usual class rules being thrown aside, you should always follow these three principles:

*Practice with a calm, conscious breath.*

*Include a variety of movements.*

*Stay mindful of the full yogic experience, following your inner teacher.*

Once you know what your needs are, consider these options:

*Begin with centering.* Sit still, close your eyes, and connect with your body. Drop your sit bones, lift your spine, and relax your face. Breathe, connecting with your physical and mental consciousness. Wait for your inner cue to begin movement.

*Include all the movements of the spine.* Moving the spine in all directions requires forward bends, backbends, right-side bends, left-side bends, twists to the right, twists to the left, and elongating the spine.

*Move slowly, letting your breath be your guide.* You'll be amazed at how much you learn about yourself by simply slowing down.

*Challenge yourself to grow.* Set your intention for daily progress.

*Fall in love with taking care of yourself.* You are awesome.

*Give thanks.* At the end of your practice, take a few minutes to sit in gratitude for your body, your health, your loved ones, and all the gifts in your life.

## Obstacles to Practice

We all find excuses for not practicing. We're too tired, we'll do it later, or we just don't have time. If you're looking for more excuses, the *Yoga Sutras* of Patanjali are way ahead of you. According to the ancient text, written some 1,800 years ago, the main obstacles to practice are as follows:

| | |
|---|---|
| *Illness* | *Dullness* |
| *Misperceptions* | *Laziness* |
| *Mental and physical pain* | *Failure* |
| *Unsteadiness of the body* | *Sadness and frustration* |
| *Doubt* | *Irregular breath* |
| *Cravings* | |

In today's world, these obstacles can translate to pets, children, room-mates, monkey mind, depression, anxiety, and chores or errands. To break free from the land of excuse, the Sutras recommend this universal remedy: Develop a one-pointed mind. When the mind is focused on the *positive* outcome of practice, it's less likely to get entangled in the obstacles.

**Keeping Your Home Practice Interesting**

If you have 10 minutes (and who doesn't?), you can have a healthy daily yoga ritual at home. (For a great start, try the 8 Minutes to Awesome Practice in this chapter.) Once you've established the habit of practicing every day, try the following to keep your routine feeling new.

*Add pranayama.* Start out strong with bhastrika breath to elevate your energy and productivity of your practice. In a seated pose, exhale and pull the navel center and pelvic muscles in and up; inhale and release the muscles in the pelvic region, widening the belly and back. Continue for 8 to 10 breaths. Within a few breaths, you'll feel the heat turn on from the solar plexus, the body's power source.

*Learn about the eight limbs of yoga.* When you realize that asana is only one of eight limbs on the yogic path, you'll see your practice—and your life—in a whole new light.

*Add music.* If you already use music in your practice, try a different kind of music, or subtract the music all together and listen to your breath.

*Select a special corner or room to practice.* A different practice space changes your viewpoint.

*Add incense or essential oils.* The scent of your environment can alter your emotional state by triggering a pleasant memory. Coconut takes you to an exciting island adventure, vanilla conjures up images of childhood, and lavender calms the nerves before bedtime. Do some research on other scents, and have fun experimenting.

*Choose one type of pose.* Dedicate your practice to one type of pose such as seated poses, lunge variations, or navel-center work.

# 8 MINUTES TO AWESOME

## Intention

To ignite an active energy state in 8 minutes.

## Lesson

You can produce more of almost anything in this world except one thing—time. Once it's over, it's gone for good, and you can never get it back. That's why it's essential to know that if you want to live a better life, learn to be the master of your own time. The quality of your minutes is all that matters.

The moment you wake up is the beginning of the rest of your day. What you choose to do with your day and the choices you make can be significantly altered when you live in an active energy state. The way you feel is in direct relation to how content, empowered, patient, and loving you are. The fact is, when you feel good, you live a better life.

Kick off your day by using your first-thing-in-the-morning time to commit to this high-energy 8-minute practice. Place it on the list of daily rituals you already do in the morning, such as drink a cup of coffee, brush your teeth, and check your email.

This 8-minute practice will rock your mind and body, and help you become aware of how you spend each precious moment.

### Practice Tips

Practice on an empty stomach. A cup of coffee or a glass of water is OK, but skip any solid foods till after your practice.

Use a timer for each movement.

Prepare to get fired up for the day. Let the exercise reward you with a strong body, an open heart, a calm mind, and a positive outlook.

Focus on every breath. Use your muscles to encourage clear decisions, release stale energies, and feel gratitude for this amazing new day.

### 5 Movements in 8 Minutes

This practice is packed with five powerful movements that offer sustainable mind–body improvements far beyond the 8 minutes it takes to complete them.

○ *Uddiyana bandha (2 minutes).* It's said that if you only do one practice a day, it should be uddiyana bandha. This ancient exercise stimulates the internal agni (fire), helps relieve constipation, and strengthens the will. Plus, it lights the fire in the belly, giving you the confidence to accomplish anything!

1. From a standing position, bend your knees and rest your hands just above them as you lean forward.

2. Exhale completely, and pull your belly back toward your spine; hold your breath.

3. Squeeze your pelvic floor muscles and lift your belly up behind your ribs to hollow out your torso, and tuck your chin in toward your chest, holding uddiyana bandha.

4. Inhale when needed, and release the pelvic floor, belly, and chin.

5. Repeat this exercise several times for 2 minutes.

○ *Downward dog (2 minutes).* Downward dog is a buffet of delicious full-body stretches. From squatting to back stretching to twisting, there's a dog that suits your home style. Used as an inverted posture, it brings fresh blood flow to the brain. If holding the pose for 2 minutes seems like too much to handle, mix it up by moving the hips left and right, lifting one leg, or bending the knees.

○ *Seated twist (2 minutes; 1 minute per side).* The twist lengthens the muscles around the spine, spreads the wide muscles of the back, and ignites the hip flexors. It is also the perfect remedy to erase internal tension.

○ *Bridge (1 minute).* Bridge connects the top of the head to the soles of the feet as the entire front of the body unfolds. With skillful breathing, bridge ignites the chakras, stimulates the sexual organs, connects the mind to the heart center, and massages the thyroid.

○ *Inverted action (1 minute).* One minute in this pose delivers all the benefits of inversions, including draining the feet, ankles, and legs from stuck energy.

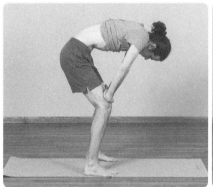
Uddiyana bandha

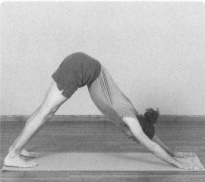
Downward dog

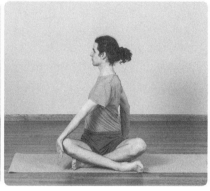
Seated twist

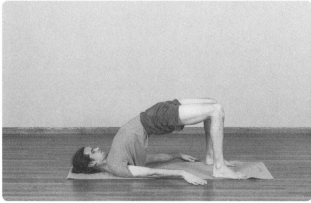
Bridge

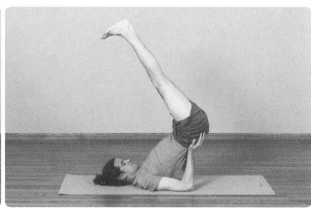
Inverted action

## Intention

To make the most of your practice time.

## Lesson

To encourage a daily practice and discourage excuses, select how much time you want to devote to your home yoga. While the amount of time you have may change from day to day, it's your *commitment* to the practice that builds discipline. Remember to focus on the positive results of the practice, not the time or effort it takes to get it done. This lesson outlines a 10-, 20-, and 60-minute time pledge to your health and wellness. Set a timer so you won't be looking at the clock, and enjoy taking care of your inner and outer worlds.

### 10-Minute Revival

Any time that you a need quick dose of energy, try this fast, stimulating revival practice.

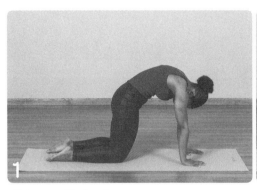

Cat–cow with fanning

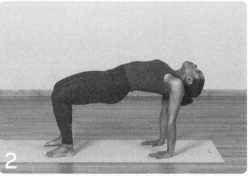

Reverse table

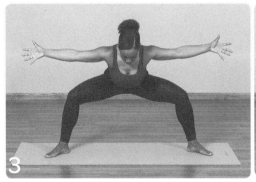

Bear squat

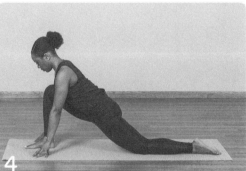

Low lunge

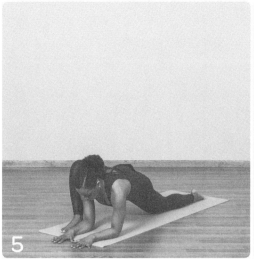

5

Dragon

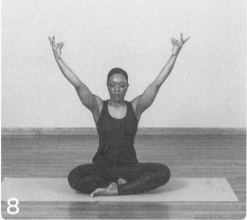

6

High lunge twist

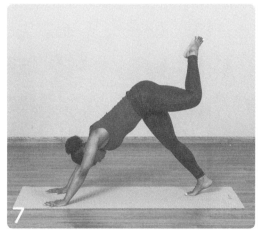

7

Downward dog with hip circles

Bhastrika pranayama with knowledge mudra

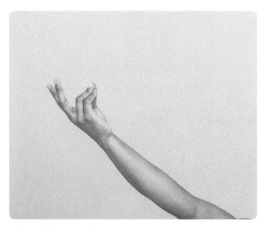

Knowledge mudra

## 20-Minute Force Within Mini-Class

*Yoga is the practice of tolerating the consequences of being yourself.*

—Bhagavad Gita

The energy that you're feeling at any given moment, even now, is your current identity. If you're feeling lethargic, why not take 20 minutes to restore your endurance?

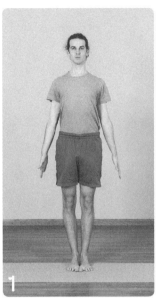
Mountain

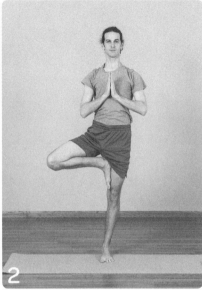
Tree

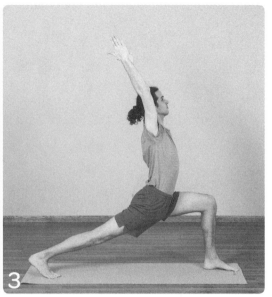
Crescent lunge

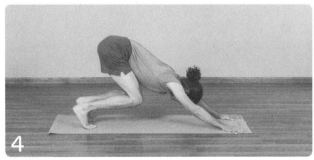
Downward dog squat

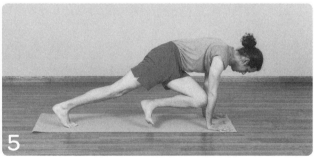
Downward dog with knee to opposite elbow

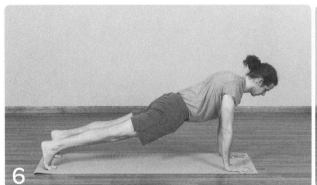
Plank

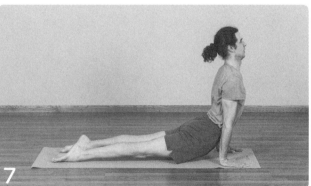
Upward dog

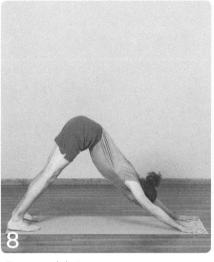

8

Downward dog

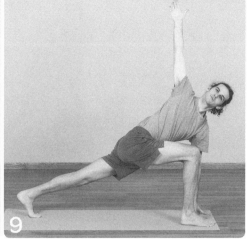

9

High lunge twist

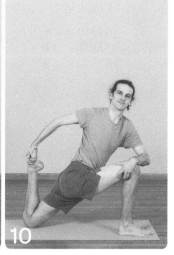

10

Low lunge twist with back foot hold

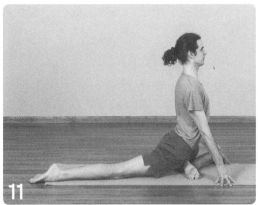

11

Pigeon

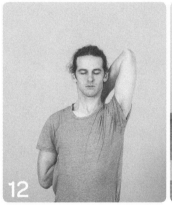

12

Cow face

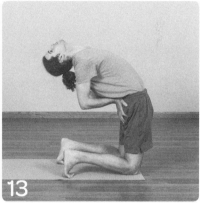

13

Camel

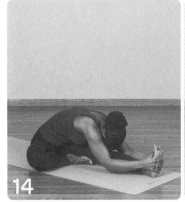

14

Head to knee

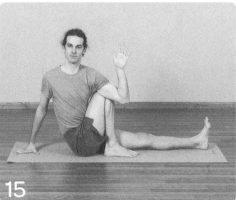

15

Extended-leg twist

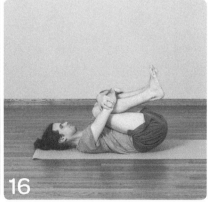

16

Knees to chest

## 60-Minute Progress Practice

With a longer practice, you can take a pose to a new level, the spot where you feel most challenged. What doesn't challenge you won't change you.

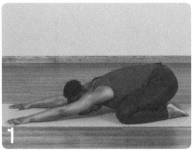

1

Child's pose

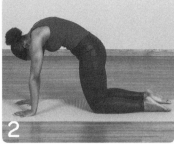

2

Cat-cow

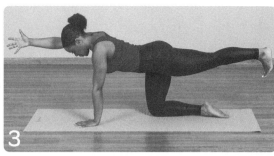

3

Table balance

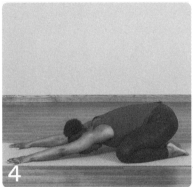

4

Child's pose

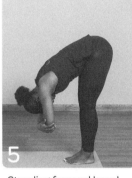

5

Standing forward bend with elbow grab

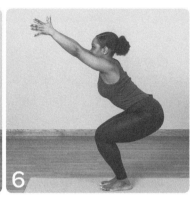

6

Chair squat

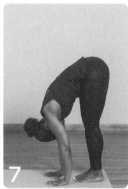

7

Standing forward bend

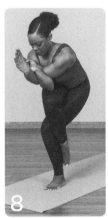

8

Eagle

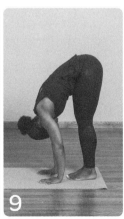

9

Standing forward bend

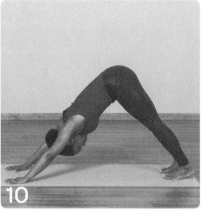

10

Downward dog

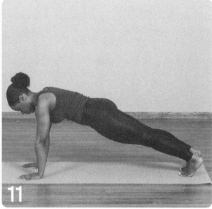

11

Plank

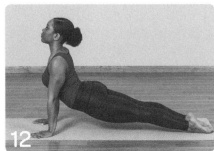

12

Upward dog

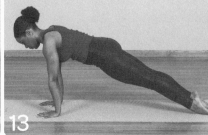

13

Pointed plank

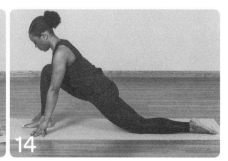

14

Low lunge

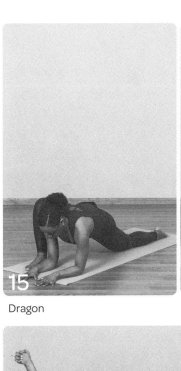

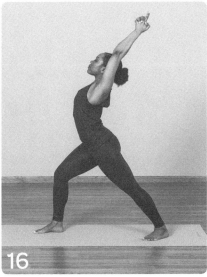

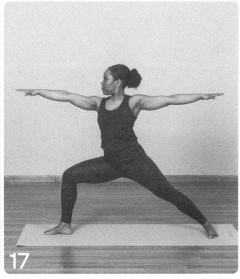

15

Dragon

16

Warrior I

17

Warrior II

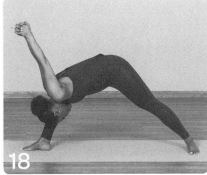

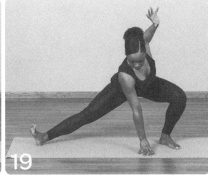

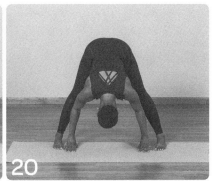

18

Humble warrior

19

Extended leg squat

20

Wide-leg forward bend

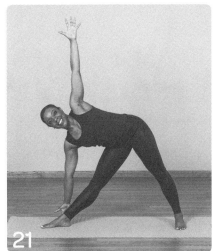

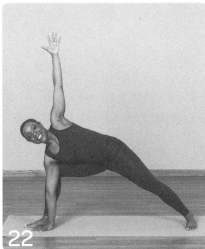

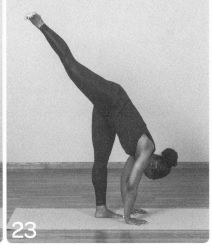

21

Triangle

22

Side angle

23

Standing splits

*(continued)*

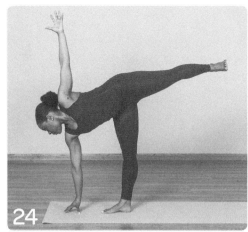

24

Half moon

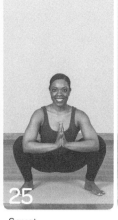

25

Squat

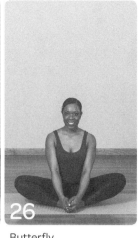

26

Butterfly

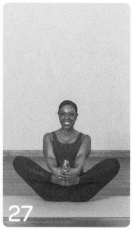

27

Butterfly balance

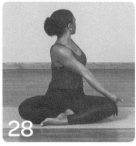

28

Seated twist

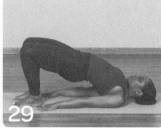

29

Bridge

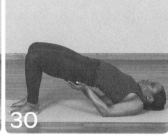

30

Bridge with palms to low back

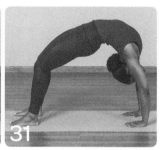

31

Wheel

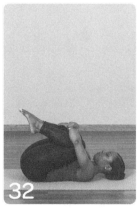

32

Knees to chest

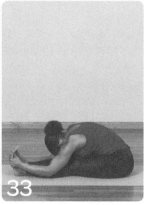

33

Seated forward bend

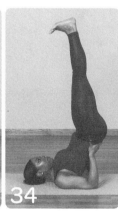

34

Shoulderstand

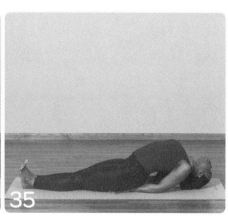

35

Fish

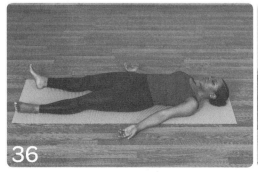

36

Savasana

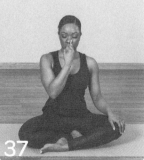

37

Nadi shodhana

# BUSTING THROUGH ANXIETY

## Intention

To accept, embrace, and release anxiety.

## Lesson

The first step to easing anxiety is to become aware of how it manifests in your body. Feel the physical sensation, then instead of *resisting* the anxiety, use the following practices to accept, embrace, and release it.

### Seated Lion's Breath

This technique is a fast and effective way to expel tension and dark matter.

*In a seated position, stretch your arms out as you take a deep breath in. Exhale while sticking out your tongue, and roar like a lion with a HA! sound. Repeat the sequence for 10 to 15 breaths.*

### Mindful Meditation

Meditation helps you become aware of the space between anxiety triggers and your reactions to them. With a dedicated practice, meditation produces the clarity to see things for what they are, instead of worse than they are. Because anxiety is caused by fear of the future, many practitioners find the *Be here now* approach to meditation quite grounding, helping them prevent panic attacks before they start.

Find a comfortable spot in your home that you can claim for your meditation practice. Start with 5 minutes a day, gradually lengthening the time of your meditation.

*Close your eyes. Notice the weight of your body and its points of contact with the ground. Listen to the sounds around you, then bring attention inside your body and do a quick scan, pausing to observe how your physical body feels. Bring your attention to your breath. Where is the breath moving as you inhale and exhale? How quickly or slowly are you breathing? Take the next few moments in stillness to observe, feel, and listen to your breath.*

If your meditation is unsuccessful as a result of a scattered mind, stay with it by dedicating your practice to a loved one who needs your full and loving attention. If being better for yourself isn't enough, do it for someone else.

### Restorative Reclining Butterfly

Deep-rooted lingering anxiety can stem from unspoken feelings of sadness which forge a barricade around the heart center. Relaxing into passive heart-opening poses unlocks these deep-rooted feelings, inviting them to rise to the surface and leave.

*Sit in front of a bolster placed vertically along the spine. Slowly lie back onto the bolster with the arms relaxed next to you, palms facing up. Place a block under each knee for support. If your head is not on the bolster, use a blanket or block under your head. Bring the soles of the feet together in butterfly. Close and rest your eyes for 5 to 10 minutes.*

*Become aware of the emotions that rise to the surface. Greet them with gratitude as if you've finally discovered the cause of your melancholy. Thank the emotions for emerging, then ask them to leave your heart center; their purpose for being there has come to an end. Say goodbye, closing the door to the pain they've caused, choosing peace over anxiety and freeing yourself from the weight of your own thoughts.*

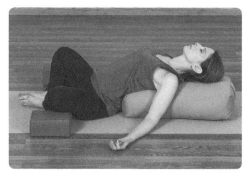

Reclining restorative butterfly (*add bolster and blocks*)

### Anxiety Rescue Breath

If you're in the middle of a panic attack, try this simple breath technique to bring you back to center. (Learn this breath *before* you have a panic attack to ensure you understand the instructions.)

> Begin in a seated position. Be aware of the sensation of the breath as it enters and leaves the nostrils. If the inhale is strained or you can't take a complete breath, concentrate on the exhalation to induce a relaxation response.
>
> Place one hand on your belly and the other on your chest.
>
> Take a deep breath in for a count of 4.
>
> Hold the breath in for a count of 3.
>
> Exhale for a count of 4.
>
> Count to 10 uninterrupted breaths.

# BEDTIME YOGA

## Intention

To release stress before bedtime.

## Lesson

Yoga asana is a natural way to settle the mind and ease muscular tension, both of which inspire a restful night's sleep.

The final pose, savasana, promotes a refreshing, dreamless experience, beneficial for those who struggle with a restless sleep.

### Practice for Deep Sleep

Prior to practice, put on your pajamas, and get ready for bed. The goal is to fall asleep in savasana.

Asana should be practiced on your bed.

- *Butterfly fold.*
- *Seated forward bend.*
- *Happy baby.*
- *Reclining hamstring stretch.*
- *Knees to chest.*

- *Reclining twist.*
- *Child's pose.*
- *Left-nostril breathing.*
- *Savasana.*

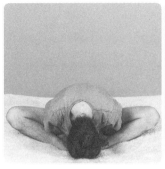

Butterfly fold

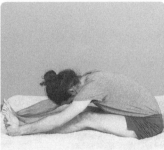

Seated forward bend

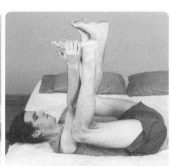

Happy baby

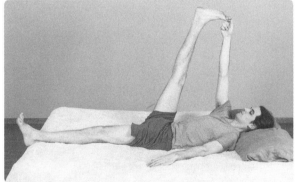

Reclining hamstring stretch

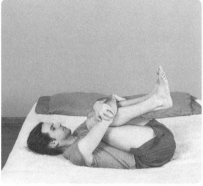

Knees to chest

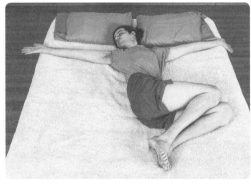

Reclining twist

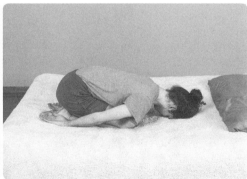

Child's pose

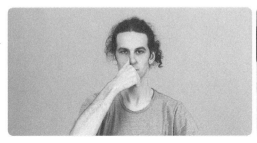

Left-nostril breathing

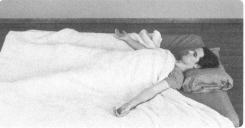

Savasana

# GOOD MORNING BED YOGA

## Intention

To set a harmonious tone for the day ahead.

## Lesson

Morning rituals awaken the senses and prepare the mind to accept the challenges of the day with ease. This practice is ideal for starting the day before you even leave the comfort of your bed.

Focus on gratitude. Be grateful you're here to live another day. When you start the day in gratitude, a cheerful attitude is sure to follow.

○ *Wide-legged child's pose.*

○ *Reclining butterfly.*

○ *Happy baby.*

○ *Reclining twist.*

○ *Reclining pigeon.*

○ *Seated pelvic tilts.*

○ *Out, up, and back shoulder stretches.* Interlace the fingers. Press the palms out in front of your chest, and lift the arms up over your head. Press the hands with palms facing the floor downward behind the head, squeezing the shoulder blades together.

○ *Cow face arms.*

○ *Gentle yoga bicycles.*

○ *Bridge.*

○ *Head to knee.*

○ *Belly massage.*

○ *Three-part breath.* Inhale in three parts. First, move breath from pelvic floor to navel center; next, navel center to heart; finally, heart to third eye. Exhale completely. Practice 8 to 10 breaths.

## Teacher Tip

Starting your day with yoga twists and self-massage followed by a glass of lukewarm water with lemon will awaken your sleepy internal organs and give your elimination system a morning nudge.

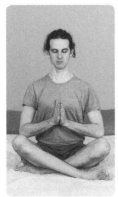
Gratitude focus

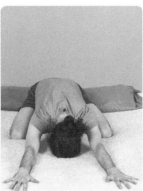
Wide-legged child's pose

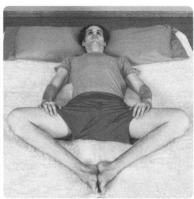
Reclining butterfly

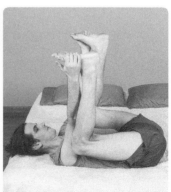
Happy baby

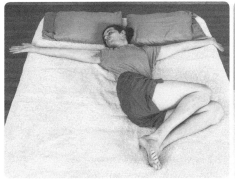

Reclining twist

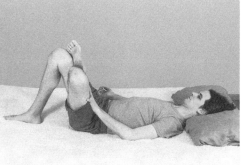

Reclining pigeon

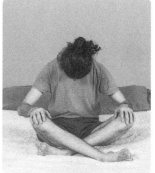

Seated pelvic tilts

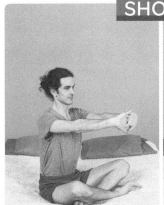

Out

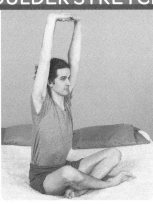

Up

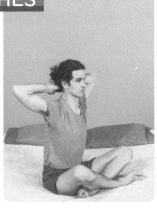

Back

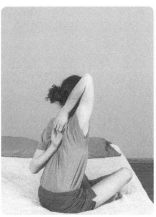

Cow face arms

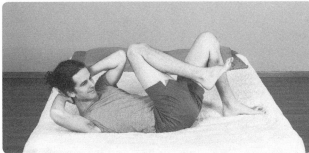

Gentle yoga bicycles

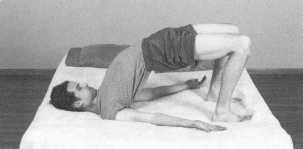

Bridge

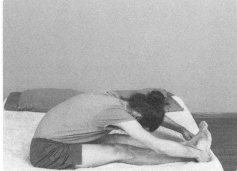

Head to knee

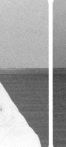

Belly massage

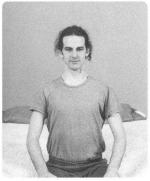

Three-part breath

## Intention

To increase energy flow during the work day.

## Lesson

While the 60 to 90 minutes you may spend on the yoga mat a few days a week helps flexibility, it's no match for the chronic stress and tension that a desk job places on the body every day.

Sitting at a desk for hours on end places unnecessary strain on the lumbar spine, overstretches the mid- to upper back, and shortens the chest and hips. Luckily, a quick fix like a short chair practice energizes the body and mind, and gets you back to productivity.

**Yoga at Work**

- ○ *Seated side stretch.*
- ○ *Shoulder rolls.*
- ○ *Neck stretches.*
- ○ *Seated cat-cow.*
- ○ *Ankle rolls.*
- ○ *Wrist rolls.*
- ○ *Cow face arms.*
- ○ *Eye exercises.*
- ○ *Seated pigeon.*
- ○ *Seated leg bend.*

- ○ *Forward bend.*
- ○ *Open chest and shoulder stretch.* Interlace fingers behind the back.
- ○ *Seated triangle.*
- ○ *Chair squat.*
- ○ *Chair twist.*
- ○ *Plank at desk.*
- ○ *Upward dog at desk.*
- ○ *Downward dog at desk.*

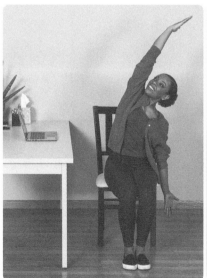
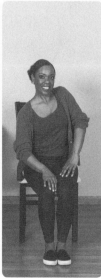
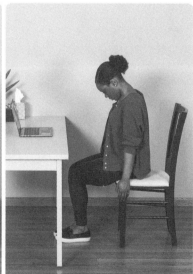

Seated side stretch          Shoulder rolls          Neck stretches

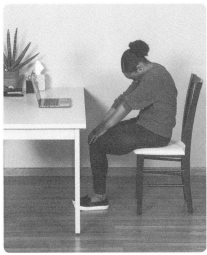

Seated cat–cow

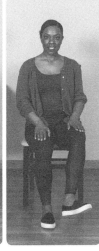

Ankle rolls

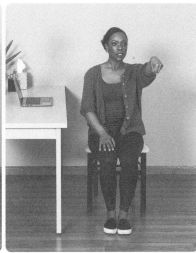

Wrist rolls

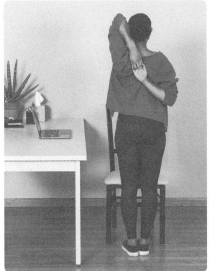

Cow face arms

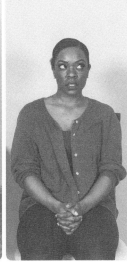

Eye exercises

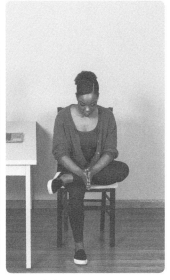

Seated pigeon

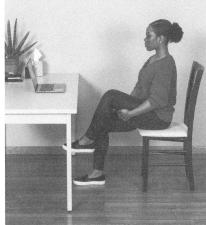

Seated leg bend

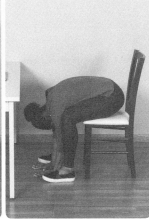

Forward bend

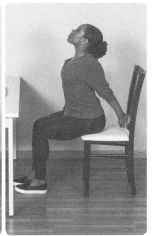

Open chest and shoulder stretch (Interlace fingers behind the back)

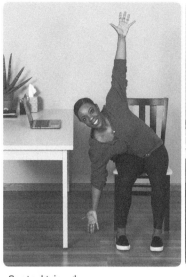
Seated triangle

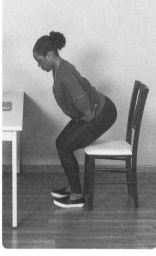
Chair squat

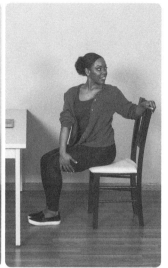
Chair twist

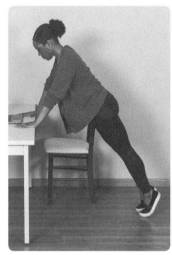
Plank at desk

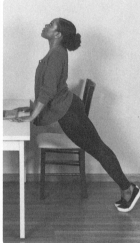
Upward dog at desk

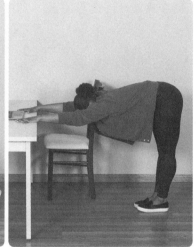
Downward dog at desk

# Guided Relaxation

*What you are is what you have been. What you'll be is what you do now.*

—Buddha

A post-asana relaxation practice provides the opportunity to clean, clear, and allow unwanted thoughts and negative energies to vanish. Relaxation polishes the mirror to the soul, opens the heart, and awakens the inner teacher. Yet, its most valuable payoff is the blessing of a relaxed consciousness. Curiously, the pose of the corpse, savasana, is the yogi's quintessential wake-up call.

This chapter covers an array of methods to slay physical pain and toxic thought patterns. The lessons ask that you practice only one asana—savasana—for all the others have prepared you for this final and most important pose.

## SAVASANA VARIATIONS

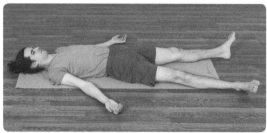

Basic savasana

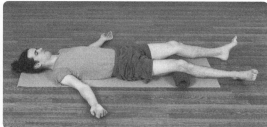

Towel or mat beneath knees

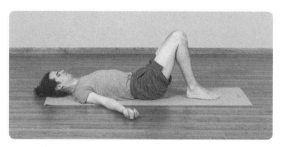

Knees bent

# BE A CORPSE

## Intention

To release toxins and wastes that rise to the surface during asana.

## Lesson

Lie in savasana. Savasana, the corpse pose, is part of your daily sadhana. Like many Eastern practices, it's a way of preparing for death. This idea encompasses the death of the body, as well as the surrender of ego attachment, adverse emotions, and physical disease, all of which are uprooted during asana.

*Gently close the eyes. Rock the head from side to side. Separate the feet hip–width apart. The palms face upward; fingers are naturally curled.*

*Make yourself comfortable, and remain in this position throughout relaxation. Constant adjusting and fidgeting hinder the effects of deep relaxation. If you have any discomfort in your lower back, place a rolled yoga mat or blanket beneath your knees, or keep your knees bent with the feet flat on the mat.*

*Bring your attention to your smooth, serene flow of breath. The exhalation is cleansing and relaxing. The inhalation is nourishing and energizing. Turn your attention inward, and consider all the adverse elements in your body, mind, and spirit that you'd like to dissolve. Perhaps it's an incident at work, a chronic pain in the shoulder, a worry about someone you love—anything that you'd like to release.*

*Mentally scan the body from head to toe and back up again, pausing briefly to become aware of each area, releasing any tension you feel there. Go slowly; tension is habitual, so it may take a while to recognize when you're holding on to it. When you identify discomfort, imagine sending the breath to that precise part of the body, soothing that area with a warm, deep breath.*

*Honor the areas in your body that need extra healing. Pause if you have pain, limitation, or emotional injury. Clear your mind of the past and the future; keep your listening thoughts in the now. When the mind wanders, simply bring it back to the breath. The body feels soft, heavy, and easy as it melts into the earth. With each exhalation, observe and feel the tension leave the body. The inhalation is full, soothing, and peaceful. Feel the space inside and around your body as anxiety and stress disappear.*

*Relax the crown of the head and the muscles around the skull, allowing both sides of the brain to fall toward the floor. Drop the muscles of the forehead, eyebrows, eyes, eye sockets, the space between the eyebrows, and your cheeks and chin. Soften the temples, the jaw, the neck, and the throat center.*

*Relax from the shoulder joints to the elbows, wrists, and fingertips. Feel the energy in the palms of your hands, and let the movement of your breathing loosen the shoulder blades, mid-back, and lower back. Invite the wide muscles of the back to release to the ground completely, letting go over and over again.*

*Soften the heart center, rib cage, abdominal organs, and pelvis. With a long, slow, deep exhalation, dis-ease is being pushed out of the body. Now with a long, slow, deep inhalation, accept the fresh prana entering your consciousness.*

*Soften the hips in and around their sockets, and breathe down the thighs, knees, calves, ankles, feet, toes, tips of the toes, and soles of the feet. Continue releasing any remaining issues with your breath until there's nothing left to let go of. Breathe as though you're inhaling from the tips of the toes up to the top of the head.*

*You are now washed in a warm healing light. This healing energy seeps into your body, filling you with generous amounts of boundless power. Feel it move through the layers of your body, deeper and deeper into every organ, all the way down to the bones.*

*Experience the light in every cell, dissolving any barriers and correcting imbalances.*

*Now it's just you and your mind. Detach from your thoughts, receiving the serenity of the pose and the flow of the moment.*

[Pause for 5 to 10 minutes.]

*When you're ready to come out of relaxation, wiggle the fingers and toes. Rock the head from side to side. Roll to the right side of the body. At your own pace, come to a seated position. Sit tall, feeling happy, spacious, and energetic. Be grateful for your experience. Notice your tranquil state of mind. Make a commitment to take this feeling with you as you move through your day with joy, serenity, and kindness.*

## Motivation Off the Mat

When the mind feels overwhelmed by drama or worry, pause. Take a moment to visualize how it feels to be in savasana with the mind clear, present, and tuned into the flow of life.

Live in a tension-free body. Several times during the day, stop what you're doing, scan your body, drop the shoulders, relax the jaw and forehead, and notice whether you're still holding tension.

## WISE WORDS

Give yourself permission to relax.

Practice relaxation as you'd practice asana—with joy, devotion, and an inquiring mind.

Slowing down through relaxation provides the opportunity to prioritize and tackle the most important work needed.

Relaxation is cumulative. The more you practice, the better you get at it.

*Words have the power to both destroy and heal. When words are both true and kind, they can change our world.*

—Buddha

# EXPANDING THE LIGHT

## Intention

To amplify the energy from your inner light.

## Lesson

*Please lie in savasana. Close your eyes and focus on each part of the body. Start from the feet and work your way upward. Progressively relax until you reach the crown of the head, giving special attention to stiff or painful areas.*

*Imagine a tiny ball of white light drifting a few inches above your head. The light is bright, clear, and filled with miraculous rejuvenating powers. You feel its energy as it floats above your head. Open your crown chakra and receive the gift from this sphere of white light, feeling relaxed, at ease, and wide awake.*

*Draw the white light energy down into your forehead, eyes, nose, cheeks, and chin. Watch the light travel into your throat, shoulders, elbows, wrists, and hands. Feel it in your fingertips, and witness the light force as it moves into your chest, back, belly, pelvic floor, hips, thighs, knees, calves, ankles, and feet. Feel the toes tingle. Visualize the light filling your entire body from the inside out.*

*Now expand the white beam of light to include the entire room. Sense your consciousness expanding, the light illuminating the entire room, and going even farther,*

*radiating through the whole building, the beam of energy breaking through the dark-*
*ness, shining out in every direction. Finally, broaden the light so that all the people*
*you love can absorb this light. Imagine them glowing with peace, wellness, and love.*

*Slowly move your attention back to your physical body, concentrating the mind's*
*eye on your heart center. When you're ready, roll to one side and come to a seated*
*position. Gently open the eyes and sense the inner light that naturally radiates from*
*your being. Know that you carry this light wherever you go.*

## Motivation Off the Mat

Create a fresh start. Upon waking, sit up in bed, open the curtains and, if weather permits, open the window. While breathing out, imagine all your negative energies and fears
of the day leaving your body with the breath. Visualize the energy as black smoke, per-
meating out into space until it disappears. Breathe in, and imagine the universe's positive energy, love, joy, and compassion embracing your soul. Accept this energy as pure
white light that enters from the pores, pervading every cell within.

## WISE WORDS

Relax and connect to the universal spirit, inviting life to flow organically.

Practice guiding your own light, so that you'll become more adept at sensing the
light in others.

# FAVORITE PLACE

## Intention

Visualizing your peace and tranquility.

## Lesson

We're going to take a short trip to your favorite place in the whole world. It can be imaginary, a place you've been to, or a place you'd like to visit. It could be inside or outside, it
could be your home, a vacation spot like a beach or mountaintop, or a setting of fun and
fantasy.

*Close your eyes. Take several slow, deep breaths, exhaling completely on each round.*

*Imagine yourself in your favorite place—a place where you feel safe, comfortable,*
*and at peace. It might be real or hypothetical, a place from your past, or somewhere*
*you've always wanted to visit. Design it exactly as you want it to be—the right tem-*
*perature, the right sounds and smells, and the right surroundings. Are you alone or*
*are there others with you?*

*Take your time, and allow this special place to take shape just as you want it. As*
*your place begins to appear, look around. What do you see? Observe the colors, tex-*
*tures, and shapes.*

*Listen. What do you hear? Waves, birds, music? Or is this place silent?*

*Take a deep inhalation, observing the smell of your special space. It might be the scent of a pine forest, or the ocean, or your favorite foods.*

*What do you feel on your skin? A breeze, raindrops, heat, the warm sun on your cheeks?*

*Take a walk through your special place. Notice a small object on the ground and pick it up. What is it? Is it smooth or rough, natural or man-made? Why have you found this? What does it mean to you?*

*Relax and enjoy the peace, comfort, and contentment within your special place where nothing can harm you. You are thankful and happy to be here. Everything is right, just as it should be.*

[Pause 5 to 10 minutes.]

*When you're ready to return to your mind and body in this physical space, take a deep breath in, exhale fully, and roll to your right side. At your own pace, rise to a seated position.*

*Envision your special place and the object you found. You can return to your favorite place whenever you need to de-stress and take a 5-minute vacation.*

## Motivation Off the Mat

Check in with your environment. Where you spend time has a substantial influence on your state of mind. Notice that it's easier to relax and be at peace in some rooms than in others. Look around the room or space where you practice. Piles of clutter act as constant reminders of things you need to do, countering your efforts to stay grounded and clear in your journey.

Powerful imagery crosses many disciplines. The most effective images are the ones that have meaning to you.

If you have a health issue, imagine that healthy cells are plump, juicy, and active, while diseased cells are shrinking until they evaporate entirely.

## WISE WORDS

Imagery can relieve pain, speed healing, and help the body conquer hundreds of ailments.

Visualization is the brain's method of communicating to the other organs.

Strong leaders are visionaries, able to spot potential as well as flaws. They see every detail in their minds before acting.

## Teacher Tip

Give your students permission to experience their imaginary place as a favorite memory such as reliving a significant childhood experience.

# DARK CLOUD

## Intention

To dissolve the dark cloud surrounding your consciousness.

## Lesson

*Tonglen* is Tibetan for "sending and taking" and refers to an ancient Buddhist meditation practice to awaken compassion by connecting to the suffering of the world.

> *Bring your awareness to your open heart center, awakening the wisdom and love within you. Feel free to call on the presence of a divine being. Visualize this being sending rays of compassion and wisdom directly to you.*
>
> *Imagine that sitting next to you is a loved one who is suffering. Open yourself to this person's suffering, feeling your heart connect with their heart. Call upon your loving spirit to help you liberate your loved one from pain.*
>
> *Now breathe in the other person's suffering, visualizing it as a dark cloud entering your heart center. As you exhale, transform the darkness, sending warm, healing light and pure love to the other person.*
>
> *Continue this breathing gift as long as you'd like. At the end of the practice, imagine that your intentions of love and compassion have released your loved one from suffering. Now see that person glowing with renewed joy, contentment, and love.*
>
> *Next, envision others who may also be suffering—friends, relatives, or neighbors. Practice taking in their pain and sending it back transformed with healing love, clarity, and understanding. Explore the joy that stems from freeing others of their pain. Finally, offer your happiness to all beings, dedicating the power of your pure intentions to everyone in your personal universe, including yourself.*

## Motivation Off the Mat

Create a morning celebration. When you wake up, celebrate! You're here, alive for another day to enjoy your loved ones, have a new experience, and another opportunity to achieve something meaningful.

Know that you're not alone. With each inhalation, visualize taking in and transforming the suffering of others who are experiencing the same loss, sadness, illness, or emotional anguish as you. This visualization helps you accept your own circumstances with more awareness and self-compassion.

## WISE WORDS

Don't avoid your own negative circumstances. Instead, extend acceptance and compassion toward your suffering and fears.

*The wound is the place where the light enters you.*

—Rumi

# JOURNEY THROUGH THE CHAKRAS

## Intention

To tour and balance the seven major energy centers.

## Lesson

*Find your center here in this moment, in this body. Follow the breath as it enters your nose and fills your lungs. Breathe from the abdomen, thoroughly filling up on the inhalation and emptying out on the exhalation.*

*Observe each of your chakras spinning along the spine, from your pelvis to the crown of your head. As you breathe in, imagine that you are breathing red, earth energy from the soles of your feet, up your legs, and into your root chakra at the tip of the spine. With each new breath, allow more red energy to move up your legs, filling and balancing your root chakra, the center of survival. Imagine the whole room glowing red; feel its strength and power, resonating as the root energy travels up your feet and legs into your root.*

*With your next breath, move your awareness up to your second chakra, the center of pleasure in the lower belly. Observe the red earth root energy rise up into the orange energy at the pelvic center. Feel the space around the body glowing with an orange current. Watch as your orange chakra grows and spins until it extends out from your body.*

*Move your awareness to your third chakra, the center of will and power. Allow the red and orange energy to lift into the yellow chakra at the solar plexus. Imagine a pulsating golden glow beaming from the solar plexus, fortifying you with its strength, will, and the power to achieve your goals, as its vibrant rays stream through each part of your body.*

*On your next breath, focus your awareness on your fourth chakra, the heart center. Sense the red, orange, and yellow energies escalating into an emerald-green point at the center of your chest, your spiritual heart. The heart is your connection between the physical and spiritual states of consciousness. The heart chakra is the ruler of love, compassion, and wisdom. Slowly let go of tensions, imperfections, and impurities. Open your heart with the glowing emerald-green force that generates compassion for all living beings.*

*Guide your awareness to your throat, the center of communication, the fifth chakra. The red, orange, yellow, and green vibrations gracefully climb into the electric-blue space in your throat chakra. Watch the electric-blue rays extend outward from your throat, communicating with all that is around you.*

*On the next breath, move your awareness to the sixth chakra, the third eye, your center of intuition. This chakra vibrates to the bold color indigo and is the home of your inner vision and intuition. Allow the red, orange, yellow, green, and blue vibrations to move up into the indigo pulse at the eyebrow center. See the purity of your thoughts as you wash away toxic images, cleansing and soothing your inner view. Psychic energy is available to you now. The third eye is open, and the color indigo is streaming from the space between your eyebrows.*

*With your next breath, shift your awareness to your crown center, the seventh chakra, your connection to the divine. Watch the red, orange, yellow, green, blue, and indigo vibrations surge upward into the vibrant, violet energy in your crown. Reflect on your spirit and enjoy the presence of the violet force flowing in as it surrounds your inner and outer body.*

*Now, imagine a golden white aura pouring out from the crown chakra, blanketing your entire body. You're completely refreshed, calm, and peaceful. You're balanced on all levels of your consciousness, full of vitality and lifeforce. Enjoy.*

## Motivation Off the Mat

Feed the chakras. When one or more of your chakras is out of balance, add chakra-specific foods to your diet that nourish and fuel your energy centers.

○ *Root (survival):* Root vegetables, proteins, and spices such as horseradish, hot paprika, chives, and cayenne pepper.

○ *Sacral (pleasure):* Sweet fruits such as melons, mangos, strawberries, passion fruit, and oranges; honey, almonds, and spices such as cinnamon, vanilla, carob, and sesame seeds.

○ *Solar (will):* Granola and grains, pastas, breads, cereal, rice, flax seed, and sunflower seeds; dairy, including milk, cheeses, and yogurt; spices, including ginger, turmeric, cumin, and fennel.

○ *Heart (love):* Leafy vegetables such as spinach, kale, dandelion greens, broccoli, cauliflower, cabbage, celery, and squash; spices such as basil, sage, thyme, cilantro, and parsley.

○ *Throat (communication):* Liquids such as water, fruit juices, herbal teas; lemons, limes, grapefruit, kiwi; lemongrass, peppermint, and spearmint.

○ *Brow (intuition):* Dark-colored fruits such as blueberries, red grapes, blackberries, raspberries, grape juice, pomegranate juice; spices such as lavender and poppy seed.

○ *Crown (connection to divine):* Burn incense and smudge herbs such as sage, copal, myrrh, frankincense, and juniper in your home, car, and workspace.

## WISE WORDS

Let yourself be guided by intuition instead of what a book, guru, or teaching tells you.

Be your own guru, and practice svadhyaya (self-study).

What you feel in a chakra can only be seen through the inner eye.

The subtle body speaks the language of inner wisdom.

# SILENT CHANTING

## Intention

To silently purify the emotions.

## Lesson

It's tempting to fall mindlessly into distraction, filling the silence with music or visual entertainment. Like children afraid of the dark, our modern culture has become afraid of quiet.

When the mind is absorbed in chant, it experiences a cleansing. Chant develops our concentration and strength of mind, as it purifies unfriendly emotions. The intentional sound of chant, unlike the noisy fillers in your life, enhances the silence around you, balances your inner and outer worlds, and takes you back to your true nature.

Silent chanting is the practice of integrating chanting into your personal silence and can be practiced anywhere at any time.

> *Using a three-part exhalation, silently repeat the three seed syllables found in* Om *in unison with your breathing.* Oh *is the seed sound of divine body.* Ah *is the seed sound of divine speech.* Mm *is the seed sound of divine thought.*
>
> *To practice silent chanting, exhale the first third of your breath from the third eye to the heart center, and mentally say* Oh. *Exhale the second third of your breath from heart to navel and mentally say* Ah. *Finally, exhale the last third of your breath from navel to public bone and mentally say* Mm, *until the last bit of breath is released. Follow this long exhalation with an equally long inhalation.*

Repeat this sequence 10 times, then let the silent chant dissolve into relaxed breathing.

## Motivation Off the Mat

Silently chant any word or phrase that has meaning for you. For example, if you want to change a stale attitude, thinking *I can do anything* can reframe your thoughts and provide the confidence needed to renew your attitude.

## WISE WORDS

Within the silence, listen for the voice of reason, your inner self, and the divine.

With practice and persistence, become the master of your words and thoughts.

# Glossary

**agni sara** (AHG-nee SAH-rah)—Yogic fire ignited by breathing practices.

**ajna** (AHJ-nah)—Sixth chakra, located at the eyebrow center.

**ahimsa** (Ah-HIM-sah)—Nonharming; first of the five yamas.

**anahata** (Ahn-ah-HAH-tah)—Fourth chakra, located at the heart center.

**anjali mudra** (Ahn-JAHL-ee MOO-drah)—The gesture of hands in prayer at the heart center.

**anuloma krama** (Ahn-ah-LOH-mah KRAH-mah)—Segmented inhalation.

**aparigraha** (Ah-PAH-ree-GRAH-hah)—Nonpossessiveness.

**asana** (AH-sah-nah)—Postures or yoga poses; the third limb of raja yoga.

**ashtanga** (AHSH-tahn-gah)—The eight limbs of yoga as described by Patanjali.

**asteya** (Ah-STAY-ah)—Nonstealing.

**avidya** (Ah-VEED-yah)—Literally "not knowing" or "ignorance;" spiritual tunnel vision.

**bhastrika** (Bah-STREEK-Kah)—The bellows breath practiced by rapidly exhaling and inhaling.

**boat pose**—Navasana (Nah-VAH-sah-nah).

**bow pose**—Dhanurasana (Dohn-your-AH-sah-nah).

**bridge pose**—Setu bandha sarvangasana (SAY-too BAHN-dah SAHR-vahn-GAH-sah-nah).

**butterfly pose**—Baddha konasana (BAH-dah Koh-NAH-sah-nah).

**camel pose**—Ustrasana (Oohs-TRAH-sah-nah).

**chakra** (Shah-KRAH)—Spinning vortex of subtle energy.

**cobra pose**—Bhujangasana (BOOJ-ahn-GAH-sah-nah).

**concentration**—Dharana (Dah-RAH-nah). The sixth limb of raja yoga.

**cow face**—Gomukhasana (Goh-moo-KHA-sah-nah).

**crocodile pose**—Makarasana (MAHK-ah-RAH-sah-nah).

**downward dog pose**—Adho mukha shvanasana (AH-doh MOO-kah shvah-NAH-sah-nah).

**dukha** (DOO-kah)—Suffering.

**eagle pose**—Garudasana (Gah-roo-DAH-sah-nah).

**easy pose**—Sukhasana (Soo-KAH-sah-nah).

**firefly pose**—Tittibhasana (Tit-tee-BHA-sah-nah).

**fish pose**—Matsyasana (Mahtz-YAH-sah-nah).

**focus point**—Drishti (DRISH-tee).

**four limbs**—Chaturanga (Chaht-uh-RAHN-gah)

**half-bound lotus posterior stretch**—Ardha baddha padma paschimottanasana
(AHR-dah BAH-dah PAHD-mah PASH-ee-moh-tah-NAH-sah-nah).

**half-lotus twist**—Ardha padma Bharadvajasana (AHR-dah PAHD-mah Bah-ROD-vah-jah-sah-nah).

**half-moon pose**—Ardha chandrasana (AHR-dah Shahn-DRAH-sah-nah).

**ham (Hum)**—Seed sound of the fifth chakra.

**hatha yoga (HAH-tah YOH-gah)**—The physical practice of balancing the solar and lunar currents of human consciousness, representing the dual nature of man.

**headstand**—Sirsasana (Sher-SHAH-sah-nah).

**head-to-knee pose**—Janu shirshasana (JAH-noo Shur-SHAH-sah-nah).

**hero pose**—Virasana (Vir-AH-sah-nah).

**horse mudra**—Asvini mudra (AHS-vee-nee MOO-drah).

**ida** (EE-dah)—The main energy channel that ends in the left nostril, embodying the moon, and connecting to right-brain activity.

**ishvara pranidhana** (ISH-var-ah PRAH-nee-DAH-nah)—Surrender to divine consciousness.

**kapalabhati** (Kah-pah-lah-BHA-tee)—Shining skull breath using controlled but forceful exhalations.

**king dancer pose**—Natarajasana (Nah-tah-raj-AH-sah-nah).

**kundalini** (KOON-dah-lee-nee)—Dormant energy at the base of the spine, awakened through various yoga practices.

**lam** (Lum)—Seed sound of the first chakra.

**lion pose**—Simhasana (Sim-HAH-sah-nah).

**locust pose**—Salabhasana (Shah-lah-BAH-sah-nah).

**lotus pose**—Padmasana (PAHD-mah-sah-nah).

**lotus shoulder stand**—Sarvanga padmasana (SAHR-vahn-GAH PAHD-mah-sah-nah).

**manipura** (Mahn-ah-PUR-ah)—Third chakra, located at the solar plexus.

**mantra** (MAHN-trah)—Sacred sound used in meditation.

**meditation**—Dhyana (Dee-YAH-nah). The seventh limb of raja yoga.

**moon salutation**—Chandra namaskara (Shan-drah Nah-mahs-KAH-rah).

**muladhara** (MOO-lah-hah-rah)—Root chakra, located at the perineum.

**nadi** (NAH-dee)—Subtle energy channel.

**nadi shodhana** (NAH-dee SHOH-dah-nah)—Alternate-nostril breathing.

**namaste** (Nah-mah-STAY)—Greeting interpreted to mean "The light in me bows to the light in you."

**niyamas** (Nee-YAH-mahs)—Observances; the second limb of raja yoga.

**om** (Ohm)—Divine sound of the universe.

**Patanjali** (Pah-TAHN-joh-lee)—Hindu sage and author of the *Yoga Sutras*.

**pigeon pose**—Kapotasana (Kah-POH-tah-sah-nah).

**pingala** (Peen-GAH-lah)—The main energy channel that ends in the right nostril, embodies the sun, and is connected to left-brain activity.

**plow pose**—Halasana (Hah-LAH-sah-nah).

**prana** (PRAH-nah)—Universal energy that animates all living things.

**pranayama** (PRAH-nah-YAH-mah)—Control of lifeforce; also referred to as breathing practices; the fourth limb of raja yoga.

**pratyahara** (PRAH-tyah-HAH-rah)—Withdrawal of the senses; fifth limb of raja yoga.

**pyramid pose**—Parshvottanasana (Par-shvot-TAH-nah-sah-nah).

**raja yoga** (RAH-jah YO-gah)—The royal path; eight-limbed path of yoga.

**ram** (Rum)—Seed sound of the third chakra.

**reclining easy pose**—Supta sukhasana (Soop-TAH Soo-KAH-sah-nah).

**revolved head-to-knee pose**—Parivrtta janu sirsasana (Par-ee-vrit-ah JAH-noo Shur-SHAH-sah-nah).

**revolved triangle pose**—Parivrtta trikonasana (Par-ee-vrit-ah Trik-cohn-AH-sah-nah).

**root lock**—Mula bandha (MOO-lah BAHN-dah).

**sahasrara** (SAH-ha-sah-rah)—Seventh chakra, located at the crown of the head.

**samadhi** (Sah-MAH-dee)—The superconscious state, a state of bliss; the eighth limb of raja yoga.

**santosha** (San-TOH-shah)—Contentment.

**satya** (SAHT-yah)—Truth.

**saucha** (Soh-shah)—Purity.

**savasana** (Shah-VAH-sah-nah)—Corpse pose; the final relaxation pose of the asana practice.

**seated angle pose**—Upavistha konasana (Oo-pah-VEESH-tah Kohn-NAH-sah-nah).

**seated forward bend**—Paschimottanasana (POSH-ee-moh-tah-NAH-sah-nah).

**seated twist**—Marichyasana (MAH-rih-si-AH-sah-nah).

**shanti** (SHAHN-tee)—Peace.

**shoulderstand**—Sarvangasana (SAHR-vahn-GAH-sah-nah).

**side angle**—Parshvakonasana (Par-shvah-KOH-nah-sah-nah).

**side plank**—Vasistha pose; Vasisthasana (Vah-shish-TAHS-ah-nah).

**splits**—Hanuman pose; Hanumanasana (Hah-new-mahn-AHS-ana).

**standing forward bend**—Uttanasana (OOH-tah-NAH-sah-nah).

**standing spread-leg forward fold**—Prasarita padottanasana (Prah-sa-REE-tah Pah-doh-tahn-AH-sah-nah).

**supine twisted leg lifts**—Jathara parivartanasana (Jah-TAH-rah Pah-ree-var-TAHN-ah-sah-nah).

**sun salutation**—Surya namaskara (SOOR-yah Nah-mahs-KAH-rah).

**sushumna** (Soo-SHOOM-nah)—The central and main nadi that runs along the spine and ends at the crown chakra.

**svadhisthana** (SVAHD-hiss-tahn-ah)—Second chakra, located at the lower abdomen.

**svadhyaya** (Svahd-YAH-yah)—Self-study.

**tadasana** (Ta-DAH-sah-nah)—Mountain pose.

**tapas** (TAH-pahs)—Determined effort.

**tree pose**—Vrikshasana (Vrik-SHAH-sah-nah).

**triangle pose**—Trikonasana (Trik-cohn-AH-sah-nah).

**tortoise pose**—Kurmasana (Koohr-MAH-sah-nah).

**twisted chair pose**—Parivrtta utkatasana (Par-ee-vrit-ah OOT-kah-sah-nah).

**uddiyana bandha** (OO-DEE-anna BAHN-dah)—An energy lock that includes a forceful exhalation followed by a sharp lifting of the intestines and diaphragm into a vacuum created in the thoracic cavity.

**ujjayi** (OO-JAH-yee)—A breathing practice that uses an audible vibration by gently closing the glottis in the throat.

**upward dog pose**—Urdhva mukha shvanasana (OORD-vah MOOK-hah Shvah-NAH-sah-nah).

**vam** (Vum)—Seed sound of the second chakra.

**vinyasa** (Vin-YAH-sah)—A series of asanas that link movement with breath.

**visuddha** (Vah-SHOO-dah)—Fifth chakra, located at the throat center.

**vrittis** (Vrit-EEZ)—Fluctuations of the mind.

**warrior pose**—Virabhadrasana (Veer-ah-bah-DRAH-sah-nah).

**wheel pose**—Chakrasana (Shah-KRAH-sah-nah).

**yamas** (YAH-mahs)—Five restraints; first limb of raja yoga.

**yoga** (YOH-gah)—To join or yoke.

***Yoga Sutras*** (YOH-gah SOOT-rahs)—A series of aphorisms relating to the practice of yoga as codified by Patanjali.

# Recommended Reading List

My favorite yoga and meditation books have stayed with me long after I've finished them. The books listed here are a select few, a mere drop in the literary ocean of yoga knowledge, that have influenced my practice, teaching, and my life.

*Autobiography of a Yogi* by Paramahansa Yogananda

*Beyond Power Yoga: 8 Levels of Practice for Body and Soul* by Beryl Bender Birch

*The Breathing Book: Good Health and Vitality Through Essential Breath Work* by Donna Farhi

*The Complete Illustrated Book of Yoga* by Swami Vishnu-devananda

*Fierce Medicine: Breakthrough Practices to Heal the Body and Ignite the Spirit* by Ana T. Forest

*Full Catastrophe Living* by Jon Kabat-Zinn

*Hatha Yoga Pradipika* by Swami Vishnu Devananda

*Journey of Awakening: A Meditator's Guidebook* by Ram Dass

*Light on Pranayama* by B.K.S. Iyengar

*Light on Yoga* by B.K.S. Iyengar

*Living Your Yoga: Finding the Spiritual in Everyday Life* by Judith Lasater

*Meditation and Its Practice* by Swami Rama

*Meditations From the Mat* by Rolf Gates and Katrina Kenison

*Meditation Is Boring: Putting Life In Your Spiritual Practice* by Linda Johnsen

*Old Path White Clouds: Walking the Footsteps of the Buddha* by Thich Nhat Hanh

*Philosophy of Hatha Yoga* by Usharbudh Arya

*The Power of Now: A Guide to Spiritual Enlightenment* by Ekhardt Tolle

*Science of Breath* by Swami Rama, Rudolph Ballentine, and Alan Hymes

*The Shambhala Encyclopedia of Yoga* by George Feuerstein

*The Upanishads* by Eknath Easwaran

*Wheels of Life: A User's Guide to the Chakra System* by Judith Anodea

*When Things Fall Apart: Heart Advice for Difficult Times* by Pema Chodron

*Wherever You Go, There You Are: Mindfulness Meditation in Everyday Life* by Jon Kabat-Zinn

*The Yamas & Niyamas: Exploring Yoga's Ethical Practice* by Deborah Adele

*Yoga for Wellness* by Gary Kraftsow

*Yoga: Mastering the Basics* by Sandra Anderson and Rolf Solvik

*Yoga: The Path to Holistic Health* by B.K.S. Iyengar

*Yoga: The Spirit and Practice of Moving Into Stillness* by Erich Schiffmann

*The Yoga Sutras of Patanjali* by Georg Feuerstein

*Zen Mind, Beginner's Mind* by Suzuki Shunryu

# Asana Index

# About the Author

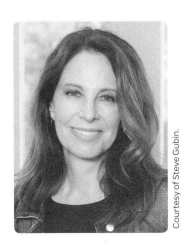

Courtesy of Steve Gubin.

**Nancy Gerstein** is a yoga teacher, author, speaker, and entrepreneur. She is the creator of Motivational Yoga, a yoga style that empowers life decisions, goals, and results. Nancy's teachings incorporate spiritually strengthening practices that bolster personal growth and self-motivation. Her classes feed the body and the mind, encouraging students to make conscious choices about how they direct thoughts, energy, and physical focus to live the best live they can. It's Nancy's belief that a genuine yoga practice begins within.

A Himalayan Institute–certified yoga teacher, Nancy is a frequent contributor to yoga publications and websites, including *Elephant Journal*, *Yogi Times*, *Yoga Magazine*, and *Yoga and Health Magazine*, and she is the author of *Guiding Yoga's Light* (Human Kinetics), a go-to reference book for yoga teachers and students. *Motivational Yoga* is Nancy's third book.

Nancy resides in Morton Grove, Illinois. In her free time she enjoys hiking, traveling, and trying most things at least once.

# You read the book—now complete an exam to earn continuing education credit!

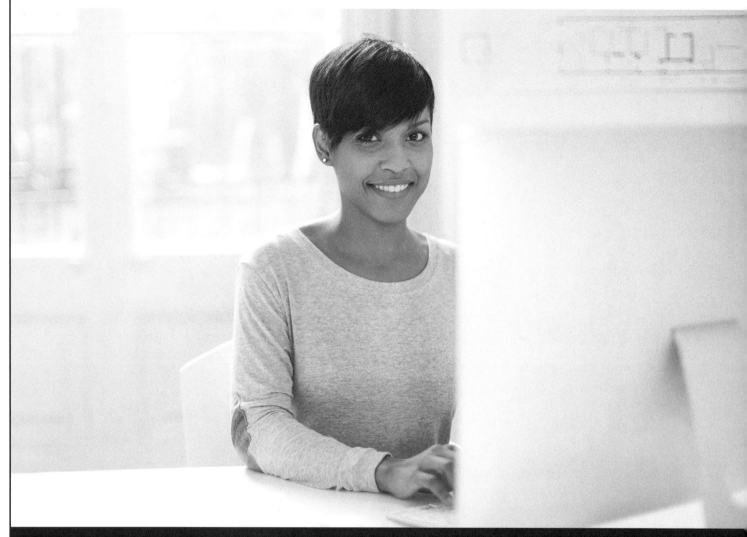

## Congratulations on successfully preparing for this continuing education exam!

If you would like to earn CE credit, please visit

**www.HumanKinetics.com/CE-Exam-Access**

for complete instructions on how to access your exam.
Take advantage of a discounted rate by entering
promo code **MY2020** when prompted.

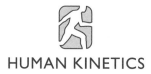